W9-BES-142

# Head and Neck Oncology

# Controversies in Cancer Treatment

Harvey A. Gilbert, M.D.
Series Editor
Chief, Department of Radiology
Presbyterian Intercommunity Hospital of Whittier
Whittier, California

# Head and Neck Oncology

## Controversies in Cancer Treatment

Edited by
A. Robert Kagan, M.D.

Department of Radiation Therapy
Southern California Permanente Medical Group
Los Angeles, California

John W. Miles, M.D.

Department of Otolaryngology
Southern California Permanente Medical Group
Los Angeles, California

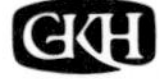

G. K. Hall Medical Publishers
Boston, Massachusetts

G. K. Hall Medical Publishers
70 Lincoln Street
Boston, MA 02111



81 82 83 84 / 4 3 2 1

Head and neck oncology.

(Controversies in cancer treatment)

Bibliography.
Includes index.
Contents: The impact of radiation biology on patient management / Amos Norman—Diagnosis, follow-up, and treatment of carcinoma in situ of the vocal cord / Alden H. Miller—The management of carcinoma in situ of the larynx / Patrick J. Doyle—[etc.]
1. Head—Cancer—Therapy. 2. Neck—Cancer therapy. 3. Head—Cancer. 4. Neck—Cancer. I. Kagan, A. Robert (Arthur Robert), 1936– . II. Miles, John, 1930– III. Series. [DNLM: 1. Head and neck neoplasms—Therapy. WE 707 H432]
RC280.H4H39 616.99'491 81-2908
ISBN 0-8161-2169-9 AACR2

The authors and publisher have worked to ensure that all information in this book concerning drug dosages, schedules and routes of administration is accurate at the time of publication. As medical research and practice advance, however, therapeutic standards may change. For this reason, and because human and mechanical errors will sometimes occur, we recommend that our readers consult the *PDR* or a manufacturer's product information sheet prior to prescribing or administering any drug discussed in this volume.

# CONTRIBUTORS

Alando J. Ballantyne, M.D.
Department of Surgery
M.D. Anderson Tumor Institute
Houston, Texas

J. P. Bataini, M.D.
Institut Curie
Paris, France

François Beland, Ph.D.
School of Public Health
University of Michigan
Ann Arbor, Michigan

John Beumer III, D.D.S., M.S.
Department of Maxillofacial Surgery
UCLA School of Dentistry
Los Angeles, California

William C. Constable, M.B., Ch.B., D.M.R.T.
Division of Radiation Oncology
University of Virginia Hospital
Charlottesville, Virginia

Patrick J. Doyle, M.D.
Division of Otolaryngology
University of British Columbia
St. Paul's Hospital
Vancouver, British Columbia, Canada

Frederick R. Eilber, M.D.
Department of Surgery
Division of Oncology
UCLA School of Medicine
Los Angeles, California

David Elkon, M.D.
Division of Radiation Oncology
University of Virginia Hospital
Charlottesville, Virginia

François Eschwege, M.D.
Institut Gustave-Roussy
Villejuif, France

Juan V. Fayos, M.D.
Division of Radiation Therapy
University of Miami School of Medicine
Jackson Memorial Hospital
Miami, Florida

Peter J. Fitzpatrick, M.D., F.R.C.P. (C), F.R.C.R.
Department of Radiation Oncology
The Princess Margaret Hospital
Ontario Cancer Institute
Toronto, Ontario, Canada

Jack L. Gluckman, M.D., F.C.S. (S.A.)
Department of Otolaryngology and Maxillofacial Surgery
University of Cincinnati Medical Center
College of Medicine
Cincinnati, Ohio

Richard H. Jesse, M.D.
Department of Surgery
M.D. Anderson Tumor Institute
Houston, Texas

A. Robert Kagan, M.D.
Department of Radiation Therapy
Southern California Permanente Medical Group
Los Angeles, California

John A. Kirchner, M.D.
Department of Head and Neck Surgery
Yale University School of Medicine
New Haven, Connecticut

Walter Lawrence, Jr., M.D.
Division of Surgical Oncology
Medical College of Virginia
Virginia Commonwealth University Cancer Center
Richmond, Virginia

William Lawson, M.D., D.D.S.
Department of Otolaryngology
The Mount Sinai Medical Center
New York, New York

B. Luboinski, M.D.
Institut Gustave-Roussy
Villejuif, France

John W. Miles, M.D.
Department of Otolaryngology
Southern California Permanente Medical Group
Los Angeles, California

Alden H. Miller, M.D.
Department of Otolaryngology
USC School of Medicine
Los Angeles, California

Amos Norman, Ph.D.
Departments of Radiation Oncology and Radiological Sciences
UCLA School of Medicine
Los Angeles, California

Robert G. Parker, M.D.
Department of Radiation Oncology
UCLA School of Medicine
Los Angeles, California

Samuel L. Perzik, M.D.
Department of Surgery
Loma Linda University School of Medicine
Loma Linda, California

Harry C. Schwartz, D.M.D., M.D.
Division of Otolaryngology
Southern California Permanente Medical Group
Los Angeles, California

Donald A. Shumrick, M.D.
Department of Otolaryngology and Maxillofacial Surgery
University of Cincinnati Medical Center
College of Medicine
Cincinnati, Ohio

Max L. Som, M.D.
Department of Otolaryngology
The Mount Sinai Medical Center
New York, New York

F. Kristian Storm, M.D.
Department of Surgery
Division of Oncology
UCLA School of Medicine
Los Angeles, California

Elliot W. Strong, M.D.
Department of Surgery
Head and Neck Service
Memorial Sloan-Kettering Cancer Center
New York, New York

Barry S. Tepperman, M.D.
The Princess Margaret Hospital
Ontario Cancer Institute
Toronto, Ontario, Canada

Jose J. Terz, M.D.
Department of General and Oncologic Surgery
City of Hope National Medical Center
Duarte, California

Paul H. Ward, M.D., F.A.C.S.
Department of Surgery
Division of Head and Neck Surgery
UCLA School of Medicine
Los Angeles, California

We would like to dedicate this book to
Alden Miller, M.D.
Clay Whitaker, M.D.
William Simpson, M.D.
Juan del Regato, M.D.
Chahin Chahbazian, M.D.
in appreciation for their training and friendship.

*John W. Miles, M.D.*
*A. Robert Kagan, M.D.*

# CONTENTS

# SERIES PREFACE

The impetus for this series came from the intellectually and emotionally difficult experiences my colleagues and I have encountered when attempting to make decisions about the best treatments for patients who have cancer. The patient's and physician's anxiety about the disease and the toxic treatments necessary for its eradication hamper reasoned discussions and charge the atmosphere with hidden messages. The physician's own fears of death and failure to cure enhance the intensity of this interchange. Unfortunately the resultant decision in each patient's case often only partly rests on scientific doctrine. Science deals predominantly with measurable quantities such as survival, but the quality of life as it is perceived in each situation is equally important. Therefore discussion of controversy in cancer is not and should not be only a cataloging of scientific facts but also must contain intuitive and affective measurements of human value.

Each of the books in this series is unique. Some editors chose to explore a vast range of topics; others chose to narrow down the number of issues and explore them in greater depth. Not all sides of each issue are presented, for the editor felt in some cases that only one or two points of view should be elaborated. For some, only one point of view was thought necessary, in which instances the contributor included a discussion of the standard, accepted opinion in addition to setting forth his or her position. The series was conceived of as a whole; as a result some issues are discussed in only one book because of space constraints, but would have been appropriate for other books in the series as well. On the other hand, other controversies are included in more than one book and are addressed by a different group of discussants in each; these controversies were repeated because of their universal appeal and current interest.

The editors for these books were selected because they possessed the following attributes:

1. a high level of expertise in the fields;
2. respect of their colleagues as fine clinicians;
3. continual questioning of the standard dogmas, and spending their professional lives attempting to improve the standard of medical practice; and
4. they are kind, caring individuals who value the patient-physician relationship.

Controversy is inherent in oncology; I am hopeful that the reader will gain significant insights toward making better decisions in managing patients.

I would like to acknowledge Dolores Groseclose for editorial assistance and Deanne, Jason, and Jill Gilbert for their support.

Harvey A. Gilbert
Series Editor

# INTRODUCTION

Legitimate differences of opinion exist in many aspects of the management of head and neck tumors. One's appraisal of tumor size, the absence or presence of adjacent tissue (including bone) infiltration, adenopathy, and histologic grading may differ from that of one's colleagues. The morbid residue of curative treatment affects the quality of survival. Individualization and clinical judgment are important for proper management decisions. Unfortunately, clinical judgment cannot be quantified. Statistical evaluation rarely deals with patient selectivity, intellectual prejudice, or technical competence.

Terz and Lawrence have shown that the fashionable desire for radiations combined with surgery cannot be supported by numbers. Elkon and Constable are more optimistic concerning combined therapies. Fayos and Beland have vividly demonstrated that sometimes skillful treatment in the wrong patient ends in unnecessary morbidity. Ballantyne questions the superiority of radiations over surgery for lesions of the anterior tongue and floor of the mouth. Need the reader be reminded that Ballantyne's institution, M. D. Anderson Tumor Institute, is internationally recognized for its proficiency in radiation therapy as well as in surgery?

The authors selected for this book are all experts in the field of head and neck cancer. Each was asked to take a point of view, rather than review the literature and present an overview for patient management. We have asked the authors to present their data and their opinions, while anticipating that their respected colleagues will do the same. The format of this book is not that of a debate, but an information center to provide medical opinions side by side. Readers are to digest and resolve controversy in the hope that their patients will profit from this experience.

Although each author's point of view is well known, we feel there is much to be gained intellectually and scientifically in soliciting these opinions side by side. In this way we hope to encourage a frank presentation and representation of their clinical work.

The editors have supported a basic mistrust of survival percentages, which do not mediate the intuitive. Although the ability of language to communicate is at times partial, we have asked our colleagues to grapple with some of the major problems in head and neck cancer in a personal manner.

The expression of experiential data is usually neglected because they cannot be assigned numbers. We believe that experiential descriptive data are as worthwhile as numerical, statistical data and can be expressed clearly and simply. Judgment and opinion will always be controversial since they are largely perceptual and unsystematic, limited by disciplinary boundaries.

Self-education is possible either by making one's own mistakes or by learning from the misfortunes of others. The knowledge gained from books can mature our judgment and prepare us, without causing actual danger to our patients as a result of errors in clinical decisions.

As students our training was rich in a now lost oral tradition. The patient with head and neck cancer needs a physician who can understand the empiric and analytic difficulties largely ignored in our scientific journals and books. Ward's chapter elegantly supports the necessity of the oral tradition for comprehensive education.

The question as to whether the incidence of radiation-induced cancer should influence clinicians' choice of therapy is addressed first by Lawson and Som and then by Parker.

What manner of treatment, if any, should follow the histopathologic diagnosis of carcinoma in situ of the vocal cord (see Doyle and Miller)?

Intensive histopathologic examination of the larynx after laryngectomy has enriched our knowledge of the causes of vocal cord fixation. Radiation therapy continues to compete for management with salvage surgery (Bataini), partial laryngectomy (Kirchner), total laryngectomy (Shumrick and Gluckman), and postoperative radiation (Eschwege and Luboinski). Perhaps computed tomography (CT) will help to define the different anatomic causes of cord immobility or limited mobility and thereby lend strength unintentionally to radiation, surgery, or combined treatment. Controversy in this area, however, will indubitably continue.

Perzik formulates the view that the biologic potential of melanoma is seen at its inception, with a positive lymph node dissection merely indicating disseminated disease. Storm and Eilber propose that the removal of positive lymph nodes markedly improves survival. Have we not been "entertained" by similar arguments in adenocarcinoma of the breast?

Beumer and Schwartz address extremely important matters. The cured patient with mandibular necrosis or severe functional disability is scored as NED by the surgeon or radiation therapist. (The concept of NED—no evidence of disease—implies that the patient is alive and well.) This is an incorrect assessment because the quality of life is equally important to these patients. Clinicians should take a more active interest in a patient's sense of dignity. To be alive and robbed of self-worth because of morbidity cannot be tabulated as a success, except by the most shallow clinician. To emphasize that life at any functional level is better than death should not be tolerated in the intellectual spirit of a multidisciplinary head and neck cancer conference.

Jesse and Strong discuss the issue of how extensive a neck dissection should be. Fitzpatrick and Tepperman demonstrate that radiation therapy of neck nodes can be successful but presents a complex biologic problem. Finally, Norman reviews the impact of research on our treatment. Must he destroy our illusions?

Controversy will continue in fields of medicine in which there are advances and progress. It is our purpose to explore some of these controversial areas in a constructive manner. Whether or not we have been successful is left to you, the reader, to judge.

# Chapter 1

# *The Impact (?) of Radiation Biology on Patient Management*

# Amos Norman

In the 1920s Regaud's classic experiments led directly to Coutard's clinical studies of fractionated dose schedules for the treatment of head and neck cancer, which culminated in the fractionated dose radiotherapy techniques in use today. In 1970 Henry Kaplan wrote, "Although we tend to think of these experiments as having been crude and at best only semiquantitative, it is an ironic fact that they are the only radiobiological experiments to date that have had a lasting and universal impact on the practice of radiotherapy." Surveying the same field 10 years later must we come to the same melancholy conclusion? Is it possible that the considerable progress in radiation therapy, particularly in the last 30 years, owes nothing to the remarkable advances made during that time in our understanding of the actions of ionizing radiation on living cells?

If we narrow our field of view to include only routine radiotherapy protocols, then we can find little evidence for the impact of modern radiation biology. If we broaden our view to include some indirect consequences of the vast number of radiobiologic and epidemiologic studies of the late effects of radiation, then we find immediately a small, growing, and not altogether benign impact. If we broaden our view further to include experimental protocols, then we find that radiation biology has had a major effect on patient management. Furthermore, if we regard not only what we do in the clinic but what we think we are doing, then modern radiobiologic experiments have had a lasting and universal impact.

During the past half century advances in radiotherapy have come from progress in dosimetry and treatment planning, from improvements in radiotherapy equipment, and from major gains in clinical oncology in our "knowledge about the natural history of different types of neoplasms, their proclivity for and routes of metastasis, and their relative responsiveness to radiation. Collectively, there is little question that these physical and clinical contributions deserve credit for significantly widening the scope of radiotherapy and for major improvements in long-term survival ratio for several different types of cancers" (Kaplan 1970). During that time, and particularly since the introduction by Puck and Marcus of the technique of clonal culture of mammalian cells in vitro in 1956, experiments in radiation biology have provided a firm scientific foundation for radiation therapy. Ironically, the impact on the practice of radiotherapy has come not from the fundamental work carried out by radiobiologists in order to understand the action of radiation on living cells but from the very large number of studies applied to public health problems arising from the manufacture and testing of nuclear weapons and the building of nuclear power plants. These studies have raised in the public mind acute concerns for the carcinogenic, mutagenic, and teratogenic hazards of ionizing radiations.

One consequence has been to sensitize the therapists to the risks of inducing cancer in normal tissues by radiation. Thyroid cancer as a late effect of treating the thymus in children, and more recently as a result of treating tinea with x-rays, has become a textbook example of iatrogenic carcinogenesis (Pochin 1976). More pertinent here is the evidence for late effects of radiation in such slow renewal tissues as the pituitary and thyroid glands following radiation therapy for head and neck cancer (Fuks et al. 1976). This subject is treated at length elsewhere in this volume; I shall conclude, therefore, with two remarks. The very success of modern programs of radiation therapy and chemotherapy in prolonging the lives of patients has also greatly increased the opportunities for observing late effects of radiation. It is now necessary to consider the risk of inducing cancer when planning treatments to control cancer.

The fear of radiation has had a considerable impact on the management of patients. It has influenced, perhaps subconsciously, decisions to use external beam therapy in certain situations rather than the relatively more hazardous, to the therapist and allied personnel, interstitial therapy. It has made more difficult the recruitment of people into almost every position in the radiation therapy department. And it has driven up sharply the costs of radiation therapy. These costs—for shielding, for personnel monitoring, for worker's compensation and other insurance—affect decisions concerning facilities and equipment and so influence directly the availability and quality of radiation therapy clinics. As the legitimate concern for radiation safety turns into hysteria in the United States, government regulations become more onerous, and the cost of compliance soars. This is an altogether dismal and familiar story. I shall pursue it no further except to remark that public safety is a political issue and therefore, quite properly in a democracy, subject to political action and political passion.

The model of Gray and associates (1953) showing the failure of radiation therapy to control tumors has stimulated more clinical trials in radiation therapy than all the other work combined in radiation biology since the classic experiences of Coutard. The model may be summarized in three statements:

1. Tumors contain foci of chronically hypoxic cells.
2. Hypoxia renders cells resistant to radiation.
3. Tumor recurrence is due to the proliferation of the hypoxic cells.

The first statement appears to rest solidly on histologic and biophysical evidence. Tumors grow in cords. As the result of anoxia, cords with a radius greater than 200 microns—the approximate distance that oxygen can diffuse through respiring tissues—contain necrotic centers. Between the actively growing rim of cells and the necrotic center there is, presumably, a thin ring of chronically hypoxic cells. The second statement rests on the universal observation in radiation biology of the "oxygen effect": every cell from whatever tissue and from every form of life exhibits a radiation sensitivity about three times greater in the presence than in the absence of oxygen. The third statement appears to be a logical consequence of the first two.

I think it fair to say that Gray's model has become the conventional wisdom in radiation therapy; the failure of local control is due to proliferation of clonogenic cells that become hypoxic and hence radioresistant because of their distance from the blood supply.

Gray's model stimulated a large amount of work in radiation biology. Single-dose survival curves on cell populations irradiated as solid tumors and assayed as single cells revealed a resistant fraction—presumably the hypoxic cells of Gray's model—with a range of values centering around 15%. These results quickly turned the question "Why does radiation sometimes fail to control tumors?" into "Why does it succeed in controlling tumors with doses that are clearly inadequate to sterilize the large numbers of radioresistant cells?" Further work revealed the familiar answer, "reoxygenation" (Kallman 1972). During a course of fractionated doses the fraction of radioresistant cells did not increase, as would be expected if the surviving cells remained radioresistant. Instead the radioresistant fraction remained more or less constant during the treatments. This was explained by postulating a rapid reoxygenation of the hypoxic cells. Such a mechanism provides a satisfying rationale for fractionated dose schedules in the clinic. It also contradicts the first statement in Gray's model, for if reoxygenation of hypoxic cells commonly occurs during fractionated dose therapy, then the tumor effectively is freed of hypoxic cells. The second statement in Gray's model has also become dubious. After prolonged exposure to hypoxia, cells lose the relative radioresistance they exhibit after short exposures, and may even become more sensitive than the well-oxygenated cells (Berry, Hall, and Cavanaugh 1970). Finally the third statement, the critical one for understanding failure in radiation therapy, has been challenged by the recent direct observation in experimental tumors that regrowth in heavily irradiated tumors occurred not in the area close to necrotic regions but from foci in the peripheral, well-vascularized regions of the tumor (Yamaura and Matsuzawa 1979). If the oxygen effect plays any role in the success or failure of radiation to control tumors, the evidence now suggests it may be because of "acutely hypoxic cells"—cells rendered hypoxic by temporary interruptions in the blood flow of well-vascularized regions of the tumor—rather than because of the chronically hypoxic cells postulated in Gray's model (Brown 1979).

While radiation biologists were accumulating evidence that Gray's model failed to account for the results of laboratory experiments, radiation therapists were meeting failure in clinical trials of two strategies based on Gray's model. One, the "chemical strategy," sought to increase the relative radiosensitivity of the hypoxic cells by introducing hypoxic cell sensitizers into the tumor. The other, the "physical strategy," attempted to reduce the relative radioresistance of the hypoxic cells by using high linear energy transfer (LET) radiations, against which hypoxia affords little protection.

The simplest and most effective hypoxic cell radiosensitizer is oxygen, and the most direct way to get oxygen into the hypoxic cells is by placing the patient in a chamber containing pure oxygen at two to three atmospheres of pressure. The great expectations attending the early clinical trials of hyperbaric oxygen (HBO) treatment led to great disappointment when the trials failed to reveal any significant improvement in survival or, in most instances, even in local control of several different types of cancer. These clinical results, taken together with the findings in radiation biology, seemed to me to have created the conditions for the rejection of Gray's model. We were in a state described by Kuhn (1970) when he wrote: "Scientific revolutions are inaugurated by a growing sense, again often restricted to a narrow subdivision of the scientific community, that an existing paradigm has ceased to function adequately in the exploration of an aspect of nature to which that paradigm itself had previously led the way." Gray's paradigm, which had led to a vigorous exploration of the role of chronically hypoxic cells in the radiocurability of tumors, had ceased to function adequately.

It is an easy jump from the rejection of Gray's model to the rejection of the notion that the oxygen effect plays any significant role in radiation therapy. That jump is premature. The recent reports (Dische 1979) of the results of extensive and well-controlled trials of HBO in radiotherapy of tumors at four sites—the head and neck, uterine cervix, bladder, and bronchus—are encouraging. In particular Henk and colleagues (1977a, 1977b) have obtained an increase in the local control of head and neck cancer in one series of 276 patients from 30% for tumors treated in air to 53% for those treated in HBO. In a second series of 103 patients the local control rate increased from 47% in air to 65% in HBO. In the former group there was no difference reported in the overall patient survival, but in the latter group the two-year survival of patients treated in HBO was 71%, a significantly higher rate than the 50% for patients treated in air. I expect that we shall come to agree with Henk and Smith (1977b) "that radiotherapy in HBO can probably offer patients with advanced laryngeal carcinoma a better chance of survival with preservation of a normal voice than any other treatment" and "that HBO when available will improve the results of radiotherapy in head and neck cancer and that it should not too readily be discarded."

It may be that the increased radiocurability of head and neck cancer in HBO is not due simply to the sensitization of chronically or acutely hypoxic cells in the tumor. The fact that HBO even at daily dose increments as small as 200 rad appears to increase the effects of radiation upon both tumor and normal tissues is not consistent with a simple radiobiologic model of the oxygen effect (Dische 1979). Nevertheless, the simplest hypothesis for the differential effect of HBO on normal and tumor tissues is still that oxygen sensitizes hypoxic cells in the tumor. Thus the results of recent trials of HBO encourage not only the wider use of HBO but also the continued investigations of other hypoxic cell sensitizers.

Two nitroimidazoles, metronidazole (Flagyl) and misomidazole (Ro-070582), are the best studied of the new hypoxic cell radiosensitizers. They are free, of course, of the special hazards involved in using oxygen at high pressure, but they have serious neurologic side effects. In trying to assess their eventual impact on patient management it is best not to consider them simply as substitutes for HBO. For example, their distribution in tumors and hence their ability to sensitize both chronically and acutely hypoxic cells may be quite different from that of oxygen dissolved in the blood under high pressure (Brown 1979). Whatever the eventual outcome, the development of the new radiosensitizers provides a fine illustration of the impact of careful work in radiation biology on the development of experimental protocols in radiation therapy (Fowler 1979).

The encouraging results of HBO have also made me a little less skeptical of the clinical results with fast neutron therapy. At first glance the results of Catterall and associates (1975, 1977) on treating advanced tumors of the head and neck are impressive. With neutrons they obtained local control in 54 of 71 cases (76%), whereas with photons they achieved local control in only 12 of 62 cases (19%). Some of the photon patients, however, received rather low doses of radiation. Moreover, the neutron patients had a severe complication rate of 17% versus 4% in the photon series. The data suggest that much of the difference between results achieved in the two groups is due to variations in the dose and dose distributions between the neutron beams and the x- and gamma-ray beams. The trials, therefore, do not provide a clear answer to the question of whether fast neutron therapy is capable of increasing the curability of head and neck tumors. There are now several cyclotrons designed for radiation therapy under construction or already operating in Europe, Japan, and the United States. The combined results of clinical trials will, within the next decade, establish the role of fast neutrons in radiation therapy.

So far I have been discussing strategies that have originated in radiation biology to deal by chemical or physical methods with hypoxic cells which may be responsible for the lack of radiocurability of some tumors. Are there any other ideas that have crossed over from radiation biology to the clinic? One idea flowed naturally from the demonstration by radiation biologists that radiosensitivity varies with the stage in the cell cycle. This has led to some attempts to increase the curability of tumors by arresting the cycling tumor cells in a radiation sensitive stage. In one such effort Esser and colleagues (1976) irradiated squamous cell carcinomas of the oral cavity and oropharynx after arresting the cells with bleomycin. Measurements of the DNA distributions with a flow cytofluorometer showed that the drug treatment increased the number of tumor cells in the radiosensitive $G_2$ stage from an average of 6.7% to 13.6%. They could not demonstrate a correlation, however, between tumor regression and the fraction of cells in $G_2$. It seems to me that the manipulation of the cell cycle for therapy is at the heart of chemotherapy. Certainly the chemotherapist has a large array of cycle specific drugs that can be applied in virtually unlimited combinations in order to exploit differences in the cell cycle of normal and cancer cells. It seems prudent to leave strategies based on the partial synchronization of tumor cells to the chemotherapist.

Is there anything else going on in radiation biology that may affect patient management? Certainly many radiation biologists are now working hard to investigate the effects of hyperthermia on normal and cancer cells, and certainly some of their results have directly influenced current clinical trials of hyperthermia. Hyperthermia, however, has a history going back long before the birth of radiation therapy, and its modern development as a clinical tool is going on in several areas of clinical oncology. It seems best, therefore, to consider hyperthermia, like chemotherapy, as an independent modality rather than as an adjunct to radiation therapy.

We have become accustomed to the idea that progress in science leads to new or improved technology; advances in understanding nature lead to better control over nature. Radiation therapy, after all, owes its birth to the discovery of x-rays by a physicist, and the development of the latest radiologic marvel, the CT scanner, can be traced back to advances in solid-state physics that made possible the small computer. Science has another function, however: it sets limits on what we can do. Since the establishment of thermodynamics, for example, only charlatans and crackpots claim the ability to extract more energy from a machine than is fed into it. Furthermore, every engineer knows that the temperature differences in the working cycle of an engine place absolute limits on its efficiency. It seems to me that radiation biology has placed certain limits on what can be done in radiation therapy. It did so when it showed, after extensive investigations, that cancer cells are not intrinsically more radiosensitive than normal cells. Let me be precise. If you show me a single-cell survival curve, I cannot tell you whether this was obtained with a population of normal or cancer cells. Moreover, both sets of cells respond almost identically to such dose-modifying factors as anoxia. This is not surprising, for cancer cells can arise as the result of very small changes in the normal cells, perhaps nothing more in some instances than the loss of a few receptors for inhibitors of cell division. There is no reason to expect that the radiation damage in chromosomes which results in cell sterilization will be affected significantly by the subtle differences between normal and cancer cells. There are significant differences, however, in radiosensitivity among populations of both cancer and normal cells derived from various tissues, and there may be large differences among various cell lines derived from a single cell line. The implications are clear: there may be radioresistant or radiosensitive—I use the term here to mean radiocurable—tumors embedded in radioresistant or radiosensitive normal tissues, and tumors that appear identical in type, site, and extent may differ in radiosensitivity. In other words, there are tumors that are not good candidates for control by radiation therapy. It can be argued that this idea grew directly out of clinical experience. I am arguing only that radiation biology, which has inspired new strategies for improving cure rates in the clinic, has also shown the limitations of radiation therapy. These limitations are set by the intrinsic differences in the radiosensitivities of various cell populations—differences resulting in the large variation in the parameters, Do, Dq, n—that are commonly used to describe single cell survival curves. These differences undoubtedly are accentuated by differences in the architecture of individual tumors, that is, by subtle differences in the blood supply and other features of the solid tumor.

It seems to me, then, that the most dramatic increase in the cure rates achieved by radiation therapy of head and neck cancer will come by excluding from the clinic those patients who are poor candidates for success. I am not trying to be flippant. I want only to emphasize my conviction that a great deal more attention should be paid by biologists and therapists to identifying the poorly responding tumors either before or at least early during the course of radiation therapy. What has been done recently to this end? Sobel and associates (1976) have shown that if tumor clearance occurred within one to three months following completion of treatment, local control could be predicted in cancers of the oral cavity, oropharynx, and hypopharynx with approximately 80%, 70%, and 50% reliability, respectively. Clearly, rates of tumor clearance are not useful predictors of local control. A more promising approach appears to be through the study of tumor cell kinetics. Nervi and colleagues (1978), however, have shown that cell kinetics parameters could not be correlated with the response to treatment of head and neck cancer even when the cancers were grouped according to their clinical growth characteristic. We badly need to identify a marker substance or a new measurement that will improve our ability to predict the radiation curability of head and neck cancers.

Looking back over the past 30 years we must admit that radiation biology has had little direct impact on patient management. Looking forward into the near future we see some prospect of an impact when and if HBO, fast neutrons, and hypoxic cell sensitizers find a modest place in radiotherapy of head and neck cancer. I say "modest" because dramatic effects would have been evident many years ago. Moreover, radiation biology will continue to influence experimental protocols, particularly those involving combinations of radiation, drugs, and hyperthermia, and thus will play a modest role in clinical advances. The indirect influence of radiation biology is more difficult to trace, although it certainly has altered our view of the complex factors that determine success or failure in the clinic and thus has made us aware of the limitations of radiation therapy. This awareness in turn has contributed to the current drive to seek improvements in cancer cure rate through the appropriate combination of surgery, chemotherapy, hyperthermia, and radiotherapy. To the extent that radiation biology can help determine the optimal combinations for the individual patient it will directly influence patient management.

## References

Berry, R. J.; Hall, E. J.; and Cavanaugh, J. Radiosensitivity and the oxygen effect for mammalian cells cultured in vitro in the stationary phase. *Br. J. Radiol.* 43:81–90, 1970.

Brown, J. M. Evidence for acutely hypoxic cells in mouse tumors, and a possible mechanism of reoxygenation. *Br. J. Radiol.* 52:650–656, 1979.

Catterall, M.; Bewley, D. K.; and Sutherland, I. Second report on results of a randomized clinical trial of fast neutrons compared with x or gamma rays in treatment of advanced tumors of head and neck. *Br. Med. J.* 1:1642–1643, 1977.

Catterall, M.; Sutherland, I.; and Bewley, D. K. First results of a randomized clinical trial of fast neutrons compared with x or gamma rays in treatment of advanced tumors of the head and neck. *Br. Med. J.* 2:653–656, 1975.

Dische, S. Hyperbaric oxygen: the Medical Research Council trials and their clinical significance. *Br. J. Radiol.* 51:888–894, 1979.

Esser, E.; Schumann, J.; and Wannenmacher, M. Irradiation treatment of inoperable squamous cell carcinomas of the oral cavity and oropharynx after partial synchronization. *J. Maxillofac. Surg.* 4:26–33, 1976.

Fowler, J. F. New horizons in radiation oncology. *Br. J. Radiol.* 52:523–535, 1979.

Fuks, Z. et al. Long-term effects of external radiation on the pituitary and thyroid glands. *Cancer* 37:1152–1161, 1976.

Gray, L. H. et al. Concentration of oxygen dissolved in tissues at time of irradiation as a factor in radiotherapy. *Br. J. Radiol.* 26:638–648, 1953.

Henk, J. M.; Kunkler, P. B.; and Smith, C. W. Radiotherapy and hyperbaric oxygen in head and neck cancer. Final report of first controlled clinical trial. *Lancet* 2:101–103, 1977a.

Henk, J. M., and Smith, C. W. Radiotherapy and hyperbaric oxygen in head and neck cancer. Interim report of second clinical trial. *Lancet* 2:104–105, 1977b.

Kallman, R. F. The phenomenon of reoxygenation and its implications for fractionated radiotherapy. *Radiology* 105:135–142, 1972.

Kaplan, H. S. Radiobiology's contribution to radiotherapy: promise or mirage? Failla memorial lecture. *Radiat. Res.* 43:460–476, 1970.

Kuhn, T. S. *The structure of scientific revolutions.* Chicago: University of Chicago Press, 1970.

Nervi, C. et al. The relevance of tumor size and cell kinetics as predictors of radiation response in head and neck cancer. *Cancer* 41:900–906, 1978.

Pochin, E. E. Malignancies following low radiation exposures in man. *Br. J. Radiol.* 49:577–579, 1976.

Puck, T. T., and Marcus, P. I. Action of x-rays on mammalian cells. *J. Exp. Med.* 103:653–666, 1956.

Sobel, S. et al. Tumor persistence as a predictor of outcome after radiation therapy of head and neck cancer. *Int. J. Radiat. Oncol. Biol. Phys.* 1:873–880, 1976.

Yamaura, H., and Matsuzawa, T. Tumor regrowth after irradiation: an experimental approach. *Int. J. Radiat. Biol.* 35:201–209, 1979.

# Chapter 2

# *Diagnosis, Follow-up, and Treatment of Carcinoma in situ of the Vocal Cord*

# Alden H. Miller

Carcinoma in situ of the vocal cord is a relatively new histopathologic diagnosis and a newer clinical entity. Since it has only recently been accepted as a disease entity, at least a few controversies about it still exist. Some of these are the characteristic histologic features of carcinoma in situ, its association with the development of invasive cancer, and the most appropriate initial and subsequent treatment.

The term carcinoma in situ was introduced by Broders in 1932 to describe an early preinvasive stage of intraepithelial carcinoma that is recognized by the profound alteration in intact surface epithelium (Broders 1940). The realization of the true, potentially malignant nature of this lesion was expressed by this early term of intraepithelial carcinoma, and dates back at least to the observations of Bowen in 1912. Many studies since then have shown that not all carcinoma in situ has gone on to the invasion stage, but an overall average of about one in six treated cases has.

Controversy has existed as to the terms to be used and their definition and the histologic description of the hyperplastic changes in the larynx associated with the early development of laryngeal carcinoma.

Terms such as "premalignant," "leukoplakia," "squamous cell hyperplasia, with or without keratosis," "epithelial hyperplasia," "epithelial hyperplasia with atypia," "keratosis with atypia," "epithelial dysplasia," and "keratosis with dysplasia" have all been used recently.

At the Centennial Conference on Laryngeal Cancer in Toronto in 1974 (Alberti and Bryce 1976), a panel of seven pathologists, nine laryngologists, and one radiotherapist accepted the following four conditions as indicating hyperplastic changes in the larynx:

1. Keratosis.
2. Keratosis with atypia.

3. Carcinoma in situ.
4. Carcinoma in situ with microinvasion.

All seven pathologists agreed on the recognition of these entities as proliferative lesions. The first two conditions were considered benign.

Every pathologist agreed that the term "premalignant" should no longer be used for laryngeal lesions, and the term "leukoplakia" should be abandoned as a diagnostic pathologic term; at best it is a descriptive clinical term without specificity as to pathologic significance.

## Keratosis

Four pathologists and all 10 therapists agreed with the use of this term. Two pathologists preferred to call this change "squamous cell hyperplasia with or without keratosis." One wanted to call it "epithelial hyperplasia."

Histologically, keratosis was described as an epithelial hyperplasia with an orderly maturation sequence, with normal cellular cytology and architecture and some degree of surface keratinization, be it orthokeratotic or parakeratotic. This picture of simple keratin production could be called simple keratosis.

## Keratosis with Atypia

Three pathologists and eight laryngologists agreed with the use of this term and its definition. One pathologist preferred to use "epithelial hyperplasia with atypia." Two pathologists preferred to use "squamous cell hyperplasia with atypia or with dysplasia" and one preferred the term "epithelial dysplasia." Two therapists substituted dysplasia for atypia, as in "keratosis with atypia."

Keratosis with atypia is one demonstrating some degree of either cellular atypism or disturbance of maturation sequence. The atypia may vary in degree from slight to great and could be graded mild, moderate, or severe. The terms atypia and dysplasia have been used synonymously by some. Atypia usually refers to cell (cytology) abnormalities while dysplasia usually relates to tissue and/or architecture. Both keratosis and keratosis with atypia are benign. Statistically, however, keratosis with atypia has a poor prognosis with respect to being associated with later developing carcinoma.

## Carcinoma in situ

One of the high points of the workshop was the unanimous acceptance of the third term, carcinoma in situ. All 7 pathologists and all 10 therapists accepted this term and considered it a clinical entity. It seems that it should be accepted worldwide.

The histologic features of carcinoma in situ of the larynx are seen in the squamous epithelium. The epithelium appears hyperchromatic and basophilic and the normal stratiform differentiation of the epithelium is lost. The normal layers are indistinct or missing and the regular progression from basal cell layer to surface is no longer present. The basal cells vary in size and shape and their type is abnormally extended up through the more superficial layers, so that the normal single-cell layer, where the intercellular bridges have usually disappeared, tend to be rounded or irregularly polyhedral; the nuclei vary in size and shape and large "bird's eye" nuclei with large nucleoli are present. The absence of a distinct and uniform basal cell layer and the occurrence of anisonucleosis throughout the thickness of the epithelium are the most arresting and convincing features to the observer. Mitotic figures are usually numerous and can always be found in the area involved. These figures may be normal or atypical and multipolar in appearance. Irregular foci of keratinization can be found in any portion of the epithelial layer. In some cases this occurs near the surface, and occasionally the entire surface is covered by a keratotic or parakeratotic layer of considerable thickness. The appearance of the process of carcinoma in situ, either with or without accompanying well-defined hyperkeratosis, suggests that this profound change can occur either in previously normal epithelium or in epithelium which is the seat of keratosis.

Some define carcinoma in situ as a proliferative disorder of the epithelium in which all of the generally accepted cytologic criteria of malignancy are manifest, except one: invasive beyond the squamous epithelium. Others insist that there must be a full-thickness replacement of the epithelium by cells with malignant cytologic features, a disorderly and faulty maturation sequence with minimal differentiation and an absence of invasion.

### Carcinoma in situ with Microinvasion

Again, 4 pathologists and 10 therapists accepted this terminology and its definition. Two pathologists preferred to term this pathologic change "squamous cell carcinoma with microinvasion." One pathologist called it "carcinoma with superficial invasion."

Microinvasion implies violation of the basement membrane with histologic evidence of early invasion. It may be only a few cells in depth.

## Clinical Presentation

Most clinicians agree with pathologists that the term "leukoplakia" should not be used, but rather that "keratosis" or "keratotic membrane" or "thick," "thin," "smooth," or "shaggy white spots," "plaques," or "areas" should be used descriptively. Keratosis and keratosis with atypia cannot be differentiated clinically but must be determined microscopically.

The criterion for our selection of carcinoma in situ of the larynx was the demonstration of carcinoma in situ, without invasive or infiltrating carcinoma, in the initial and the early subsequent biopsies in each case. The histologic features found in the epithelium to support this pathologic diagnosis are (1) loss of differentiation; (2) altered polarity of cellular orientation; (3) hypercellularity; (4) cellular atypism; (5) micronucleosis and anisonucleosis; (6) altered staining reaction; and (7) mitotic figures that are atypical in polarity and/or are in the upper layers of the epithelium.

## Treatment

More than 30 years of study of more than 350 patients with carcinoma in situ of the larynx have provided me with significant answers and clues as to its association with the development of invasive cancer and as to the most appropriate initial and subsequent treatment (Miller, Batsakis, and van Nostrand 1976).

During this period, five to six times as many patients were seen with invasive carcinoma as those with only carcinoma in situ. The ratio was 5.7 to 1 in an early five-year period and 5.8 to 1 in another five-year period 10 years later. This suggests that the relative incidence is a basic feature of the natural occurrence of these two conditions and has not been influenced either by doctor or patient education or by competence of biopsy taking.

It seems to be a general feature of carcinoma in situ that the condition appears at an earlier age than invasive carcinoma in the same organ. In our clinical laryngeal cases, in the years 1951 to 1955, the average age of the carcinoma in situ cases was 53 years, compared to an average of 60 years in invasive carcinoma of the larynx. In the 1966 to 1970 cases, the average age of the carcinoma in situ was 58 years, and of invasive carcinoma, 62 years. In this period, among men, the youngest patient seen with carcinoma in situ was 29 years old, and the youngest seen with invasive carcinoma was 37. The clinical appearance of in situ carcinoma at a somewhat younger age than invasive carcinoma is compatible with the concept that carcinoma in situ is a preinvasive predecessor of carcinoma of the infiltrating type.

Of the first 250 patients seen, 183 had a very adequate follow-up. Thirty-two of these patients, 1 in 6 plus, developed invasion, attesting to the invasive potential of the lesion.

The initial treatment has been (1) the complete stripping or restripping of one or both cords; (2) laryngofissure and cordectomy of one true cord; or (3) radiation. Treatment was predicated on the site and extent of the lesion and the procedure used in first making the diagnosis. Leukoplakic (keratotic) lesions, even if extensive, were usually completely stripped for diagnosis. If these exhibited carcinoma in situ were small in extent and seemed to have been completely removed (grossly and by microlaryngoscopy), no further treatment was instituted, but close observation was begun. Any reappearance of keratosis or induration was restripped. If now only keratosis was demonstrated microscopically, observation was continued. If residual or recurrent carcinoma in situ was proved then or later in the same limited lesion, cordectomy was performed. When carcinoma in situ was found extensively or bilaterally in repeated stripping biopsies, radiation therapy was usually employed. In patients with widespread leukoplakia, a repeated and complete stripping of all of the visible lesion was performed within a week to 10 days after an initial *limited* biopsy had revealed carcinoma in situ. The above protocol was then followed.

The nonleukoplakic lesions were usually limited in extent and were treated in the same way as were the small leukoplakic lesions; that is, if the cord did not return to a completely normal appearance after the biopsy stripping, biopsy was repeated. If residual carcinoma in situ was demonstrated in a lesion that could be removed by laryngofissure and cordectomy, these procedures were performed. Carcinoma in situ patients with diffuse injected induration of all of one cord received radiation therapy. Radiation treatment was also used in those patients in whom recurrences of carcinoma in situ were proved by repeated strippings after lengthy periods during which the larynx had remained clear and normal in appearance. In a few instances patients have elected radiation treatment rather than surgery.

The following tables demonstrate the results of treatment in the first 203 patients adequately followed for at least 10 years.

In table 2.1 the failures were the recurrences of carcinoma in situ or the first demonstration of invasive carcinoma after complete stripping and after a period of at least two and a half months or more during which time the larynx clinically had appeared to be clear.

Table 2.2 breaks down the initial treatment failures between recurrences and the beginning of invasive carcinoma. Note that the 25 failures of stripping as initial treatment resulted in an almost equal number of recurrences (12) and invasive carcinoma (13). In contrast, the 22 failures of radiation as initial treatment resulted in four and a half times as many instances of invasive carcinoma (18) as recurrences (4). It was noted that recurrence after radiation is often insidious. It may be manifested by limited motion or fixation of an arytenoid rather than by mucous membrane changes.

**Table 2.1**
Results of Initial Treatment of Carcinoma in situ

| Initial Treatment | Number of Patients | Cures | Failures |
|---|---|---|---|
| Stripping | 100 | 75 | 25 |
| Laryngofissure only | 60 | 56 | 4 |
| Radiation only | 43 | 21 | 22 |
| Totals | 203 | 152 | 51 |

**Table 2.2**
Incidence of Recurrence of In Situ versus Invasive Cancer after Failure of Initial Treatment for Carcinoma in situ

| Treatment | Failures | Recurrences | Invasive Carcinoma |
|---|---|---|---|
| Stripping | 25 | 12 | 13 |
| Radiation | 22 | 4 | 18 |
| Laryngofissure | 4 | 3 | 1 |
| Totals | 51 | 19 | 32 |

The length of time for invasive carcinoma to develop after carcinoma in situ had been demonstrated and the initial treatment was as follows: with stripping, 2 to 96 months; with laryngofissure and cordectomy, 32 and 42 months; with radiation, from 4 to 64 months. The spread in elapsed time before invasion was practically the same after stripping as after radiation treatment. After laryngofissure and cordectomy for in situ, invasive carcinoma did not occur for two and a half years and was uncommon.

A recapitulation as to the eventual outcome in the 32 patients in whom invasive carcinoma developed revealed that 10 were cured by laryngectomy, 10 by laryngofissure, 4 by radiation, and 2 by stripping only. Six patients (2% of the entire series) died despite all therapy, surgical or combined. One other radiation failure treated by laryngectomy has residual disease. There has been only 1 death in the 100 patients whose carcinoma in situ was treated initially by a vocal cord stripping.

Of the 43 patients who received radiation as the initial treatment, 21 were cured. Carcinoma in situ recurring after stripping was cured by radiation in 7 patients, but radiation failed in 4 such patients. Invasive carcinoma developed in 18 patients receiving radiation as the initial therapy. Five of these 18 patients died.

Stripping away of the mucosa of the involved cord as the initial treatment resulted in a 75% cure rate. This procedure appears to be the treatment of choice if the patient can be observed closely for evidence of residual or recurrent disease. This is especially true in small, localized, single, or unilateral lesions. It has been successful in some patients with microinvasion.

Radiation as initial treatment has the highest rates of recurrence and development of invasion. But it must be stated that after the first few years, radiation as initial treatment was selected only for those patients with bilateral involvement or with total involvement of one cord in the nonkeratotic type.

In summary it should be stated that while carcinoma in situ does not have a typical clinical picture for identification, it should be suspected whenever there is keratosis over an underlying, indurated, thickened base. It must be immediately added, however, that a nonkeratotic but deeply reddened, indurated area of a vocal cord may also be the site of carcinoma in situ.

# References

Alberti, P. W., and Bryce, D. P., eds. *Centennial conference on laryngeal cancer.* New York: Appleton-Century-Crofts, 1976.

Bowen, J. T. Precancerous dermatoses. *J. Cutan. Dis.* 30:241–255, 1912.

Broders, A. C. The microscopic grading of cancer. In *Treatment of cancer and allied diseases,* vol. 1, eds. G. T. Pack and E. M. Livingston. New York: Paul B. Hoeber, 1940.

Miller, A. H.; Batsakis, J. C.; and van Nostrand, W. P. Premalignant laryngeal lesion carcinoma in situ superficial carcinoma: definition and management. In *Centennial conference on laryngeal cancer,* eds. P. W. Alberti and D. P. Bryce. New York: Appleton-Century-Crofts, 1976.

# Chapter 3

# *The Management of Carcinoma in situ of the Larynx*

Patrick J. Doyle

Carcinoma in situ of the larynx is a malignant neoplasm. It is almost always confined to the true vocal cords and histologically lies between dysplastic leukoplakia and invasive squamous cell carcinoma.

Untreated, this condition will frequently progress to invasive carcinoma, and for this reason must be treated vigorously.

It is also significant that carcinoma in situ is frequently seen involving both vocal cords or in conjunction with dysplastic leukoplakia either on the same or the other cord or in conjunction with invasive squamous cell carcinoma of the same or the other cord. This diffuse presence of carcinoma in situ should be interpreted as various stages of the same disease, but it must also be realized that we are faced with "field disease." It is in only rare circumstances, therefore, that localized or surgical treatment of the carcinoma in situ lesion is indicated.

The treatment of choice for the vast majority of patients with carcinoma in situ of the vocal cords is radiotherapy. Supervoltage radiotherapy should be used in a full tumoricidal dose.

## Incidence

There has been an increase in the incidence of carcinoma in situ of the vocal cords over the past 20 years. At the Cancer Control Agency of British Columbia the incidence increased from 1% of all laryngeal cancer patients seen during the sixth decade to 12.7% of new laryngeal cancer patients seen between 1970 and 1972 (Doyle and Flores 1977). This increase, however, is apparent rather than real. It is related to a greater awareness of the condition by both otolaryngologists and pathologists, to the routine use of microlaryngoscopy for more accurate removal of involved tissue, and to the improved anesthetic methods that have made careful microlaryngoscopy and biopsy possible. The Cancer Control Agency of British Columbia (CCABC) series has also shown a high incidence of associated abnormal histology. Of 586 patients with invasive carcinoma of the larynx, 20 had an associated carcinoma in situ and 26 an associated dysplastic leukoplakia. In 4 instances carcinoma in situ was under observation prior to the diagnosis of invasive carcinoma, and in 15 instances leukoplakia was under observation prior to the diagnosis of invasive carcinoma.

## Treatment

These findings substantiate the previous statement that carcinoma in situ is frequently part of malignant and premalignant disease occurring throughout the laryngeal epithelium and further substantiate the concept of field treatment rather than spot treatment of the carcinoma in situ. At CCABC almost all patients are treated with a course of cobalt 60. A source skin distance (SSD) of 80 or 90 cm is used and a tumor dose (TD) of 6000 to 6500 rad is delivered in five to six weeks in 25 to 30 fractions. The nominal single dose (NSD) equivalent ranges from 1720 to 1900 ret. Parallel and opposed fields $5 \times 5$ or $5 \times 7$ cm in size are used. Compensator filters of aluminum are used to even the dose distribution. The patient is treated in the supine position using a plastic shell to reproduce exactly the same position of the neck at all times during treatment. Thirty-seven patients were so treated between 1940 and 1972. Thirty-three of 34 patients followed for more than five years showed no evidence of recurrent disease or invasive laryngeal carcinoma—a cure of 94%. Only one patient treated by radiotherapy went on to develop invasive squamous cell carcinoma. It was determined, however, that this patient had bilateral vocal cord disease at the time of the original diagnosis, but only one vocal cord was biopsied and this showed carcinoma in situ. Eight months after completion of therapy, biopsy of the opposite cord showed invasive carcinoma and a subsequent total laryngectomy showed extensive invasive carcinoma of both vocal cords as well as the subglottic larynx and upper trachea. This undoubtedly represented an incident of missed invasive carcinoma rather than the development of a new disease. It is the author's opinion that the 51% failure for radiotherapy reported by Miller (1974) possibly represents similar errors in the original diagnosis. Miller (chapter 2) treats surgically only patients with small lesions and single lesions, whereas they use radiotherapy for bilateral, widespread, and multicentric lesions. Not only are they treating more extensive disease with radiotherapy, but coexisting invasive cancer is more likely to be present in the multicentric or widespread group. The early appearance of invasive cancer in 18 of the 22 recurrences, many of which were detected within a few months of radiation, indicates a strong possibility that coexisting invasive carcinoma was present prior to the institution of treatment. On the basis of these findings carcinoma in situ should be managed as follows.

1. Any patient found to have carcinoma in situ on laryngeal biopsy must have careful microlaryngoscopy with examination of the hypopharynx, larynx, subglottic larynx, and upper trachea.
2. If the lesion is small and confined to one cord, complete stripping of that cord is indicated.
3. If both cords are abnormal, stripping and/or careful multiple biopsies are essential.
4. If a small localized lesion is found, repeat cord stripping is performed in one month.
5. If any biopsy reveals an invasive carcinoma the patient must not be classified as a case of carcinoma in situ.
6. Radiotherapy should be withheld only if all of the following conditions exist:
   a. a small localized lesion of one vocal cord;
   b. repeat stripping of the vocal cord one month after the original diagnosis reveals no evidence of disease;
   c. the patient has stopped smoking;
   d. there is no possibility that the patient will be lost to follow-up.

If all of the conditions as listed in number 6 exist, the localized carcinoma in situ may be treated either by careful excision under microlaryngoscopy or $CO_2$ laser excision under microlaryngoscopy. I prefer the $CO_2$ laser.

If all of the conditions listed in number 6 do not exist, a full course of radiotherapy should be given. Involvement of both vocal cords is an absolute indication for a full course of radiotherapy.

# References

Doyle, P. J., and Flores, A. D. Treatment of carcinoma in situ of the larynx. *J. Otolaryngol.* 6:363–367, 1977.

Miller, A. H. Carcinoma in situ of the larynx—clinical appearance and treatment. *J. Otolaryngol.* 3:567–572, 1974.

# Chapter 4

# *Hemilaryngectomy for Cancer of the Vocal Cord with Fixation*

# John A. Kirchner

In glottic cancer, the term "fixation" implies deep invasion of the thyroarytenoid muscle (fig. 4.1). Other causes of vocal cord immobility are rarely encountered. Invasion of the cricoarytenoid joint, the recurrent nerve, or the posterior cricoarytenoid muscle is usually accompanied by extensive infiltration of the thyroarytenoid muscle and extraglottic parts of the larynx. I have not observed radiation fibrosis as a cause of vocal cord fixation in the absence of residual cancer.

The vocal cord may, however, be immobilized by cancer that has extended laterally along its entire superior surface without actually crossing the ventricle (Kirchner and Som 1971).

True fixation, then, has traditionally been regarded as an ominous feature in glottic cancer, indicating a poor result if treated by radiotherapy and requiring total rather than partial laryngectomy if treated surgically. Martensson and associates (1967) reported a five-year survival of 24% with radiotherapy as compared to 55% with surgery for such growths. Vermund, in his study of fixed cord glottic cancer (1970), reported 42% versus 61% controls in 162 patients treated by radiation or surgery, respectively. Fletcher and colleagues (1975) cite fixation of the vocal cord as a cause of failure to control glottic cancer by radiation.

Vertical hemilaryngectomy as a curative operation for fixed vocal cord lesions was initially contraindicated or undertaken with great trepidation (Figi 1955). In 1959, confronted by a 45-year-old woman with a fixed vocal cord and persistent cancer after a full course of supervoltage radiation, Som performed a hemilaryngectomy when the patient adamantly refused to have the larynx removed in toto. The patient was alive and well 13 years later at last follow-up.

**Figure 4.1**

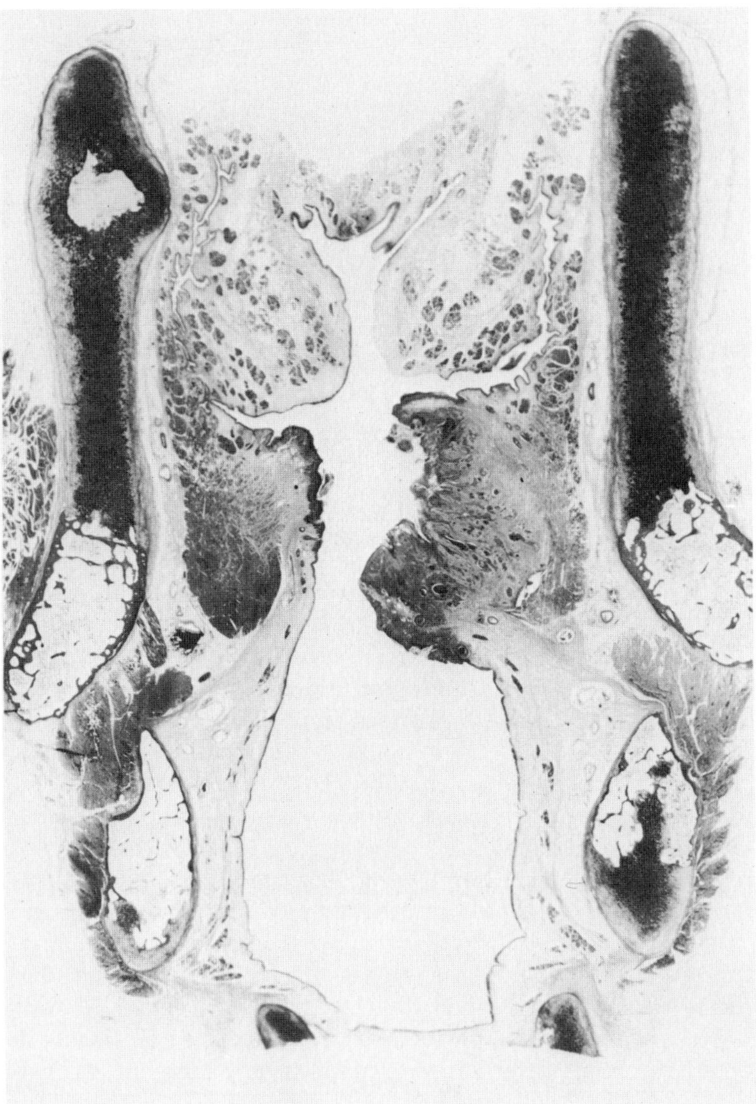

*Fixed cord lesion that might safely have been resected by hemilaryngectomy. The thyroid ala is intact, there is a good subglottic margin, and the ventricle is free of tumor. The opposite cord, however, showed keratosis and possible premalignant changes.*

**Figure 4.2**

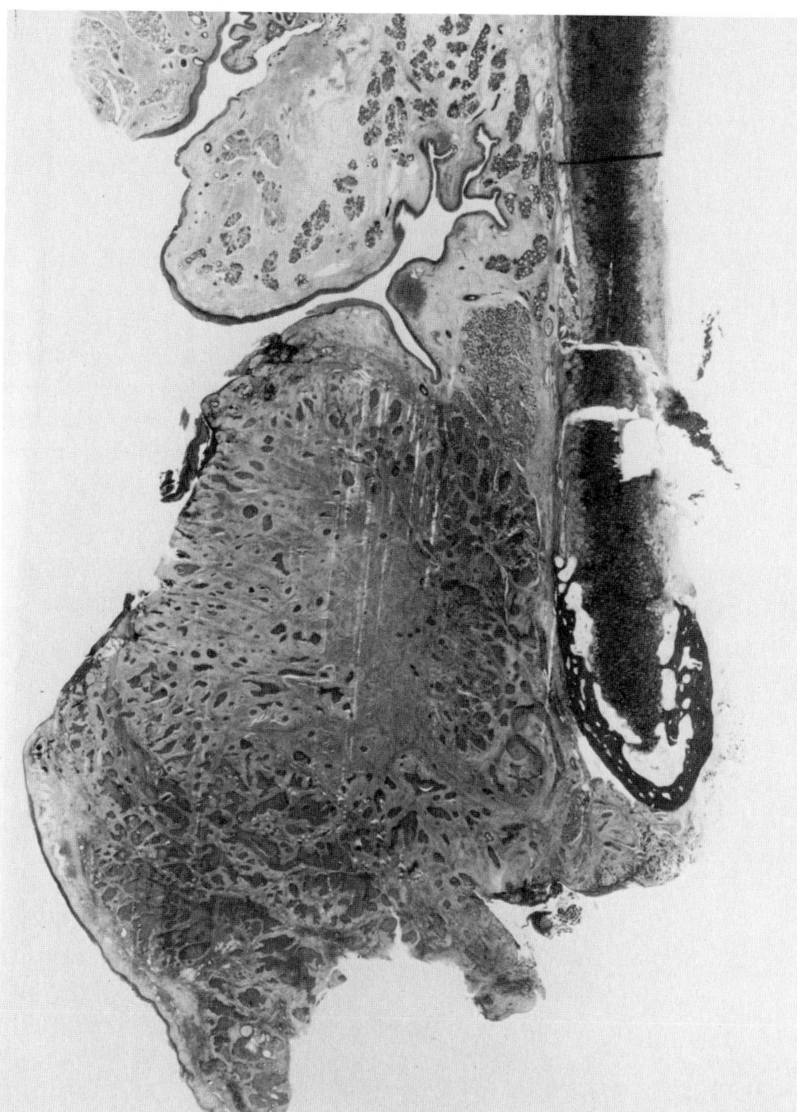

*Hemilaryngectomy specimen, sectioned through the tumor, showing cancer at lower plane of resection. The tumor extends below the level of the inferior edge of the thyroid ala and more than 1 cm below the free edge of the true cord. It is therefore not a suitable candidate for conventional hemilaryngectomy and illustrates the most frequent cause of failure with this operation.*

In 1971 Kirchner and Som reported their results with hemilaryngectomy for glottic cancer with fixation. Thirteen of 22 patients, or 60%, were alive and well 2 to 14 years postoperatively. Of the remaining 9 patients with recurrent cancer, 3 were salvaged by total laryngectomy (Kirchner and Som 1971).

Of the five lesions in which fixation was associated with subglottic extension there were four recurrences. This is consistent with our subsequent observations in serially sectioned laryngectomy and hemilaryngectomy specimens, indicating that failures are usually the result of inadequate margin at the inferior edge of the resection (Fig. 4.2). As additional evidence, Myers and Ogura (1979) report local recurrences in 26 of 238 hemilaryngectomy patients (11%), most of these with cases involving the stoma.

In the anterior and midlarynx, subglottic extension of 1 cm or more is often associated with invasion of the lower edge of the thyroid cartilage, a feature that disqualifies the lesion for hemilaryngectomy because the margins are unpredictable. Conversely, invasion of the thyroid ala has never

**Figure 4.3**

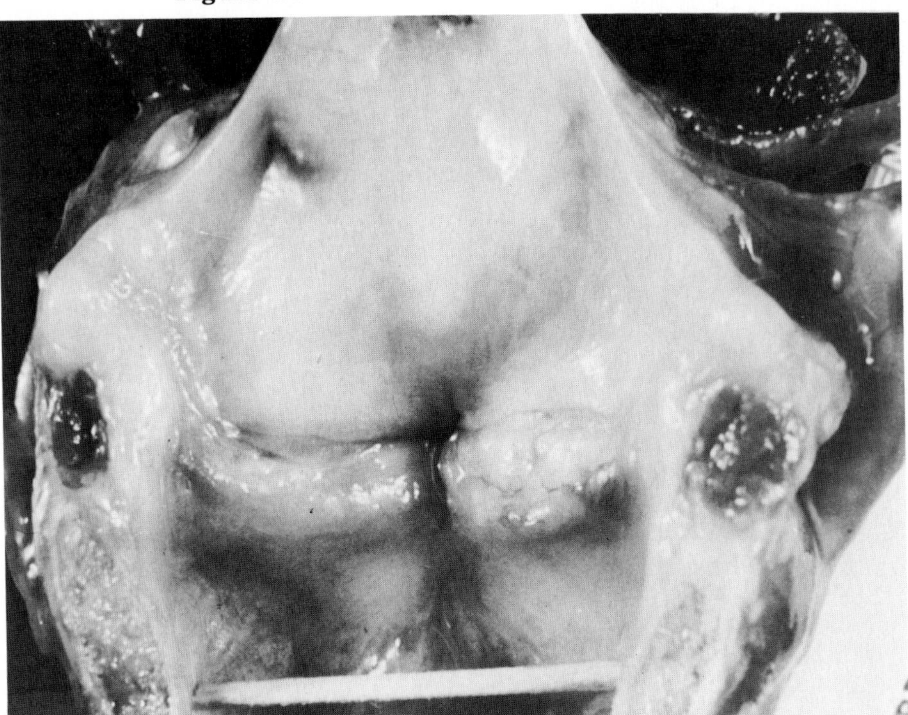

*Glottic cancer with fixation was routinely treated by total laryngectomy in our clinic in 1964. In this specimen, cancer involves the entire true cord but not the ventricular band, which is merely displaced upward (see fig. 4.4).*

been observed in our surgical specimens in which the glottic tumor did not extend more than 8 to 9 mm subglottically, as shown by preoperative tomography or contrast laryngography.

This dimension is valid only in the anterior and midlarynx. In the posterior larynx, the cricoid plate lies immediately below the level of the true cord, so that even 5 to 6 mm of infraglottic extension of cancer may allow invasion of the cricoid plate in this area (Kirchner 1977). Since this structure is usually ossified in patients with laryngeal cancer, the disease spreads readily within its marrow spaces, making it difficult to estimate the extent of invasion. It is mainly for this reason that I have not attempted to resect the rostrum of the cricoid plate in such cases. Another reason is that aspiration often complicates resection of the cricoid rostrum, even after reconstruction with a cartilage muscle flap.

I have had no experience with the technique described by Biller and Som (1977) for reconstructing this area after the cricoid rostrum has been resected. Our laboratory material leads me to believe that lesions suitable for

**Figure 4.4**

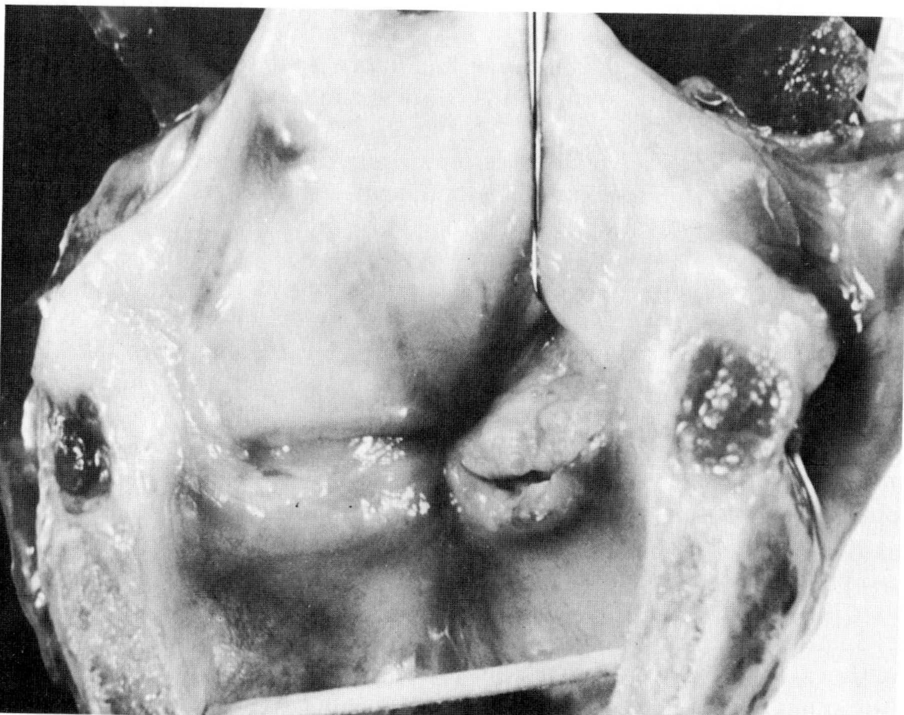

*Cancer involves the superior surface of the true cord but does not cross the ventricle. Small T3 glottic growths of this type are ideal candidates for hemilaryngectomy.*

this type of resection and reconstruction are extraordinarily rare, since invasion of the arytenoid and the cricoarytenoid joint is usually associated with extensive and unpredictable invasion into the soft tissues and adjoining laryngeal framework.

Although the subglottic extent of a vocal cord lesion is the single most important feature in determining feasibility of hemilaryngectomy, other margins must be carefully assessed because they may reflect the depth of invasion and the potential for partial rather than total laryngectomy.

The superior surface of the true cord, for example, may be involved with cancer without precluding hemilaryngectomy as the operation of choice. Fixation in this case may be due simply to extension of tumor along the superior surface of the cord, binding it to the inner surface of the thyroid ala (figs. 4.3 and 4.4). A word of caution, however: this type of lesion may extend high up into the ventricle under an intact ventricular band, and in such a case, will probably invade the thyroid ala. The upward extent may not be appreciated at laryngoscopy even if the ventricular band is pulled up by a hook. Only one such lesion has been identified in our series of 36 fixed cord glottic growths, but the possibility should be borne in mind in preoperative laryngoscopy (figs. 4.5, 4.6, and 4.7).

Lesser degrees of spread along the superior surface of the true cord are adequately managed by conventional hemilaryngectomy since the superior margin of resection traverses the false cord and includes the entire ventricle in the specimen.

In the presence of a fixed cord lesion, involvement of the inferior or ventricular surface of the false cord usually indicates invasion of the thyroid ala and contraindicates hemilaryngectomy.

Anteriorly, the tumor should not involve the opposite vocal cord. Resection of any more than a few millimeters of the uninvolved cord to obtain a safe margin may result in stenosis and an inadequate airway. Similarly, the growth must not have extended upward onto the base of the epiglottis, which usually indicates invasion of the laryngeal framework at this point (Kirchner, Cornog, and Holmes 1974).

Posteriorly, the arytenoid cartilage should be free of tumor. Although this structure is removed at hemilaryngectomy and although its bulk can be replaced by a muscle cartilage flap from the thyroid ala, the undermining and rotation of mucosa from the pyriform sinus, required to resurface the area, may result in a shallow pyriform sinus and aspiration (figs. 4.8 and 4.9).

Since the hemilaryngectomy specimen includes all or most of the ipsilateral thyroid ala, the operation provides a safe margin along the lateral aspect of the tumor, but only when this structure has not been invaded by cancer. As described above, lesions that do not extend more than 9 or 10 mm infraglottically in the anterior and midlarynx are therefore appropriately treated by hemilaryngectomy. The rare exception to this rule is the lesion shown in figures 4.5, 4.6, and 4.7. I am not sure that such a lesion is glottic in the true sense, since it may have arisen in the ventricle itself.

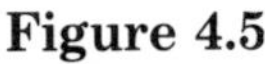

**Figure 4.5**

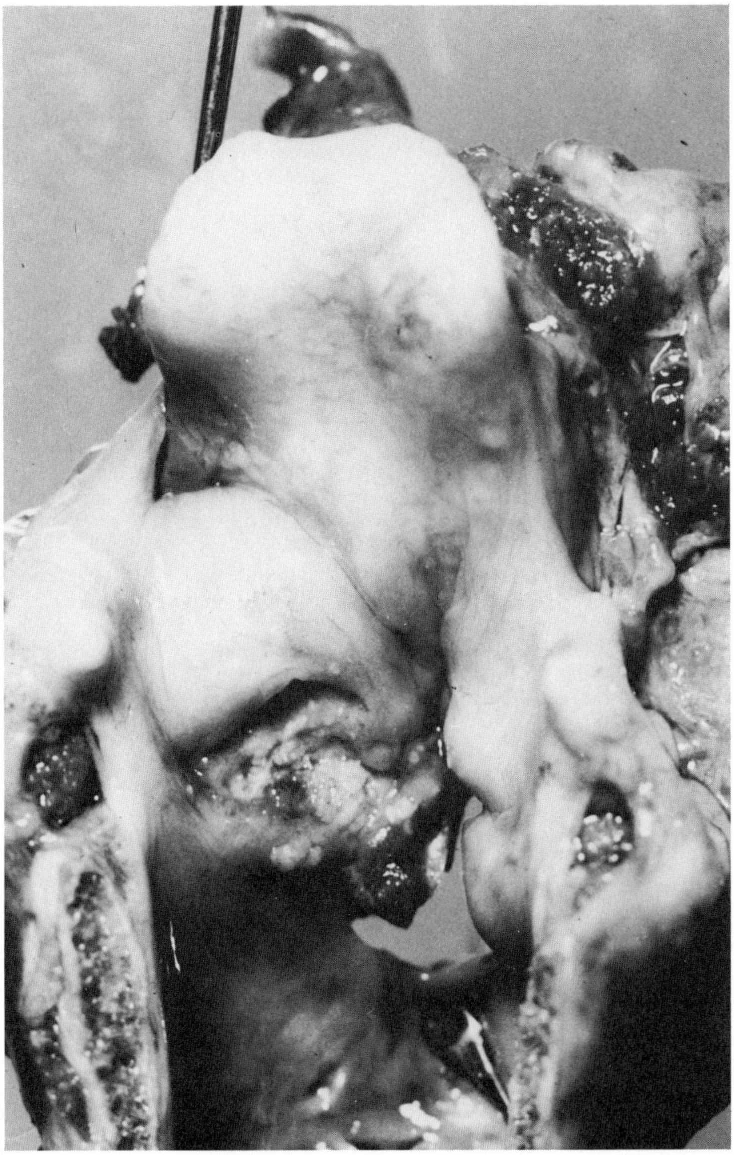

*Glottic cancer with fixation of the true cord and fullness of the ventricular band as seen on indirect laryngoscopy. Hemilaryngectomy was attempted, but cricothyrotomy revealed tumor extending high up into the ventricle (see figs. 4.6 and 4.7).*

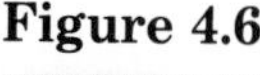

**Figure 4.6**

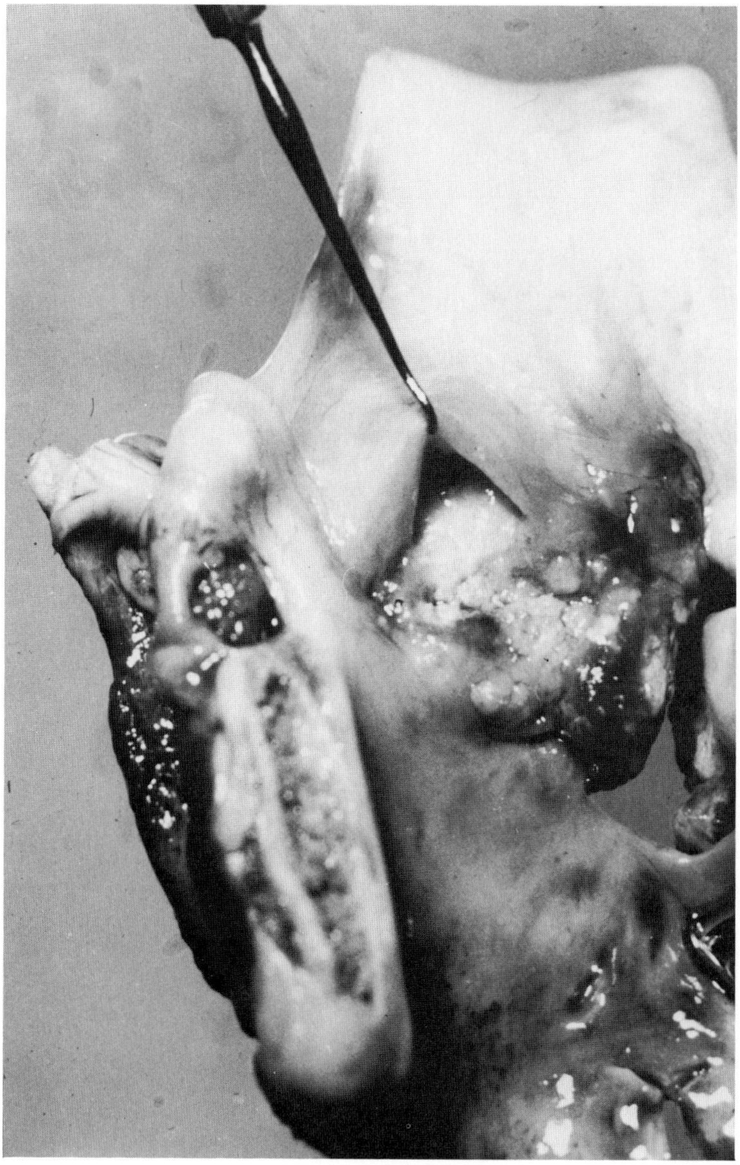

*Tumor extends high up into the ventricle, making the lesion unsuitable for hemilaryngectomy because of the likelihood of invasion into the thyroid ala (see fig. 4.7).*

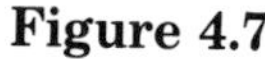

**Figure 4.7**

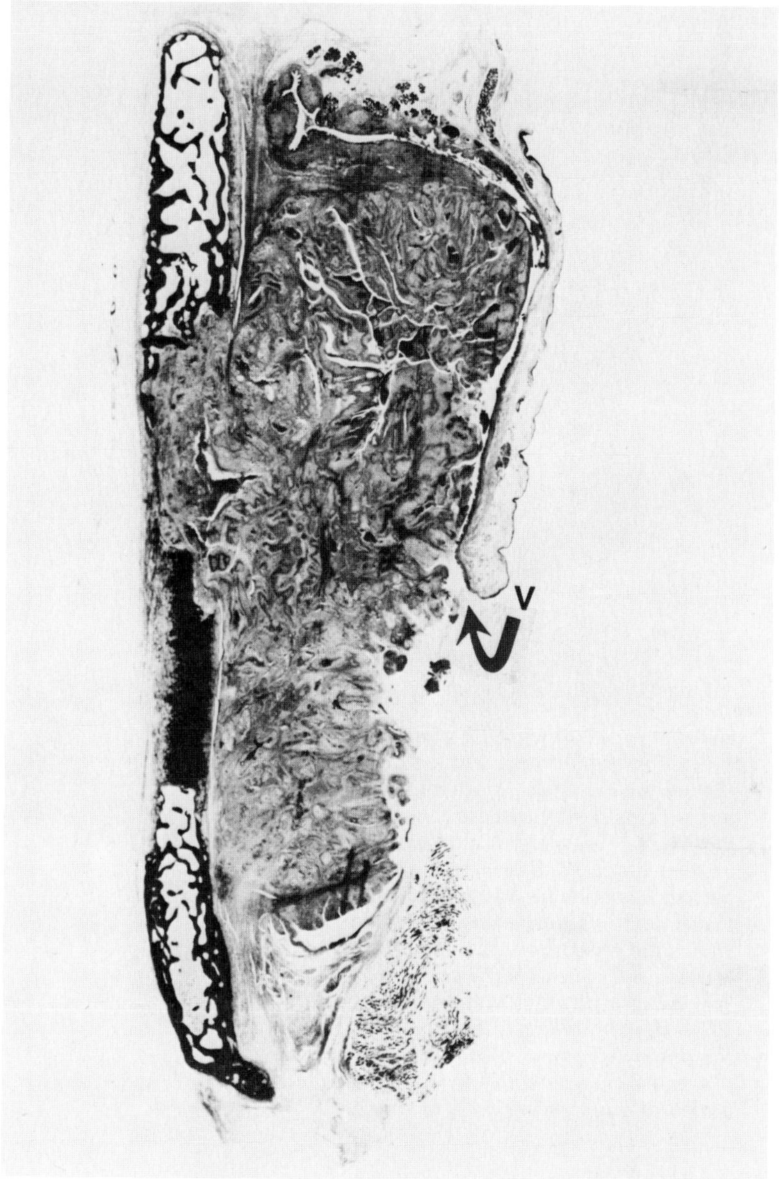

*Section of the glottic lesion shown in the two previous figures. The growth fills the ventricle but does not cross it to involve the ventricular band, which is merely displaced into the laryngeal lumen and free of cancer. Upward extension of this degree should alert the surgeon that cancer may have invaded the ala and that elevation of the external perichondrium and hemilaryngectomy is contraindicated.*

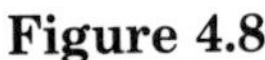
**Figure 4.8**

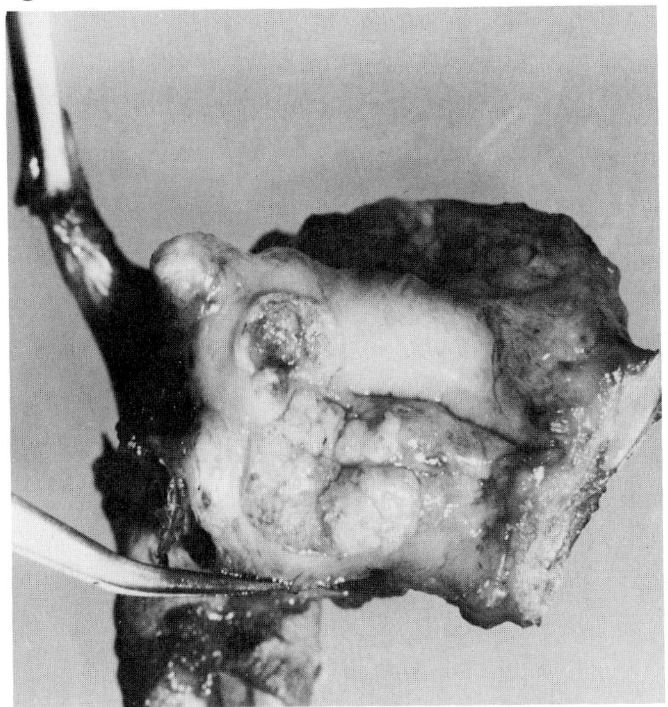

*Hemilaryngectomy for T2 glottic cancer producing limitation of motion and extending upward behind the ventricle onto the arytenoid cartilage. The patient was free of disease for more than five years, maintained his weight, and eventually died of unrelated causes. During the entire postoperative period, however, he had to swallow liquids in small amounts to prevent aspiration. The specimen shows the reason for this: the amount of adjacent mucous membrane that had to be removed for a safe margin resulted in a shallow pyriform sinus. This, in turn, allowed liquids to be directed into the posterior larynx, a complication that can be prevented only partially by the various techniques aimed at augmenting bulk in this area.*

Of the 30 total laryngectomy specimens with fixed vocal cord that we have studied by serial sections, 6 could probably have been safely managed by hemilaryngectomy.

The technical details of hemilaryngectomy are beautifully illustrated in Som's most recent report on the procedure (1975).

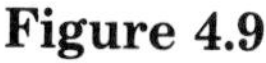

**Figure 4.9**

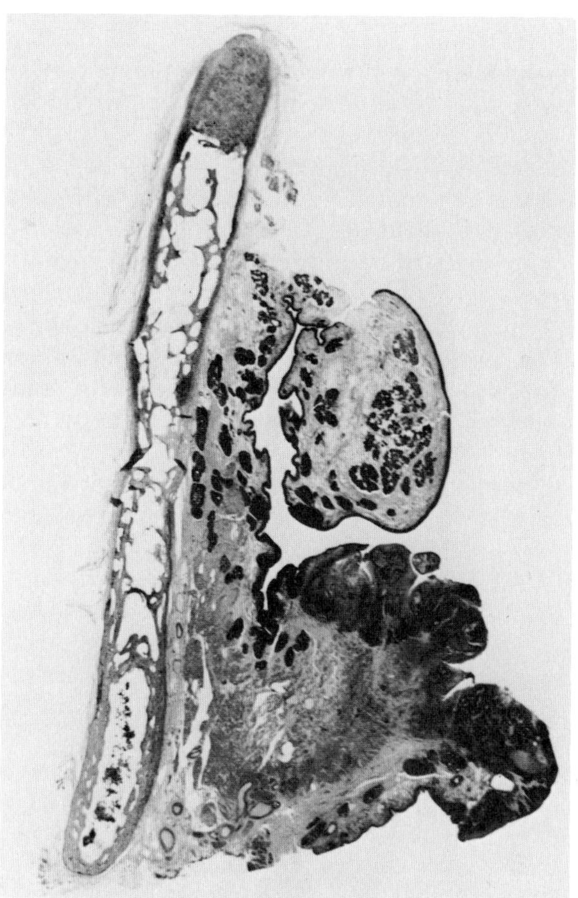

*Coronal section of lesion shown in figure 4.8. Limitation of mobility in this case was due to extension of the growth along the superior surface of the true cord without invasion of the thyroarytenoid muscle. In our experience, radiotherapy is not as effective as surgery for controlling T2 glottic lesions.*

Radiotherapy failures can be managed successfully by hemilaryngectomy, providing that the lesion was initially suitable for this operation. This is a very important provision. The surgeon who is confronted for the first time by a fixed cord glottic carcinoma that has failed to respond to radiotherapy is in a poor position to estimate the lesion's suitability for hemilaryngectomy. The surface may have healed over underlying nests of cancer cells, leaving the margins unpredictable. What is more often true is that the original extent of the lesion was underestimated by the surgeon or radiotherapist who first examined the larynx. In this case, certain physical features of the lesion that would have made it unsuitable for hemilaryngectomy may have been overlooked and are no longer present after radiotherapy. The only person capable of recommending hemilaryngectomy in case of radiation failure is the laryngologist who examined the patient initially and who has examined the larynx at short intervals after treatment.

Healing has not been a major problem in hemilaryngectomy performed for radiation failures. The reason for this, I believe, is that little if any of the thyroid cartilage (usually ossified in these patients) is exposed, since the vertically cut edge of the contralateral thyroid ala is adequately covered by the remaining true cord, ventricular band, and adjacent soft tissues. These structures are well vascularized, even after a conventional course of supervoltage radiation, and help protect the remaining framework against infection and necrosis. Nevertheless, previous radiation occasionally results in perichondritis, loss of parts of the thyroid ala, and prolonged or permanent tracheostomy.

In summary, fixation is not, of itself, a contraindication to hemilaryngectomy for glottic cancer. A survival of 60% can be expected, and failures might still be salvaged by total laryngectomy, especially if the patient has been examined at short intervals during the postoperative period.

Subglottic extension beyond 9 or 10 mm in the male larynx renders the lesion unsuitable for hemilaryngectomy. Posteriorly, the margin of safety is much smaller; in my opinion, the rostrum of the cricoid should not be excised in order to get a safe margin. Permission for total laryngectomy must be obtained in every case before operation.

## References

Biller, H. F., and Som, M. L. Vertical partial laryngectomy for glottic carcinoma with posterior subglottic extension. *Ann. Otol. Rhinol. Laryngol.* 86:715–718, 1977.

Figi, F. A. Carcinoma of the larynx and its present-day management. *Ann. Otol. Rhinol. Laryngol.* 64:136–148, 1955.

Fletcher, G. H. et al. Reasons for irradiation failure in squamous cell carcinoma of the larynx. *Laryngoscope* 85:987–1003, 1975.

Kirchner, J. A.; Cornog, J. L., Jr.; and Holmes, R. E. Transglottic cancer—its growth and spread within the larynx. *Arch. Otolaryngol.* 99:247–251, 1974.

Kirchner, J. A. Two hundred laryngeal cancers: patterns of growth and spread as seen in serial section. *Laryngoscope* 87:474–482, 1977.

Kirchner, J. A., and Som, M. L. Clinical significance of fixed vocal cord. *Laryngoscope* 81:1029–1044, 1971.

Martensson, B.; Fluur, E.; and Jacobson, F. Aspects of treatment of cancer of the larynx. *Ann. Otolaryngol.* 76:313–327, 1967.

Myers, E. M., and Ogura, J. H. Completion laryngectomy. *Otolaryngol. Head Neck Surg.* 87:342–350, 1979.

Som, M. L. Cordal cancer with extension to vocal process. *Laryngoscope* 85:1298–1307, 1975.

Vermund, H. Role of radiotherapy in cancer of the larynx, as related to the TNM system of staging. *Cancer* 5:485–504, 1970.

# Chapter 5

# *Laryngectomy for Cancer of the Larynx with Vocal Cord Fixation*

Donald A. Shumrick and
Jack L. Gluckman

In recent years there has been a dramatic alteration in the prevalence of cancer of the larynx. This condition used to be regarded as a disease affecting predominantly elderly men, but today this no longer holds true. Increasingly, younger patients and women are being diagnosed, undoubtedly reflecting a change in social habits, particularly with regard to smoking and drinking.

While carcinoma of the larynx used to be regarded as a disease with a poor prognosis necessitating mutilating surgery to obtain cure, an increasing number of early lesions are being treated by radiation and conservation surgery, that is, conservation of the function of the larynx. This trend is the result of a combination of improved surgical and radiotherapeutic skills and a greater awareness of the condition by both physicians and the public.

Unfortunately, however, the cornerstone of treatment for cancer of the larynx remains the total laryngectomy with all its sequelae, both psychological and physical. While there is no doubt that this is an excellent operation, the difficulties in successfully restoring patients to their former place in society are considerable.

For this reason there has been a trend in recent years to broaden the indications for conservation laryngeal surgery, with more advanced lesions being treated by hemi- or supraglottic laryngectomy. While there is no doubt that for specific lesions these procedures afford as good a prognosis as would be obtained by total laryngectomy, in certain situations some controversy exists as to their role. Such a situation is carcinoma of the larynx with vocal cord fixation.

## Anatomic Considerations

The single most important factor influencing our understanding of the spread of laryngeal cancer was the use of whole organ sectioning. This enabled a clear appreciation for the first time of the larynx as a three-dimensional organ and not as the two-dimensional structure perceived on indirect or direct laryngoscopy.

An appreciation of the dimensions of the paraglottic space remains the key to understanding the behavior of laryngeal cancer. Clinically, this can best be described as that portion of the larynx lying deep in relation to the mucosa of the endolarynx and is not visible to the examiner (fig. 5.1). Anatomically it is defined as bounded by the thyroid ala, conus elasticus (which separates it from the subglottis), quadrangular membrane, and anterior reflection of the pyriform sinus mucosa. This space can therefore be invaded by direct extension either from lesions arising in the endolarynx or pyriform sinuses. Interpretation of surface signs indicating tumor spread within this space is important to accurate tumor assessment. The paraglottic space communicates with, and therefore allows easy access to, the preepiglottic space, which is bounded posteriorly by the epiglottis, anteriorly by the thyrohyoid membrane and hyoid bone, and superiorly by the hyoepiglottic ligament.

## Pathologic Considerations

The spread of cancer of the larynx is determined by the site of origin and the anatomic barriers produced by the different laryngeal compartments. The cartilaginous framework is an excellent barrier to tumor spread but has certain weak points through which tumor may extend.

**Figure 5.1**

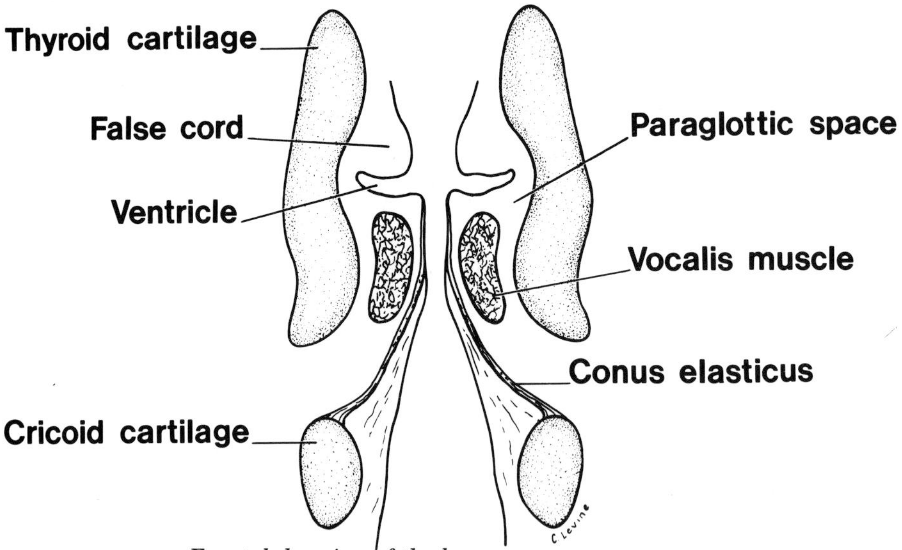

*Frontal drawing of the larynx.*

# Site of Origin

## Glottic

Most carcinomas of the larynx arise on the free margin of the vocal cord with direct spread through Reinke's space along the length of the cord. Posterior extension may occur either medially or laterally to the arytenoid cartilage. Anterior extension to the anterior commissure may result in spread from the larynx along the anterior commissure tendon. Deep extension results in infiltration of the vocalis muscle with initial limitation of cord movement and later complete fixation (fig. 5.2A). Deeper extension into the paraglottic space then occurs, with invasion of the thyroid cartilage and extension through the cricothyroid membrane being logical extensions of this process.

## Subglottic

The subglottic region is ill defined in the literature, but generally is accepted clinically as being an area commencing 10 mm below the free edge of the cord and extending to the lower edge of the cricoid cartilage. At the anterior commissure and posterior commissure its site of commencement is approximately 5 mm below the cord. Involvement of the subglottis is associated with an ominous prognosis for two reasons: (1) easy access to, and therefore early spread through, the cricothyroid membrane; (2) early involvement of the cricothyroid node, a condition regarded by many authors as having the same prognosis as a contralateral node.

While clinically this definition of the subglottic space is generally accepted, histopathologically the conus elasticus is regarded as the barrier separating the glottis from the subglottis. Should the tumor therefore penetrate this membrane it must be regarded as being subglottic, even though macroscopically it may involve only the undersurface of the cord (fig. 5.2C).

## Supraglottic

Spread of carcinoma across the ventricle from the supraglottic to the glottis, that is, a transglottic lesion, is invariably associated with extensive paraglottic space involvement and a high incidence of cartilage involvement (fig. 5.2B).

# Vocal Cord Fixation

The attending physician should be aware of the many possible causes of vocal cord fixation, bearing in mind that in any particular situation more than one factor usually comes into play. The common causes are as follows:

1. Infiltration of the vocalis muscle. This is without a doubt the most com-

**Figure 5.2**

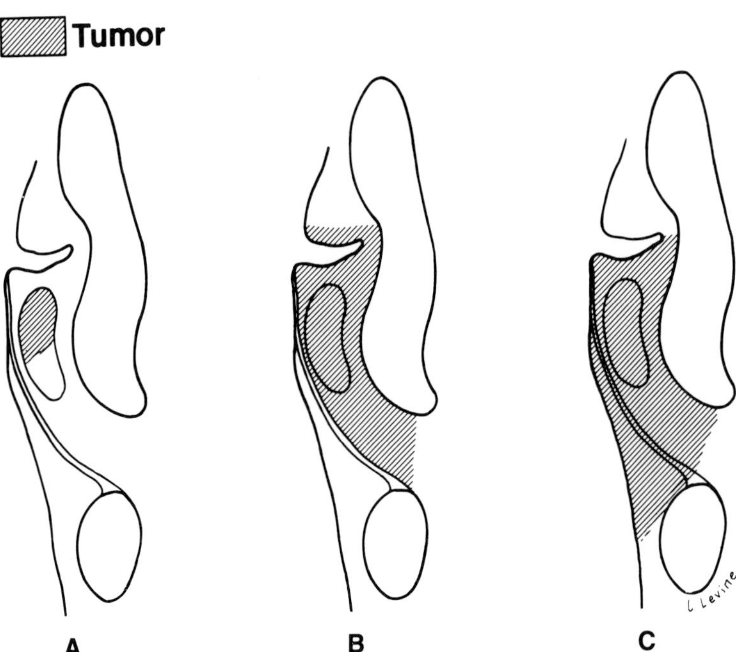


*Frontal drawing of hemilarynx.* A, *infiltration of the vocalis muscle;* B, *transglottic infiltration with invasion of the paraglottic space;* C, *penetration of the conus elasticus with invasion of the subglottic space.*

mon cause and occurs in almost every case. This condition is seen most frequently following deep infiltration by a glottic carcinoma, but may occur in transglottic, subglottic, and pyriform sinus lesions with medial extension. While there is no question that a glottic carcinoma with vocal cord fixation due to vocalis muscle infiltration alone is amenable to hemilaryngectomy, the diagnostic dilemma is whether deeper infiltration has occurred, which may render this procedure inappropriate.

2. Involvement of other intrinsic laryngeal muscles, that is, posterior and lateral cricoarytenoid and interarytenoid muscles. These are invariably invaded at a stage subsequent to involvement of the vocalis muscle.

3. Tethering of the vocalis muscle to the underlying thyroid cartilage. This generally is due to deeper infiltration after involvement of the vocalis muscle. Rarely in subglottic, transglottic, or pyriform sinus lesions the vocalis muscle may be tethered, but not infiltrated. The lower border of the thyroid

cartilage and upper border of the cricoid cartilage are usually involved, with the malignancy frequently confined to that portion of the cartilage that has undergone ossification. Occasionally, very aggressive tumors may invade the cartilage directly; this direct involvement renders the tumor no longer amenable to hemilaryngectomy.

4. Tethering of the vocal cords to the underlying cricoid plate as occurs with subglottic extension posteriorly.

5. Involvement of the cricoarytenoid joint. As an isolated occurrence, this is extremely rare and is usually associated with the other causes of vocal cord fixation.

6. Involvement of the recurrent laryngeal nerve, which is generally invaded medial to the lower border of the thyroid ala. This is involved late and rarely as an isolated entity.

7. Postradiation fibrosis without tumor invasion. The development of vocal cord fixation following completion of a curative dose of radiation should be viewed with a high index of suspicion. While this condition has been ascribed to postradiation fibrosis, the physician should be extremely wary about making this diagnosis until recurrent tumor has been absolutely excluded.

## Therapeutic Dilemma

Historically, the presence of a fixed vocal cord in laryngeal cancer was regarded as an absolute contraindication to hemilaryngectomy. This concept was supported by the clinical experience of a large number of surgeons, and has only been challenged since the advent of whole laryngeal serial sectioning, when it was noted that many of those patients who underwent total laryngectomies could have easily been treated by more conservative procedures.

There is little argument that carcinoma of the vocal cord with fixation due to vocalis muscle infiltration can be treated by hemilaryngectomy, but the dilemma exists as how to diagnose those lesions that are amenable to such therapy and to ensure that deeper extension has not occurred.

Regarding this problem, Kirchner and Som (1971) report that of 18 total laryngectomies performed for true glottic carcinoma with vocal cord fixation, all could have just as adequately been treated by a hemilaryngectomy. On the other hand, Olofsson and colleagues (1973) reported a poor correlation between the preoperative assessment and the pathologic findings, with 50% of the glottic carcinomas with vocal cord fixation being underassessed.

Certain clinical lesions with vocal cord fixation, however, have a greater chance of cartilage involvement with extension outside of the larynx and are not, in our opinion, amenable to hemilaryngectomy. These are:

1. Pyriform sinus carcinomas with vocal cord fixation. These are characterized by extensive medial infiltration with paraglottic space involvement and therefore would not be suitable for a hemilaryngectomy.

2. Transglottic carcinoma. Once the lesion has extended across the ventricle, the paraglottic space is invariably involved, and there is an increased chance of cartilage involvement and extension outside the larynx. In addition, extension upward to involve the base of the epiglottis often indicates direct invasion of the thyroid cartilage (Kirchner and Som 1971).

3. Subglottic extension. Subglottic extension has always been regarded as a contraindication to hemilaryngectomy because of the difficulty in obtaining adequate clearance of the lower extent of the tumor and its known propensity for extension through the cricothyroid membrane and early involvement of the cricothyroid nodes. Similarly any lesion that penetrates the conus elasticus has the same ominous implications and thus, even if the lesion should be merely on the undersurface of the cord, it should be regarded with suspicion.

It is therefore our opinion that in any of the above lesions no controversy should exist and total laryngectomy should be performed in preference to any conservation approach. The problem case remains the glottic carcinoma with vocal cord fixation. In this situation we know that the commonest cause is vocalis muscle infiltration alone, and this is amenable to resection by hemilaryngectomy. The difficulty lies in determining whether the lesion is truly confined to the glottis and whether any deeper infiltration has occurred that would make this lesion unsuitable for a hemilaryngectomy.

## Assessment of Patients

The evaluation of patients with a fixed vocal cord to determine whether partial or total laryngectomy should be performed is extremely complex, with subtle symptoms and signs often tipping the balance one way or the other. All facets of the investigations should be performed by experienced personnel and checked by the surgeon who is to perform the procedure. The preoperative assessment should not be delegated to an inexperienced individual. The final decision should not be taken lightly as no situation is more tragic than where cancer cure has been compromised in order to retain function. Salvage therapy, whatever the modality, is invariably associated with a poor prognosis.

### Clinical Evaluation

Palpation of the neck may be helpful, particularly palpation of the laryngeal skeleton. Expansion of the thyroid cartilage and tenderness may suggest underlying chondritis secondary to invasion. The cricothyroid membrane should be palpated for any distortion and particularly for obvious enlargement of the cricothyroid lymph nodes. Indirect laryngoscopy, in our opinion, is one of the most important methods of determining the degree of cord fixation. This appears to be more effective than direct laryngoscopy, where the larynx is often distorted by the presence of the rigid laryngoscope or ventilating tube. Subtle signs, such as fullness of the false cords, may be apparent.

# Radiology

X-ray examination of the larynx is a useful adjunct to indirect and direct laryngoscopy. Its value is to aid in determining the precise anatomic site of the lesion, as well as its size, and it may be helpful in delineating the functional alteration of the involved structures. It therefore supplements the clinical observations. While the following techniques are undoubtedly helpful, care must be taken not to misinterpret the findings, and only constant defects should be interpreted as pathologic.

## Lateral X-ray of the Neck

This is useful for gross lesions but remains valueless in deciphering the subtle signs necessary to decide what sort of therapy to institute in a particular situation.

## Xeroradiography

The supposed advantage of this technique is its ability to distinguish between structures of different intensities, particularly with regard to infiltration of cartilage. In our opinion, it does not appear to offer much more than the standard lateral view of the neck. In addition, ossification of the thyroid cartilage is variable, and normal variations may give the appearance of tumor infiltration.

## Tomography

In certain instances this technique is invaluable in determining the true extent of the disease. It demonstrates lateral spread by showing obliteration of the ventricle and fullness of the false cord, and may be able to detect early invasion of the thyroid cartilage. Its main advantage is that it is an excellent means of demonstrating subglottic extension usually manifesting as a blunting of the subglottic angle. A major drawback is its inability to show mucosal change.

## Laryngography

In our opinion, this technique, combined with cinelaryngography, is the most valuable investigative procedure available to the clinician. In our unit each patient with a suspected laryngeal carcinoma is subjected to this investigation the day prior to laryngoscopy. It is an excellent method for detecting early lesions, mucosal spread, lateral extension into the pyriform sinuses, and subglottic extension. If there is any extension of tumor anteriorly through the cartilage the contrast dye may indicate such an extension, which cannot be seen with the eye on indirect or direct examination. Its major advantage, however, remains the evaluation of laryngeal function, which can be assessed by a variety of maneuvers, including Valsalva, phonation, and inspiration.

## Direct Laryngoscopy

Direct examination of the larynx under anesthesia remains the most important means of assessing the extent of disease and determining the surgical approach. This should be done by the surgeon who is to perform the definitive surgery.

The key to this examination is an understanding of the larynx as a three-dimensional structure and interpretation of the often subtle surface signs which may indicate the true extent of the tumor. There is no substitute for experience in this evaluation.

After visualization of the endolarynx as a whole, looking carefully for any distortion of the laryngeal structures, for example, bulging of the false cords, the lesion is then examined and the subglottic and ventricles are carefully inspected. Attention should be devoted to assessing whether any submucosal spread has occurred. The cricoarytenoid joint should be inspected and palpated. Extra care must be exercised if the patient has a lesion which has recurred after radiation. Deep biopsies after initial incision of the mucosa may be necessary.

## Surgical Exploration

In many cases, even after careful evaluation by experienced personnel, a final decision cannot be made and an exploration of the larynx is necessary at the time of definitive surgery. The patient must be made aware of this eventuality and be prepared for the possibility of a total laryngectomy, including all the preoperative counseling necessary in such a situation, for example, preoperative speech therapy and counseling. It is our policy to offer all who may undergo a total laryngectomy the possibility of primary or secondary neoglottic reconstruction if feasible. The various procedures are discussed in detail with them so that they may have realistic expectations regarding these techniques. In addition, they meet with other patients who have undergone such procedures.

A tracheostomy under local anesthetic is performed and the laryngeal skeleton exposed by retraction of the strap muscles. At this stage special attention is paid to the cricothyroid membrane and thyroid cartilage at the anterior commissure looking for any gross tumor invasion. A search for enlarged cricothyroid lymph nodes should be made and if found should be sent for frozen section. The external perichondrium is then reflected, and the thyroid cartilage inspected for any suspicious areas which are then sent for histologic evaluation. If the above maneuvers are negative, the larynx should be approached as for a hemilaryngectomy.

The cricothyroid membrane is divided just above the cricoid cartilage and the subglottis carefully inspected for any tumor with emphasis on submucosal extension, particularly in failed radiation cases. Obviously, if any tumor extension outside the larynx is encountered the procedure should be immediately converted into a total laryngectomy.

After cartilaginous cuts have been made and doubt still exists as to the feasibility of a hemilaryngectomy, we have found the following maneuver useful in determining the depth of infiltration and possible involvement of the thyroid cartilage. The internal perichondrium on the affected side is stripped from the thyroid cartilage using a periosteal elevator. If the perichondrium is intact and strips easily, a hemilaryngectomy may safely be performed. If on the other hand any evidence of tumor erosion is encountered, the procedure should immediately be converted into a total laryngectomy.

The arytenoid on the affected side should be excised in lesions with a fixed cord in order to obtain improved clearance even if the vocalis muscle alone is involved.

After the surgical specimen has been removed, frozen sections are then taken from all margins to insure adequate excision. In conclusion, if any doubt exists prior to or during the procedure regarding the possibility of compromising the cancer operation by performing conservation surgery, careful thought should be given to converting the procedure to a total laryngectomy.

### Fixed Cord in Radiation Failure Cases

By far the most difficult case to evaluate for conservation surgery is the radiation failure with a fixed cord. Extreme caution should be exercised in such a case as it has been our experience that there is a tendency to submucosal spread with apparently normal overlying mucosa. For this reason the extent of the lesion is always underestimated. The approach adopted should be as described above, but with a much higher index of suspicion.

## Conclusions

1. Hemilaryngectomy is a useful operation for cancer of the larynx with a fixed vocal cord due to vocalis muscle infiltration alone.
2. Hemilaryngectomy is contraindicated in transglottic, subglottic, and pyriform sinus lesions with vocal cord fixation.

3. It is extremely difficult to evaluate clinically the true extent of a glottic carcinoma with vocal cord fixation.
4. The decision as to which procedure should be adopted should be made by an experienced surgeon after careful assessment.
5. Great caution should be exercised before recommending hemilaryngectomy in patients with radiation failure.
6. If any doubt exists prior to or during the surgery, it is better to be safe and perform a total laryngectomy, including neoglottic reconstruction if feasible.

# References

Kirchner, J. A., and Som, M. A. Clinical significance of a fixed vocal cord. *Laryngoscope* 81:1029–1044, 1971.

Olofsson, J.; Lord, I. J.; and von Nostrand, A. W. P. Vocal cord fixation in laryngeal carcinoma. *Acta Otolaryngol.* 74:496–510, 1973.

# Chapter 6

# *Radiation Therapy Alone in Advanced Epidermoid Carcinoma of the Laryngopharynx with Emphasis on the Significance of Vocal Cord Fixation*

# J. P. Bataini

Two objectives must be looked for in the management of laryngeal and pharyngolaryngeal cancer: cure of the disease and, whenever possible, preservation of laryngeal functions.

Preservation of laryngeal functions is the aim of the various conservative or reconstructive surgical procedures advocated in certain countries for early and some moderately-advanced tumors. Preservation of function is also the aim of radiotherapy, initiated in the early 1920s by Coutard at the *Fondation Curie,* which was further investigated there by Baclesse (1949).

In fact, treatment indications in squamous cell laryngeal and hypopharyngeal carcinoma show wide variations according not only to countries but also institutions and, in certain cases, among different departments of the same institution. Surgery and radiotherapy play inversely proportional roles. In certain treatment centers, radiotherapy is almost ignored or assumes an ancillary place. In others, a certain balance between surgery and radiotherapy has been achieved, thanks to an interdisciplinary approach endeavoring (not always successfully) to take into consideration the curative, functional, and cosmetic results in that order of priority. Early exophytic tumors are thus often treated by radiotherapy, and advanced cases are treated by ablative surgery alone or associated with planned radiotherapy either postoperatively or preoperatively (Cachin et al. 1979; Fletcher et al. 1970; MacComb and Fletcher 1967). Among the pioneers of this combined approach, which is used presently in many cancer institutions, were Leroux-Robert and Ennuyer (1956) in the late 1940s at the *Fondation Curie,* who used it because of the poor results obtained by conventional 200 kilovolt therapy in moderately advanced cases.

Indeed, certain factors or features in cancer of the larynx and hypopharynx such as fixation of cord, extralaryngeal spread, involvement of cartilage, and presence of cervical metastatic nodes are considered not only by surgeons but also by a fair number of radiotherapists to be unfavorable for radiotherapy, and many see them as formal contraindications to that modality. These factors influence prognosis for radiocurability, which depends, however, essentially on the number of tumor cells and the proportion of hypoxic cells in the tumor population. One has to consider that these factors also influence the results of initial surgery, although perhaps not to the same extent.

In the late 1950s, we modified the therapeutic regimens in our department at the Curie Foundation, taking into account the advantages of supervoltage radiation. All laryngeal and hypopharyngeal carcinomas, referred directly or through the ENT section, were systematically and radically irradiated, surgery being reserved for radiation failures. The objective was not only to cure the disease but to preserve function, because of the severe psychological impact of laryngectomy on the patient's social interaction and family life. The favorable results we reported at intervals since 1964 (Bataini and Ennuyer 1971; Bataini et al. 1974; Ennuyer and Bataini 1964, 1965, 1973; Ennuyer, Poncet, and Bataini 1977) stimulated us to pursue this conservative approach. Thus a large series of supraglottic and hypopharyngeal carcinomas, but relatively fewer cases of glottic carcinomas, were treated by primary radiation. Indeed, in many French centers carcinoma of the vocal cord was and is still managed by surgery, conservative in early cases, radical in extensive cases, and reconstructive in a few moderately advanced lesions. Since 1975–1976, however, thanks to a new surgical team, all glottic carcinomas have also been referred for initial radiotherapy.

The purpose of this chapter is to analyze the results of 20 years of personal experience with radical supervoltage radiotherapy in advanced cancer of the larynx and hypopharynx classically treated by ablative surgery. The influence of the unfavorable factors already mentioned on survival and on control of the disease locally and in the neck will be discussed, as will the functional results and complications, and the possibilities of salvage surgery.

Unfortunately, comparison of results of initial surgery and initial radiation is impossible. Published series vary. The variations consist of differences in staging and patient selection (Vanderbrook et al. 1979). Data collected over long periods of time are not homogeneous with respect to treatment (Smith et al. 1973). The calculation of survival from institution to institution can vary. Actual survival calculated by the life table method shows higher survival rates than absolute survival.

In laryngeal and pharyngolaryngeal tumors, prognosis differs according to the region of origin, and this holds true for all cases, early or advanced. Prognosis, which is worse for disease of the hypopharynx, improves somewhat for cancer of the supraglottis and more so for glottis. Assigning a site of origin might prove extremely difficult in advanced cases. Thus differing prognoses are due not only to different local or regional invasiveness of the carcinoma but to factors such as differences in the population involved, their smoking and drinking habits (Brugere et al. 1979a), and correlations with social status. These factors influence the general and nutritional conditions of patients and their immunologic status, perhaps favoring the appearance of distant metastases or second primaries. Patterns of survival curves thus differ in glottic, supraglottic, and hypopharyngeal carcinomas, whether treated by surgery or radiotherapy or a combination of both. Niederer and associates (1976) reviewed 163 patients with supraglottic carcinoma treated by radiation at the Ontario Cancer Treatment and Research Foundation. The overall actuarial five-year survival was 48%. The authors showed that prevention of smoking and drinking was more statistically significant in achieving 100% survival than was elimination of technical failures, radioresistance, and distant metastasis. The basis of this conclusion was that the majority of deaths occurred in patients cured of their supraglottic cancer, but dying of other diseases related to tobacco and alcohol such as arteriosclerosis, emphysema, cirrhosis, or cancer of the esophagus, lung, and oral cavity.

In this chapter, three distinct sites will be considered: (1) glottis or vocal cord; (2) supraglottis, that is, posterior surface of epiglottis, false cord, and ventricle; and (3) hypopharynx, which, in France, almost always arises in the pyriform sinus. Results concerning carcinoma of glottis and supraglottis have been published in the past years, and have not been reviewed for this presentation. A thorough analysis is planned in the near future. The analysis of the cases of carcinoma of pyriform sinus (Bataini et al. 1979a, 1979b; Brugere et al. 1979a, 1979b) is recent, and the influence of such factors as fixation of cord, extensive spread, and the different aspects of the node problem on control of the disease and survival will be discussed.

Reference will also be made to the lateral epilaryngeal carcinomas or marginal carcinomas. These arise from the lateral border of the epiglottis, the aryepiglottic fold, or the junction of lateral border of the epiglottis with the ary- and pharyngoepiglottic folds. The epilarynx, or marginal zone of the larynx, is included in the supraglottic region of the larynx in the International Union Against Cancer (UICC) and American Joint Commission (AJC) classifications. Epilaryngeal carcinomas, however, are not often dissociated from carcinomas of pyriform sinus in the published results (Vanderbrook et al. 1979).

Staging used is the UICC classification and is the following for laryngeal carcinoma:

T3: tumors limited to the larynx with fixation.

T4: tumors extending beyond the larynx, that is, extension to hypopharynx, oropharynx, cartilage, and soft tissues of the neck. In this series, extension to the preepiglottic space was staged T4.

T1 and T2 represent less advanced disease with no cord fixation.

For carcinoma of pyriform sinus, advanced cases were staged T3 when the vocal cord was fixed, whether the disease was limited to the pharyngolarynx or had already spread toward the oropharynx, cervical esophagus, cartilage, or soft tissues.

Node staging was the following:

N0: cervical lymph nodes not palpable.
N1: clinically palpable homolateral mobile cervical nodes.
N2: palpable bilateral or contralateral clinically significant mobile cervical nodes.
N3: fixed cervical lymph nodes.

Sixty percent of nodes secondary to supraglottic carcinoma (Bataini et al. 1974) and more than 80% of nodes secondary to pyriform sinus carcinoma (Brugere et al. 1979b) had cytologic examination by fine-needle aspiration. In the supraglottic series, 74% of biopsied nodes were positive for carcinoma. This indicates the high incidence of malignant involvement when a node is clinically palpable, especially when one considers that needle biopsy was often performed only when clinical doubt existed regarding possible malignancy. In the hypopharyngeal series, correlation between the clinical status of the node and the positive cytologic examination was 88% for patients with N1 and N2 stage and 99% for those with N3 stage.

## Fixation of Vocal Cord

The prognostic role of a fixed vocal cord in laryngeal and pharyngolaryngeal carcinoma has been widely discussed in the past, mainly regarding glottic cancer (Vermund 1970). Fixation is a sign of a deeply infiltrating process involving the muscular structures of the cord and the cricoarytenoid region. In certain cases, however, fixation might be caused by an inflammatory condition of the cricoarytenoid joint.

Vocal cord fixation occurs in advanced cancer of the glottis and is frequently accompanied by extension to the subglottis. In supraglottic carcinoma, the cord itself is rarely involved except when the site of origin is the ventricle, when the disease can extend rapidly to the glottis and subglottis in the so-called transglottic cases. Fixation is the rule in advanced carcinoma of the epilarynx, pyriform sinus, and retrocricoid region.

1. The reported five-year survival after total laryngectomy for advanced carcinoma of the glottis varies between 45% and 65%. Statistical study based on 1614 cases of patients with T3 disease collected from 23 centers and analyzed for the Centennial Conference on Laryngeal Cancer in Toronto in 1974 showed five-year crude survival of 45% (Till et al. 1975). The large majority of these patients were treated by surgery. Analyzed results for T4 tumors showed a five-year crude survival of 28% in a pooled series of 202 cases. In Leroux-Robert's (1975) personal surgical series concerning 620 glottic carcinomas, the crude five-year survival was 56% for T3 lesions (232 cases) and 26% for T4 lesions (31 cases). Jesse (1975) reported a four-year survival of 54% in a series of 48 patients with T4 lesions treated by surgery alone or followed by radiotherapy.

In a personal series of 45 patients staged at T3 and T4, and treated with primary radiation (Bataini et al. 1979b), absolute three-year survival was 44%: 15 of 35 patients staged at T3 N0, 2 of 3 at T3 N1, 2 of 5 at T4 N0, and 1 at T4 N1. One patient had fixed nodal disease (T3 N3) and failed. Of the 16 local failures, 12 were operated on with a resulting long-term salvage of 8 patients, thus bringing the final survival to 62%. The 9 other failures were ascribed to two recurrences in the lower part of the cervical trachea, two recurrences in the neck, two recurrences in the primary tumor and neck, and complications with one patient. Two patients died of intercurrent disease, and there was a negative postmortem examination for one of them. The 10% incidence of neck disease initially (5 of 45), the incidence of recurrence in the neck with or without recurrence in the primary (4 patients), and the risk of recurrence in the low cervical trachea (2 patients) had led us to modify our radiation technique for advanced carcinoma of the glottis along the lines followed for radiation of supraglottic carcinoma.

The five-year crude result in a small series of 27 patients was 66%, with 12 of the 18 survivors retaining a useful larynx.

2. Comparing the results of surgery and radiotherapy in advanced supraglottic carcinoma is difficult because of the node problem. The reported crude five-year survival in Toronto (Till et al. 1975) in 627 T3 and 518 T4 supraglottic carcinomas treated by surgery or radiotherapy was 34% and 24%. In a personal series of 41 patients irradiated for T3 supraglottic carcinoma, crude three- and five-year survival was 41.4% (17 of 41) and 36.5% (15 of 41), respectively. The corresponding results in a consecutive series of 94 patients staged at T4 were 43% (40 of 93) and 35.4% (33 of 93). These two series were included in the Toronto analysis.

Salvage surgery yielded rather poor results in this series, with three five-year survivors (one T3 N0, one T4 N0, and one T4 N1). Results in recent cases (T3) are definitely more encouraging and will be discussed later.

The determinate results at three years with radiotherapy only in T3 disease with or without subglottic extension showed 16 survivors out of 33 (48%). Five of 12 patients with subglottic extension (transglottic) were cured.

3. The specific influence of fixation of vocal cord was looked for in a recently studied series of 434 cases of carcinoma of the pyriform sinus treated by radiotherapy from 1958 through 1974 at the *Institut Curie* (Bataini et al. 1979a, 1979b). Results were assessed at two years, as 95% of the locoregional failures occurred by that interval. For the purposes of the study, 9 patients with bilateral nodes and 176 with fixed nodes were excluded, and the results were assessed in the remaining N0 N1 patients (table 6.1).

Local failure occurred in 28% of the cases (20 of 72) when cord mobility was normal or impaired, and increased to 36% when only the cord was fixed (63 of 177). In a determinate group, excluding patients lost to follow-up or having died of distant metastases, intercurrent disease, or second primary tumor, the local control at two years averaged 63% when the cord was not fixed versus 51% when it was.

**Table 6.1**
Radiotherapy of Carcinoma of Pyriform Sinus: Influence of Vocal Cord Mobility on Two-Year Survival and Local Control of Disease in 249 N0 N1 MO Patients

| Cord Mobility | Total Number of Patients | Two-Year Survival (No./%) | Total Local Failures (No./%) | Indeterminate Group* | Determinate Group | Local Control at Two Years in Determinate Group (No./%) |
|---|---|---|---|---|---|---|
| Normal | 33 | 15/45 | 9/27 | 10 | 23 | 14/64 |
| Impaired | 39 | 22/57 | 11/29 | 8 | 31 | 20/64 |
| Abolished | 177 | 72/40 | 63/36 | 47 | 130 | 67/51 |

*Includes patients dying of intercurrent disease, second cancer, distant metastases, or lost to follow-up within two years of radiotherapy.

Influence of fixation was also looked for in a series of 157 lateral epilaryngeal carcinomas (Bataini et al. 1979a, 1979b). Excluding patients with unfavorable node factors (5 N2 and 47 N3), the results were analyzed in the remaining 105 cases at three years after therapy, as 90% of the locoregional failures occurred by that interval (table 6.2).

Local failure occurred in 9% of patients when mobility was normal (4 of 43), in 23% when mobility was impaired (9 of 38), and in 35% (8 of 23) when it was abolished. It has to be emphasized, however, that almost all patients (31 of 36) with fixed cord already had extrapharyngolaryngeal spread; however, the three-year control in the determinate group was still 46%, against 67% and 86% when mobility was only impaired or normal.

**Table 6.2**
Radiotherapy of Lateral Epilaryngeal Carcinoma: Influence of Vocal Cord Mobility on Three-Year Survival and Local Control of Disease in 105 N0 N1 MO Patients

| Cord Mobility | Total Number of Patients | Three-Year Survival (No./%) | Total Local Failures (No./%) | Indeterminate Group* | Determinate Group | Local Control at Three Years in Determinate Group (No./%) |
|---|---|---|---|---|---|---|
| Normal | 43 | 26/60 | 4/9 | 15 | 29 | 25/86 |
| Diminished | 38 | 20/52 | 9/23 | 11 | 27 | 18/67 |
| Abolished | 23 | 8/34 | 8/35 | 8 | 15 | 7/46 |
| Unknown | 1 | 0 | 1 | 0 | 1 | 0 |

*Includes patients dying of intercurrent disease, second cancer, distant metastases, or lost to follow-up within two years of radiotherapy.

## Cartilage Involvement and Extralaryngeal or Pharyngolaryngeal Extension

For most head and neck oncologists (Cachin et al. 1979; MacComb and Fletcher 1967; Morrison 1971; Vermund 1970), cartilage involvement as well as other extralaryngeal extensions are formal contraindications to curative radiotherapy. Our personal experience indicates that cartilage involvement or extralaryngeal extensions are not contraindications to curative radiotherapy.

1. In six patients with T4 glottic carcinoma with cartilage destruction and clinical or radiologic involvement of prelaryngeal soft tissues, a three-year survival was obtained in three patients by radiotherapy alone.

2. In a series of 93 patients with T4 supraglottic carcinoma, three- and five-year survival was 43% and 35%, respectively, with two patients only being salvaged by surgery. The determinate results at three years with radiotherapy only averaged 50%. Interestingly, 16 of 32 patients with an oropharyngeal extension were cured, as were 5 out of 11 cases with definite cartilage destruction.

3. The specific influence of the extension of the disease beyond the pharyngolarynx and the influence of cartilage involvement on local control were again analyzed in the series of carcinomas of pyriform sinus without unfavorable node factors (table 6.3). When the disease was limited to the hypo-

**Table 6.3**
Radiotherapy of Carcinoma of Pyriform Sinus: Influence of Extension of the Disease on Two-Year Survival and Local Control in 249 N0 N1 MO Patients

| Extension | Total Number of Patients | Two-Year Survival (No./%) | Total Local Failures (No./%) | Indeterminate Group* | Determinate Group | Local Control at Two Years in Determinate Group (No./%) |
|---|---|---|---|---|---|---|
| ± Epilarynx or larynx | 120 | 63/52.5 | 34/28 | 27 | 93 | 59/63 |
| Opposite retrocricoid and hypopharyngeal wall | 40 | 16/40 | 14/35 | 11 | 29 | 15/52 |
| Oropharynx | 58 | 21/36 | 23/39 | 16 | 42 | 19/45 |
| Soft tissues and cartilage | 23 | 6/26 | 9/39 | 9 | 14 | 5/36 |
| Cervical esophagus alone or associated | 8 | 3/37 | 3/37 | 2 | 6 | 3/50 |

*Includes patients dying of intercurrent disease, second cancer, distant metastases, or lost to follow-up within two years of radiotherapy.

pharynx with or without involvement of the neighboring epilarynx or larynx (120 patients), failure in controlling the disease locally occurred in 28%, whereas it occurred in 39% of the 58 patients when oropharyngeal extension was present, and also in 39% of the 23 patients when cartilage and soft tissues were involved. Local failure occurred in three of the eight patients having extension to the cervical esophagus. In the determinate group, the two-year local control was 63% when the disease was limited to the pharyngolarynx (59 of 93), 45% when there was extension to the oropharynx (19 of 42), and 36% when there was cartilage and soft tissue involvement (5 of 14).

In the parallel series of 105 carcinomas of the epilarynx, local failure at three years was 18% when the disease was limited to the laryngopharynx (11 of 62), and 26% when there was extension to the oropharynx (11 of 43), the local control in the determinate group being 74% (32 of 43) and 62% (18 of 29), respectively (table 6.4).

## Metastatic Cervical Nodes

Radiotherapy is said to be much less efficient than surgery in the control of clinical disease in the neck (Cachin et al. 1979; Vermund 1970). This has not been our experience.

1. It is well known that even in advanced glottic carcinomas, nodal involvement is rare. Indeed, nodes were present only in 5 out of the 45 patients with advanced glottic carcinomas. Out of the four patients staged N1, three were cured by radiotherapy. The single patient at N3 failed.

2. In supraglottic carcinoma (Bataini 1974; Ghossein 1974), the absolute three- and five-year survival did not change significantly in the absence or presence of mobile nodes in a series of 218 cases. The three-year survival was 56.5% in patients with N0 disease (65 of 115) versus 53.5% with N1 disease (30 of 56) and 57% (16 of 28) with N2 tumor. The five-year survival was

**Table 6.4**
Radiotherapy of Lateral Epilaryngeal Carcinoma: Influence of Extension of Disease on Three-Year Survival and Local Control in 105 N0 N1 MO Patients

| Extension | Total Number of Patients | Three-Year Survival (No./%) | Total Local Failures (No./%) | Indeterminate Group* | Determinate Group | Local Control at Three Years in Determinate Group (No./%) |
|---|---|---|---|---|---|---|
| Limited | 26 | 15/58 | 5/19 | 7 | 19 | 14/74 |
| Extension to pyriform sinus or larynx | 36 | 20/56 | 6/17 | 12 | 24 | 18/75 |
| Oropharynx | 43 | 19/46 | 11/26 | 14 | 29 | 18/62 |

*Includes patients dying of intercurrent disease, second cancer, distant metastases, or lost to follow-up within two years of radiotherapy.

48.6% in N0 disease (56 of 115) versus 49% (27 of 56) in N1 disease and 43% (12 of 28) in N2 carcinoma. Survival for patients with positive mobile unilateral and especially bilateral nodes (Cachin 1979; Till 1975) compares favorably with those for surgery. Five of 19 and 3 of 19 patients with fixed nodes survived three and five years. All nodes less than 2.4 cm in diameter were controlled, whereas only half of those of more than 5 cm in diameter were controlled.

3. In carcinoma of pyriform sinus (Bataini 1979a, 1979b), the crude three- and five-year survival also did not change significantly in the absence or presence of mobile homolateral nodes. The three- and five-year survival was 36% (44 of 123) and 27% (29 of 108), respectively, for N0 tumor and 34% (43 of 126) and 23% (28 of 123) for N1b cancer. The survival for patients with $N2_b$ disease was 1 of 9 at three years and 1 of 7 at five years. Survival for patients with N3 disease was 15% (26 of 176) at three years and 10% (15 of 146) at five years. Nonetheless, when the primary tumor was controlled, the incidence of nodal failure at two years in N3 disease was as follows: Single N3 less than 5 cm, 15% (9 of 59); N3 more than 5 cm, 37% (7 of 19); multiple N3, 11% (5 of 44); bilateral N3, 19% (3 of 16).

Prognosis is evidently dismal when extensive local disease is associated with extensive nodal disease (Bataini and Ennuyer 1971; Ennuyer and Bataini 1973), as is nearly always the case in all head and neck squamous cell carcinomas. The incidence of nodal failure in N1 nodes was 8 of 42 cases (19%) receiving less than 7000 rad, and 5 of 68 patients (7%) receiving more than 7000 rad in the nodal volume.

## Functional Results and Complications

In the 20 patients cured at three years for advanced carcinoma of the vocal cord, functional results were excellent in 18 and fair in 2. None of the patients in this series had a tracheotomy during or after radiation treatment.

Of 77 patients who survived three years after radiation for supraglottic carcinoma (any T, any N, N0 M1) and did not have radical surgery, functional results were excellent in about 75% and fair with no impaired function in 16%. Five patients had a tracheotomy, and this was temporary only in two patients.

Functional results after radical radiation for carcinoma of pyriform sinus were rather good. Of the 129 two-year survivors, 7 patients only had a tracheotomy and 2 a gastrostomy.

## Salvage Surgery

Some cynical observers have said that salvage surgery is a myth. It is rarely performed and difficult. Its complications are prohibitive and its results negligible (Cachin et al. 1979). These statements have to be analyzed carefully, especially according to the site of origin of the carcinoma.

1. Salvage by secondary surgery was a real fact for advanced carcinoma of the vocal cord when it was performed in 12 of the 16 patients with local failure and was responsible for the long-term survival of 8 additional patients. Other favorable results of salvage surgery have been reported (Constable et al. 1975; Stewart et al. 1975).

2. In advanced carcinoma of the supraglottis, only three with T3 T4 and two with T2 N1 disease were salvaged (in addition to two T2 N0 cases). In the whole series, 25 patients only had salvage laryngectomy. Of these, seven (28%) survived five years free of disease after surgery. There were four fatal complications; in two of them, one with a T4 N1 and another with a T4 N2 lesion, the specimens of the primary tumor and nodes were negative. There was delayed healing in four patients. Three of these had pharyngostomes requiring secondary closure with one or more plastic procedures. In attempting to explain the small number of salvage surgery procedures attempted, one has to recall that many (94) of the lesions were staged T4 and there were fixed nodes in 19, a fair number of cases. Thus in many cases, locoregional failures were beyond surgical possibilities. Another consideration was the number (11) of isolated distant metastases and the fact that some others who died of intercurrent disease were lost to follow-up or refused surgery. Nonetheless, a much closer and more efficient follow-up could have salvaged a larger proportion of the local failures, had these patients been followed by surgery that was more effective on irradiated tissues. In fact, in a new series of patients, salvage surgery was more gratifying. In a series of 21 operated patients (Ennuyer, Poncet, and Bataini 1977), healing was normal in 11 and somewhat delayed in 8, with a single pharyngostome. One patient died from hemorrhage three months after surgery. Twelve of these 21 patients were eligible for a three-year follow-up after surgery. Six were free of disease. The failure in the six others was from local recurrence in five patients and to distant metastases in one patient.

3. Salvage surgery can cure patients with advanced supraglottic carcinoma who have failed radiation. Salvage surgery, however, is not worthwhile in patients with advanced cancer of the hypopharynx who have failed radiation. Recurrence of hypopharyngeal cancer is severe, and the patients are in poor general condition associated with cerebrovascular and cardiovascular disease.

## Discussion and Conclusions

If radiotherapy has been accepted by a large number of head and neck oncologists as the method of choice for dealing with early vocal cord carcinomas and for certain early supraglottic carcinomas, its possibilities and place have been denied in advanced carcinoma of the larynx and in carcinoma of the pyriform sinus. Fixation of cord, extralaryngeal extension with or without cartilage involvement, and presence of nodes provide almost all head and neck oncologists with deep-rooted opposition to radiotherapy. A recent publication qualifies the radiation approach when there is cartilage involvement, calling it a gross fault in management (Cachin et al. 1979).

Certainly, radiotherapy does not cure all laryngeal carcinomas and even fewer hypopharyngeal carcinomas, but neither does surgery. Moreover, surgical series are often selected: poor-risk surgical patients and well-advanced cases are treated by palliative radiotherapy and are not included in the surgical series.

In our laryngeal series, and especially in the supraglottic series, somewhat poorer results were obtained in T3 lesions as compared to T4. Curiously, there were fewer patients with T3 than T4 lesions. One explanation may be that patients in good general condition with disease still limited to the larynx were operated on, while poor-risk patients were treated with radiation. Many patients in good general condition with T4 lesions were referred for radiation, since surgeons were not keen to operate where disease was extensive and involved the base of the tongue, lateral pharyngeal wall, or the prelaryngeal soft tissues. The results were definitely better when pyriform sinus carcinoma was limited to the pharyngolarynx even when cord was fixed, as compared to cases when disease extended beyond the pharyngolarynx (table 6.3). Nonetheless, for advanced carcinoma, the control averaged 50% by radiotherapy alone.

The problem of salvage surgery has been discussed at length. It can be effective in a greater number of local or regional failures of laryngeal carcinoma if it is accompanied by closer follow-up. Thanks to better knowledge of the difficulties of surgery in irradiated tissues, complications are diminishing and long-term results are improving. Salvage laryngectomy must be performed through a direct vertical incision avoiding the carotid sheaths (Ennuyer, Poncet, and Bataini 1977; Poncet 1973). Nodal failures must be managed by enlarged adenectomies, and, should neck dissection be indicated, it should be performed neither through the same incision of laryngectomy nor at the same time.

Because of the good functional results and the definitely better salvage, we still favor radiotherapy as the treatment of choice for advanced laryngeal carcinoma with or without extralaryngeal spread. Furthermore, as the local control for T3 and T4 lesions has not been found to be dose-dependent in supraglottic carcinoma (Ghossein 1974) (as it seems to be for early cases), tumor doses of 7000 to 7500 rad in six to seven weeks are no longer exceeded, resulting in fewer complications and easier salvage surgery when needed. Such doses, however, cannot be delivered with impunity unless the patient is carefully supervised and the radiotherapist is familiar with the disease and the technique. In inexperienced hands, the complications can be prohibitive.

Carcinoma of the hypopharynx, and especially of the pyriform sinus, is more difficult to treat. The results obtained by radiotherapy in our homogeneous, consecutive series of 434 patients compare favorably with the published surgical series (Vanderbrook et al. 1979) if one takes into account that this series represented the whole population of patients with this disease treated at the Curie Foundation from 1958 through 1974, whatever their general and local conditions, and whatever the dose administered.

If the results already obtained are gratifying and justify our radiotherapeutic stand, new horizons are appearing in radiation oncology that must confirm the position and role of radiotherapy. Multiple daily fractions assume that normal tissues repair relatively more damage than do tumor tissues. This may allow us to deliver larger doses over a shorter time. Hypoxic tumor cells responsible for local failures may be destroyed by neutrons or high linear energy transfer (LET) beams or radiosensitizers. A clinical trial concerning the use of misomidazole in advanced laryngeal carcinoma and in hypopharyngeal carcinoma has already started in our institution. Better regimens of combination therapy, radiotherapy, or chemotherapy may also improve radiotherapeutic results and should be studied further.

"The voice, be it that of the actor, the singer, the poet, the politician, the protestor or just thee or me is a most cherished possession and its preservation must always remain a major consideration in the management of laryngeal carcinoma. The oesophageal voice or the artificial substitutes, though ingenious and most helpful, do not approach the spontaneous natural voice even if somewhat impaired" (Stewart et al. 1975).

Results presented here, as well as those already obtained by others (Constable et al. 1975; Jorgensen 1970), and the anticipated developments in the field of radiotherapy may indicate future trends in the management of advanced laryngeal carcinoma, namely, radiotherapy with surgery held in abeyance until recurrence.

Well-planned but also well-individualized and well-practiced, aggressive, modern radiotherapy must have a place in the primary management of advanced laryngeal and laryngopharyngeal carcinoma.

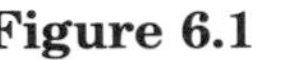

**Figure 6.1**

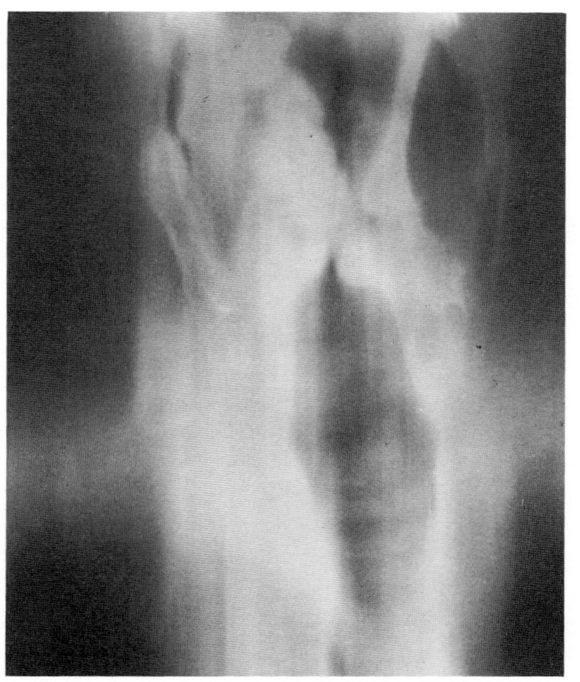

**A**

A, *58-year-old man. History of three months' hoarseness and recent earache. Moderately-differentiated squamous cell carcinoma involving epiglottis, laryngopharyngeal wall, which is deeply ulcerated down to glottis, with involvement of right pyriform sinus and fixation. Cobalt therapy April 27, 1960 to June 4, 1960. Tumor dose: 6000 rad, 32 fractions, 39 days.*

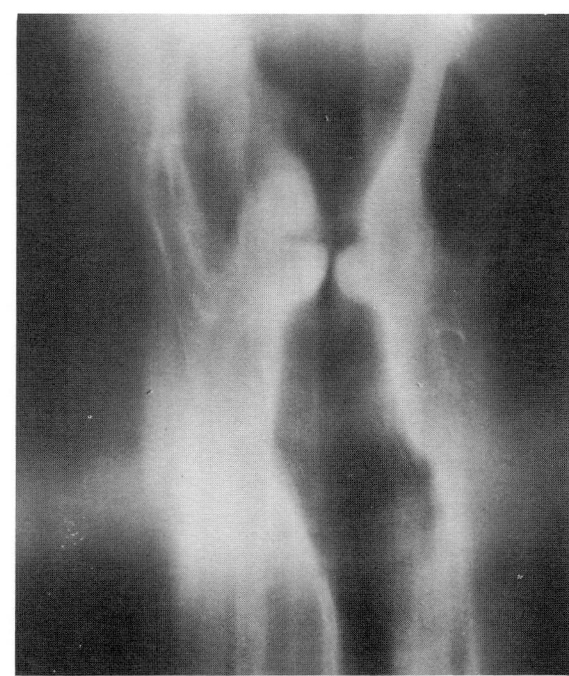

**B**

B, *Two years after, complete regression of tumor with healing of ulceration and minimal edema and normal mobility. Lost to follow-up with no evidence of disease in May 1975.*

**Figure 6.2**

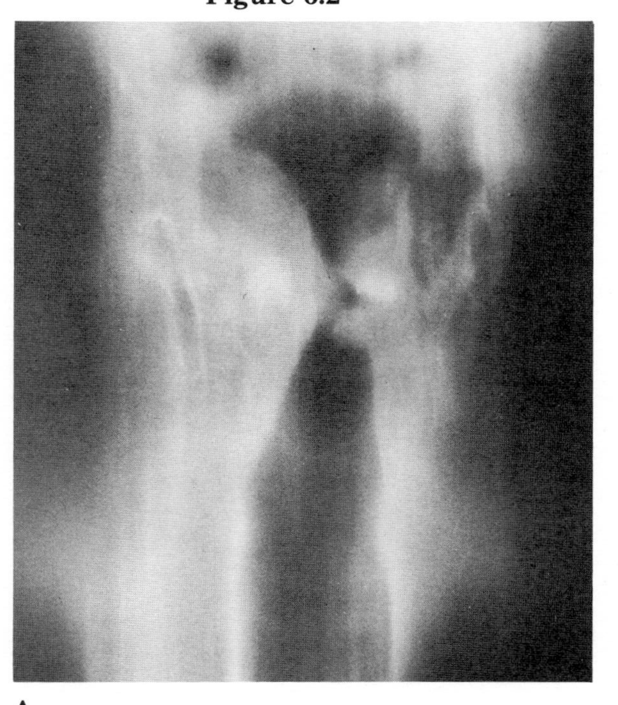

A

A, *78-year-old woman. Poorly-differentiated squamous cell carcinoma involving supraglottis, glottis, and subglottis, with involvement of right pyriform sinus. Cobalt therapy September 22, 1960 to November 9, 1960. Tumor dose: 6250 rad, 35 fractions, 44 days.*

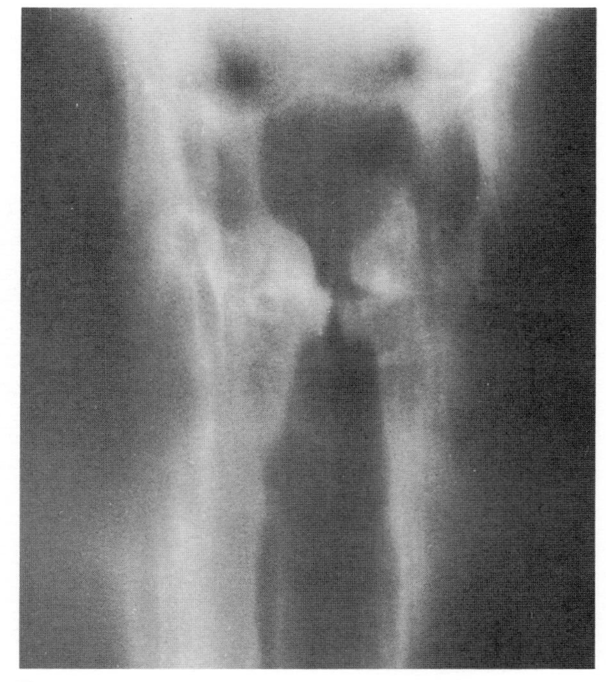

B

B, *Two years later. Excellent condition. Died in April 1966 from intercurrent disease.*

**Figure 6.3**

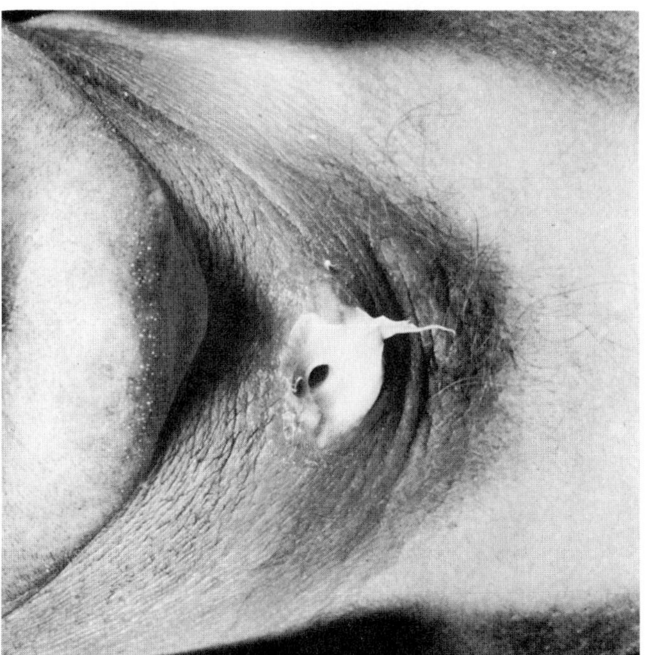

A, *42-year-old man. Increasing hoarseness for four years. Presented in August 1974 with extensive infiltration of prelaryngeal tissues, with recent ulceration. Laryngoscopy showed extensive disease involving supraglottis and anterior two-thirds of vocal cords. Laryngoceles were present on roentgenograms. Biopsy showed a well-differentiated squamous cell carcinoma.*

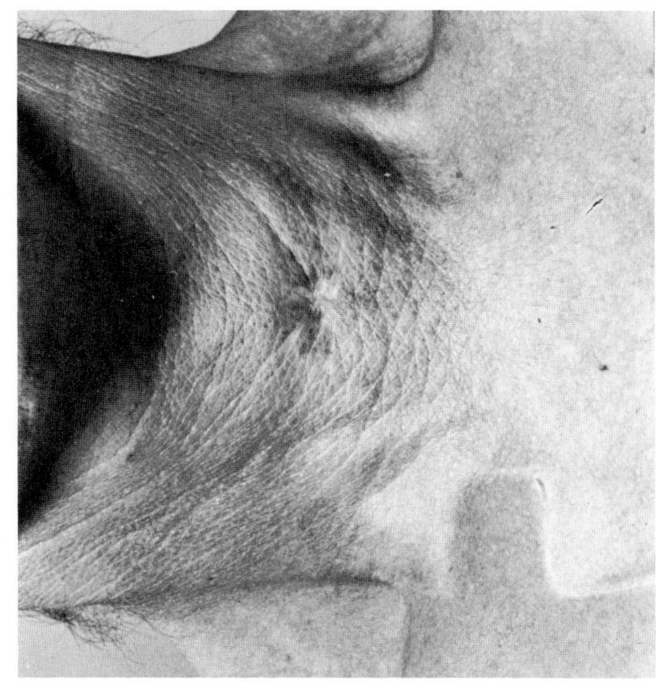

B, *Two years later after radiotherapy (cobalt 60 and electron beam) to a total of 7500 rad TD in 38 fractions over 50 days. Excellent cicatrization with minimal edema. Lost to follow-up with NED in October 1978.*

**Figure 6.4**

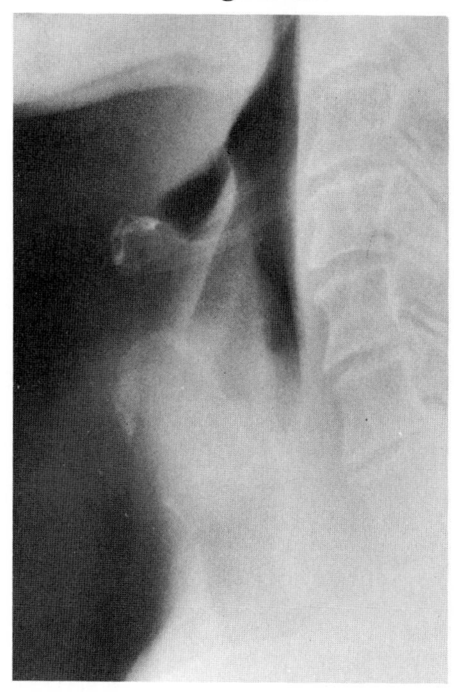

A

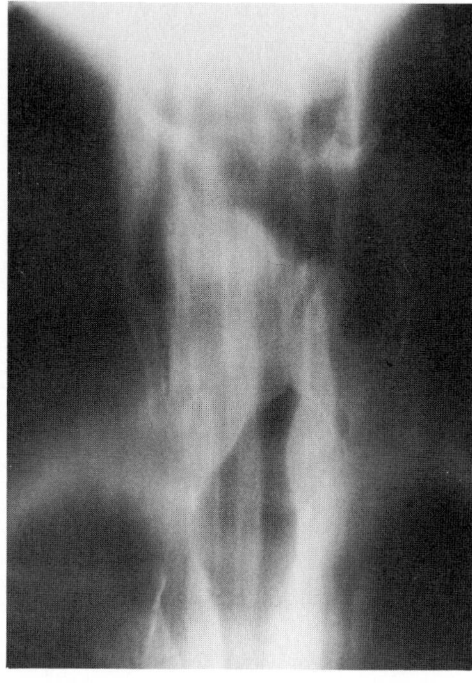

B

*A and B, 68-year-old man. Extensive laryngeal differentiated squamous cell carcinoma with six months of hoarseness and four months of dyspnea, involving supraglottis, glottis, and subglottis with fixation of right hemilarynx and important cartilage destruction. Cobalt therapy from January 10, 1973, to March 7, 1973. TD 8000 rad in 42 fractions over 56 days.*

# References

Baclesse, F. Carcinoma of the larynx. *Br. J. Radiol.* (suppl.) 3:1–75, 1949.

Bataini, J. P. et al. Treatment of supraglottic cancer by radical high dose radiotherapy. *Cancer* 33:1253–1262, 1974.

Bataini, J. P. et al. Techniques et résultats de la radiothérapie dans les cancers de l'hypopharynx et de la margelle laryngée latérale. In *Tumori della testa e del collo,* ed. P. Bucalossi. Milan: Casa Editrice Ambrosiana, 1979a.

Bataini, J. P. et al. Histoire naturelle des cancers du sinus piriforme et de la margelle laryngée latérale et causes d'échec du traitement. In *Tumori della testa e del collo,* ed. P. Bucalossi. Milan: Casa Editrice Ambrosiana, 1979b.

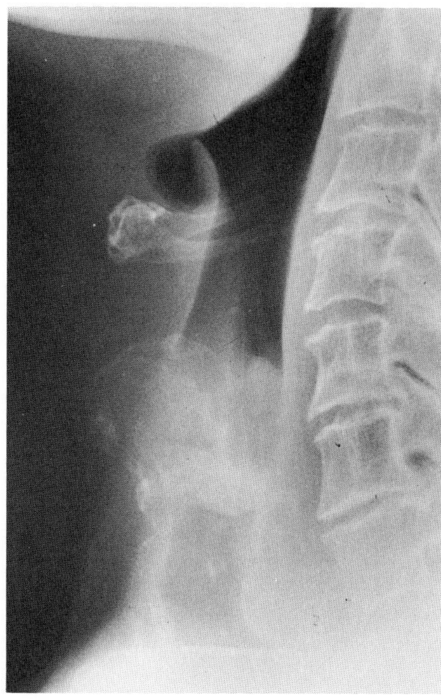

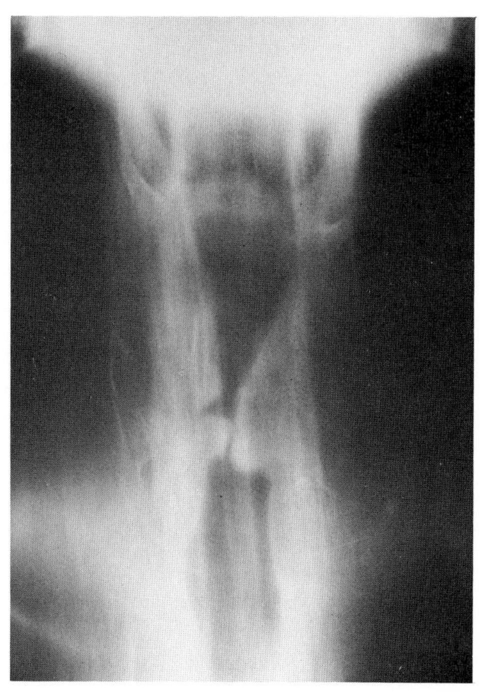

C D

C *and* D, *Four years later, no residual disease and good recalcification. NED in August 1979.*

Bataini, J. P., and Ennuyer, A. Télécobaltothérapie premiére des cancers glottiques et sous-glottiques. *J. Radiol. Electrol.* 52:753–754, 1971.

Brugere, J. et al. Epidémiologie des cancers de l'hypopharynx. In *Tumori della testa e del collo,* ed. P. Bucalossi. Milan: Casa Editrice Ambrosiana, 1979a.

Brugere, J. et al. Etude clinique et cytologique de l'envahissement ganglionaire cervical des cancers du sinus piriforme. In *Tumori della testa e del collo,* ed. P. Bucalossi. Milan: Casa Editrice Ambrosiana, 1979b.

Cachin, Y. et al. *Les cancers du larynx.* Paris: Masson, 1979.

Constable, W. C. et al. Radiotherapeutic management of cancer of the glottis, University of Virginia, 1956–1971. *Laryngoscope* 85:1491–1503, 1975.

Ennuyer, A., and Bataini, J. P. Radiocolbalthérapie dans le domaine de l'oto-rhino-laryngologie. *J. Radiol. Electrol.* 45:849–859, 1964.

Ennuyer, A., and Bataini, J. P. Treatment of supraglottic carcinoma by telecobalt therapy. *Br. J. Radiol.* 36:661–666, 1965.

Ennuyer, A., and Bataini, J. P. A propos de 1000 cas de cancers du pharynx traités par radiocobalt. Résultats á 5 ans. *J. Radiol. Electrol.* 54:7–17, 1973.

Ennuyer, A.; Poncet, P.; and Bataini, J. P. Cobalthérapie et chirurgie de rattrapage dans les cancers sus-glottiques. *Ann. Otolaryngol.* (Paris) 94:477–484, 1977.

Fletcher, G. H. et al. The place of radiotherapy in the management of squamous cell carcinoma of the supraglottic larynx. *Am. J. Roentgenol.* 108:19–26, 1970.

Ghossein, N. A. et al. Local control and site of failure in radically irradiated supraglottic laryngeal cancer. *Radiology* 112:187–192, 1974.

Jesse, R. H. The evaluation of treatment of patients with extensive squamous cancer of the vocal cords. *Laryngoscope* 85:1424–1429, 1975.

Jorgensen, K. Carcinoma of the larynx. Treatment mainly by primary irradiation. *Acta Radiol. Ther. Phys. Biol.* 9:401–418, 1970.

Leroux-Robert, J. A statistical study of 620 laryngeal carcinomas of the glottic region personally operated upon more than five years ago. *Laryngoscope* 85:1440–1452, 1975.

Leroux-Robert, J., and Ennuyer, A. Résultats de l'association chirurgie et roentgenthérapie ou de la chirurgie seule dans les épithéliomas du larynx. *Ann. Otolaryngol.* (Paris) 73:521–545, 1956.

MacComb, W. C., and Fletcher, G. H. *Cancer of the head and neck.* Baltimore: Williams and Wilkins, 1967.

Martenson, B.; Fluur, E.; and Jacobsson, F. Aspects on treatment of cancer of the larynx. *Ann. Otol. Rhinol. Laryngol.* 76:313–329, 1967.

Morrison, R. Radiation therapy in diseases of the larynx—review article. *Br. J. Radiol.* 44:489–504, 1971.

Niederer, J. et al. Failure analysis of radical radiation therapy of supraglottic laryngeal carcinoma. *Int. J. Radiat. Oncol. Biol. Phys.* 2:621–629, 1976.

Poncet, P. Laryngectomies et pharyngolaryngectomies de rattrapage aprés cobaltothérapie á doses cancéricides. *Acta Otorhinolaryngol. Belg.* 27:1005–1009, 1973.

Smith, R. R. et al. Revision of the clinical staging system for cancer of the larynx. *Cancer* 31:72–80, 1973.

Stewart, J. G. et al. The management of glottic carcinoma by primary irradiation with surgery in reserve. *Laryngoscope* 85:1477–1484, 1975.

Till, J. E. et al. A preliminary analysis of end results for cancer of the larynx. *Laryngoscope* 85:259–275, 1975.

Vanderbrook, C. et al. Association radio-chirurgicale et résultats obtenus par une chirurgie premiére suivie d'irradiation postopératoire. In *Tumori della testa e del collo,* ed. P. Bucalossi. Milan: Casa Editrice Ambrosiana, 1979.

Vermund, H. Role of radiotherapy in cancer of the larynx as related to TNM system of staging—a review. *Cancer* 25:485–503, 1970.

# Chapter 7

# *Cancer of the Larynx with Fixed Cord*

F. Eschwege and
B. Luboinski

The treatment of a cancer of the larynx with fixation of the vocal cords may differ depending on the mechanism of the fixation, that is, the different forms and degrees of invasion of the structures that participate directly or indirectly in the mobility of the normal larynx.

The discovery of vocal fixation in an extensive cancer invading the three levels of the larynx does not pose a serious problem in the choice of local therapy. On the other hand, careful clinical and radiologic analysis of a tumor involving one or two laryngeal levels may uncover fixation of the vocal cord for which the physiopathologic mechanism may not always be evident, and quite different therapeutic solutions may then be proposed.

It seemed necessary to us, therefore, to study the etiopathogenesis of the fixation, and to analyze the various management possibilities and the results of treatment in our institute to explain the therapy we currently recommend.

## Etiopathogenesis

The causes determining vocal cord fixation have a variable influence on vocal cord mobility, and thus the degree of immobility before complete fixation will vary. Recent histoclinical studies (see Kirchner, chapter 4 this volume; Micheau et al. 1976) permit us to analyze and understand these mechanisms. For us, as for Kirchner, the principal mechanism involved in fixation of the vocal cord is the tumor invasion of the thyroarytenoid muscle.

In this case the tumor extends posteriorly to involve the arytenoid cartilage, which may be partially or, more rarely, totally destroyed. Less often, the cricoarytenoid articulation alone may be involved. Fixation can also be the result of the extension of an infiltrating tumor outward toward the thyroid cartilage. The tumor may become fixed to the internal perichondrium or to the thyroid cartilage itself. This pattern of extension corresponds to the transglottic cancer of American terminology.

We have found that these tumors originate either on the vocal cord itself or in the laryngeal ventricle with secondary extension to the vocal cord by invasion of the paraglottic space.

According to Kirchner, extension into the posterior subglottic region by fixation of the vocal cord to the underlying cricoid lamina can cause immobility of the vocal cord. We feel that this posterior subglottic extension is rarely encountered.

Fixation can occur when a large exophytic tumor of the vocal cord or the mucosa covers the arytenoid. This is rare, and one must be able to differentiate clinically real fixation from apparent fixation with conservation of arytenoid mobility.

The scope of this study does not include laryngeal paralysis by involvement of the recurrent laryngeal nerve along its extralaryngeal course. The cord fixation for tumor destruction of the branches of the recurrent nerve cannot be distinguished from tumor extension to various laryngeal structures.

The problems of vocal cord fixation after radiotherapy can arise in two different circumstances.

1. Fixation of a hemilarynx may persist after radiation of a tumor of the larynx with fixation of one vocal cord. Persistent fixation in this setting is frequent and is not necessarily a sign of failure. If the tumor mass is replaced by radiation-induced fibrosis, mobility cannot be improved. Follow-up examination is difficult, and must be complete. Since superficial biopsies may be limited to a mucosa of normal appearance, tumor recurrence can pass unnoticed for long periods of time.
2. Laryngeal immobility may occur following radiotherapy of a laryngeal tumor with initially conserved vocal cord mobility. Fixation of a vocal cord should be considered (a priori) as a sign of tumor recurrence. One may take radiation fibrosis into consideration only after negative biopsy. The histologic study of surgical specimens has shown that the amount of fibrosis is directly related to the size of destroyed cancer. Residual or recurrent tumor elements may coexist with this fibrosis, and the association of radiation fibrosis and the growth of the endolaryngeal tumor will lead more or less rapidly to a nonfunctional larynx.

## Staging

The two staging systems most frequently employed are the TNM UICC (1972) and the AJC (1972). Aside from several details, these systems are identical concerning glottic and supraglottic tumors. In both, glottic and supraglottic cancers with diminished vocal cord mobility are staged T2. Tumors with fixation of one or two vocal cords are classed T3.

The only problem occurs in cases involving a large exophytic tumor of one vocal cord, when too rapid an examination could lead to the false conclusion that there is complete immobility of the hemilarynx. In fact, this diminished mobility is more often caused by the large tumor mass, and under these conditions the tumor should be staged T2 and not T3.

The diagnosis of fixation of a vocal cord is based essentially on clinical examination. In the majority of cases indirect laryngoscopy establishes fixation. Additional examinations, including direct laryngoscopy, classical radiographic examinations, and the CAT scan, make it possible to study better the exact tumor extension, and therefore the cause or causes of the fixation—important elements in the choice of treatment planning.

## Therapeutic Indications

The choice of treatment in the management of a cancer of the larynx with cord fixation is based on an understanding of the causes of the fixation and an appreciation of present therapeutic possibilities. In the last few years, the indications for treatment have been modified by the introduction of reconstructive surgical techniques.

Our treatment protocol is based on definitive laryngeal surgery and usually entails total or partial resection of the larynx with unilateral or bilateral neck dissection. The extent of this dissection and the techniques used depend on the clinical node involvement and the results of the frozen section.

After pathologic examinations of the surgical specimen, postoperative radiotherapy may be indicated.

Total surgical removal of the larynx is performed in the following situations:

Total laryngectomy is the treatment of choice for T3-T4 tumors, that is, lesions in which the fixation of the larynx is due to tumor involvement of all three laryngeal levels with or without extralaryngeal extension. On these cases decision-making is simple, for alternative treatments are considered only when there are medical contraindications for surgery. There are cases in which a subtotal or partial laryngectomy is initially considered, but when operative exploration and frozen section studies show extension to the three laryngeal levels and/or to the subglottis, total resection of the larynx must be performed. It is therefore necessary to advise the patient of the possibility of a total laryngectomy before undertaking partial laryngeal surgery.

There is still considerable controversy over the indications for hemilaryngectomy. At the *Institut Gustave-Roussy* (IGR) we prefer more extensive partial resection with reconstruction, but strict local indications must be met. Reconstructive subtotal resection removes all or parts of the glottic and supraglottic regions, the most frequent sites of tumor extension. It is therefore a cancer operation which does not completely compromise the resumption of phonatory and respiratory functions compatible with a normal life.

It is possible to perform this type of subtotal laryngectomy for tumors arising from a vocal cord, a ventricle, or the laryngeal vestibule. The tumor may involve the contralateral vocal cord under the conditions that this cord conserves its normal mobility and that its posterior third is free of disease.

True subglottic involvement is the chief contraindication for this type of surgery. Tumor extension beyond the larynx is another contraindication.

Because rupture of the lymph node capsule necessitates postoperative radiation not only of the node-bearing areas but also of the remaining larynx, the existence of a large nodal mass (3 cm or larger) is a regional contraindication for subtotal laryngeal surgery.

The patient's age and poor general condition, or the presence of clinically evident bronchopulmonary disease, also represent contraindications for this procedure, which is recommended only for patients in good physical and mental condition, capable of supporting a difficult and sometimes long postoperative period complicated by inadequate deglutition and aspiration pneumonia.

Neck dissection, whether unilateral or bilateral, is always carried out in continuity with the laryngeal surgery. The extent of the dissection is determined by the tumor invasion of the various laryngeal structures (invasion of the midline means a bilateral nodal surgery) and by the size and number of palpable nodes. If there are clinically suspicious palpable mobile nodes of less than 2 cm, we perform a modified neck dissection.

If the nodes are larger than 2 cm and/or fixed to the vessels, we carry out a radical neck dissection. If there are bilateral clinically suspicious nodes, we perform a modified neck dissection on one side and a radical neck dissection on the other side at the same time.

When no palpable nodes are found, we carry out a bilateral or unilateral dissection of the superior and middle jugular nodes, a procedure based on the study of data gathered at IGR after the pathologic examination of the surgical specimens obtained at node dissection, which show preferential invasions of these two groups, and especially the superior group. If preoperative examination and frozen section examination of the surgical specimen show no node invasion, the dissection is not carried further. If the frozen section shows node invasion, we perform a modified neck dissection (Cachin and Eschwege 1975).

# Treatment Methods

## Surgical Treatment

The surgical treatment of laryngeal tumors with vocal cord fixation is based on one fundamental principle: adequate excision.

Thorough study of the patterns of extension of cancer of the larynx has led to the development of surgical techniques that allow maximum conservation of all or one of the functions of the larynx. We now advise operative procedures that permit alternatives to total laryngectomy. Whatever the alternatives, the management of the laryngeal tumor cannot be dissociated from the management of the regional lymph nodes.

## Total Laryngectomy

Total laryngectomy remains the surgical treatment most frequently indicated for laryngeal tumors with fixation of the vocal cord. The procedure is universally established; in all cases the entire larynx is resected with the hyoid bone and with the extrinsic laryngeal muscles. Normal phonation is, of course, abolished, which necessitates vocal rehabilitation with the acquisition of esophageal speech.

The uncertain success of this rehabilitation has stimulated interest in the development of reconstructive methods including the numerous techniques of external tracheopharyngeal communication, which often necessitates a series of surgical procedures and sometimes the use of a prosthesis. We do not employ these techniques. Their success demands much time and care and are best characterized as surgical research. They are frequently complicated by salivary leakage or stenosis of the fistula.

The Stafieri internal tracheopharyngeal communication is an interesting variation. After total excision of the larynx only a tracheostomy is performed. The transected upper margin of the trachea is placed under the base of the tongue. The hypopharyngeal mucous membrane is dissected away from the larynx in the postcricoid region, and pulled over the transected margin of the trachea as a drum skin is pulled over a drum. This mucosa is incised, creating a neoglottis. Here again, the postoperative course may be complicated by stricture of the fistula and loss of phonation, or by aspiration of saliva through a gaping fistula followed by aspiration of liquids and semiliquids, giving rise to bronchopulmonary complications. Although the outcome of these fistula operations is often unsuccessful, the quality of the voice is good when they are successful.

We are presently concentrating our efforts on improving the quality of phonic rehabilitation.We attempt to use partial and/or reconstructive procedures whenever possible.

On occasion, the Hautant technique of hemilaryngectomy is used. This procedure spares more thyroid cartilage on the involved side than does the American hemilaryngectomy. The Hautant technique also removes the arytenoid, which is not the standard practice in the United States.

The Hautant technique is intended for the management of certain glottic-subglottic lesions. For us it is exceptionally indicated, for it is limited in the management of cancer by the possibility of malignant extension to the anterior commissure and/or the ventricle, thereby gaining access to the subglottic region. We feel that in the majority of cases this type of resection is limited, since the lesion often proves to be already too extensive.

Subtotal or reconstructive laryngectomies (fig. 7.1) of the Arslan-Serafini

**Figure 7.1**

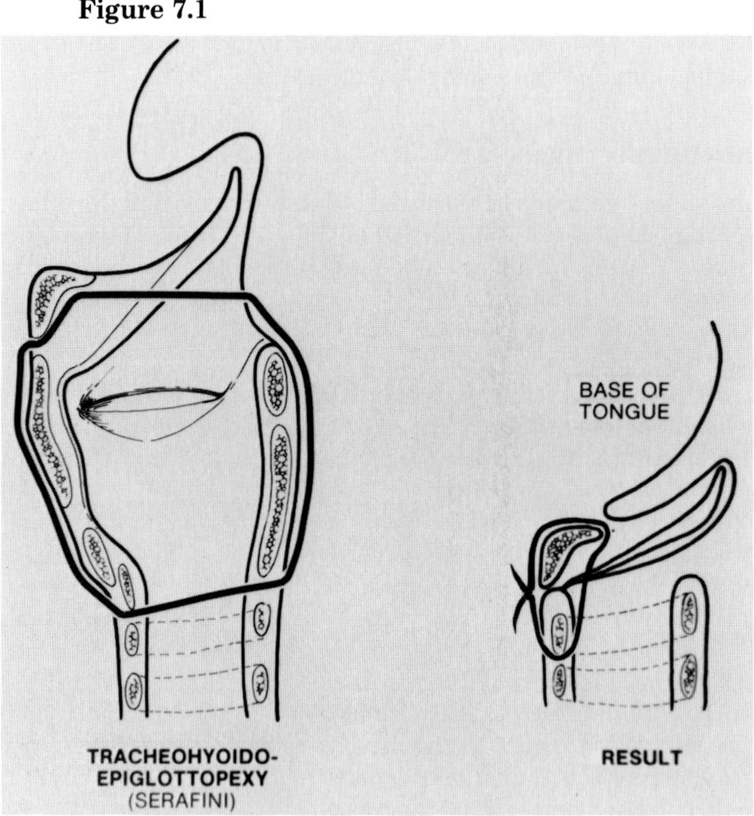


*Arslan-Serafini total laryngectomy. Note that hyoid bone is spared; first tracheal ring is sutured to the base of the tongue.*

type basically consist of total laryngectomy, sparing only the hyoid. The hyoid and the first tracheal ring are sutured to the base of the tongue. The postoperative course is complicated by inadequate deglutition for extended periods.

We prefer functional subtotal laryngectomies either with cricohyoidopexy (fig. 7.2) or cricohyoidoepiglottopexy (fig. 7.3). These procedures preserve the cricoid cartilage and one arytenoid, and thus are indicated only in cases with unilateral vocal cord fixation and, above all, only in the absence of true subglottic tumor invasion (disease spread to the level of the cricoid cartilage). Therefore these procedures may be indicated for (certain) glottic-supraglottic lesions with fixation of one vocal cord. In the majority of cases, there is eventual removal of the tracheotomy tube and restoration of the laryngeal airway. The postoperative course is complicated by inadequate deglutition which, in the majority of cases, is restored for solid foods within the first two postoperative months. This leaves only the problem of occasional as-

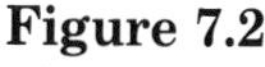

**Figure 7.2**

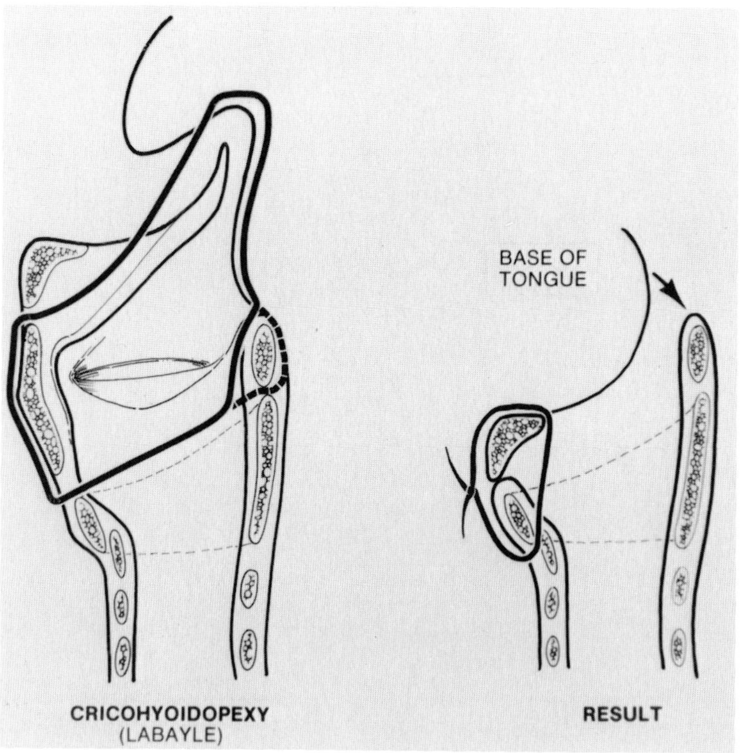


*Total laryngectomy of Labayle. Note preservation of the arytenoid, cricoid, and hyoid. The cricoid and hyoid are sutured to the base of the tongue.*

piration of liquids, which as a rule will disappear within the first postoperative year. The voice is usually low-pitched. Its quality is markedly improved by early rehabilitation. In about 20% of the cases the voice is weak and whispered.

## Treatment of the Cervical Nodes

When the laryngeal tumor is managed surgically, we feel it is always necessary to include neck dissection as part of the procedure. It may be unilateral or bilateral depending on the extension of the primary tumor. When there are no palpable nodes and the frozen section shows no signs of node involvement, we limit dissection to the superior and middle jugular nodes. If the fat pad of the frozen section is positive, we perform a modified neck dissection, sparing the sternocleidomastoid muscle, internal jugular vein, and spinal accessory nerve.

When there are clinically positive nodes, a modified dissection is per-

**Figure 7.3**

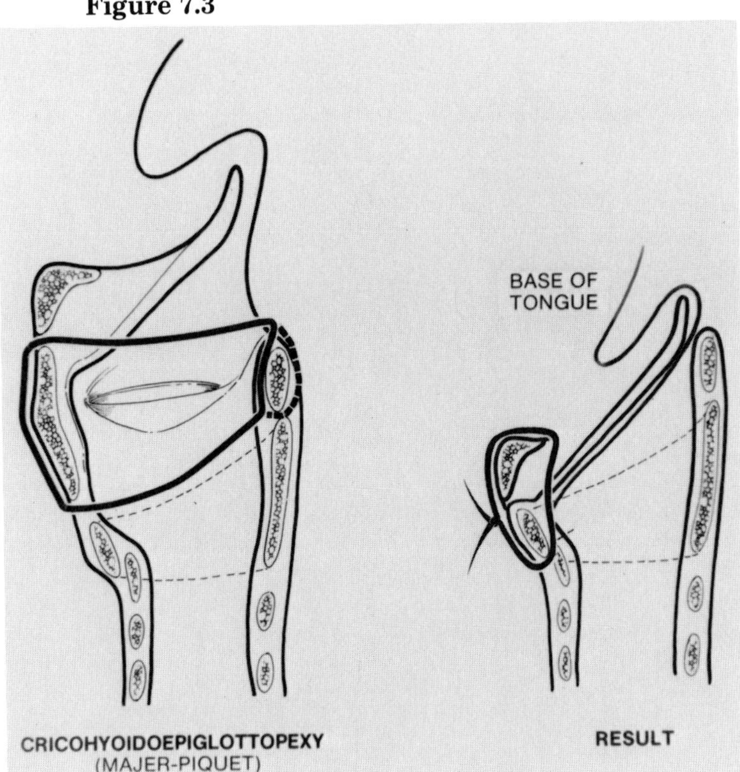


*Total laryngectomy of Majer-Piquet. Note preservation of the epiglottis as well as the hyoid, cricoid, and arytenoid.*

formed for nodes of 3 cm or less and not fixed, and a radical neck dissection is performed for nodes larger than 3 cm and/or fixed. This distinction is based on the pathologic findings in a study of 519 nodes at IGR: only 26% of nodes of 2 cm showed capsular rupture, while 71% of nodes larger than 3 cm showed capsular rupture.

When bilateral therapeutic neck dissection is necessary, we treat both sides in the same surgical procedure, beginning with the side where a functional neck dissection may be carried out.

## Radiotherapy

The radiotherapeutic management of cancers of the larynx with fixation of the vocal cords is not different in concept from the radiotherapeutic management of other laryngeal cancers. It may be definitive therapy, or elective preceding or following surgical resection. In all cases, it is necessary to assure a perfect patient set-up, with immobilization of the head and sufficient comfort to permit a strict reproducibility of the treatment session.

Two treatment techniques are commonly used, either the lateral decubitus position or the supine position with the head in hyperextension. We prefer the latter, using a head- and chin-rest system of immobilization, with a bite block. With the patient supine, we use an isocentric treatment set-up, which is particularly useful if one wishes to treat two fields a day. This technique is not readily adaptable, however, to the patient with a short neck, in which instance the lateral decubitus position seems most appropriate. In all cases, of course, only medium and high-energy treatment machines should be used.

### Tumor Volume

Even in the absence of clinical or radiologic evidence of extension to an anatomic structure adjacent to the vocal cords, when irradiating lesions with vocal cord fixation, one must keep in mind that this fixation is the result of the lesion's having extended beyond the cord. The radiotherapist does not have the advantage of exploration of the larynx for decision-making as does the surgeon. Extension beyond the cord must be assumed by the radiotherapist even when the mechanism of fixation is thought to be simple extension to the thyroarytenoid muscle or impaired mobility because of a large exophytic tumor. We feel that the inferior limit of the tumor volume should always extend below the thyroid cartilage, because of the possibility of occult submucosal extension at the level of the subglottis. Finally, even in the absence of palpable nodes, this possibility of extension to extracordal laryngeal structures (which possess a lymphatic drainage) makes it necessary in all cases to treat the cervical nodes bilaterally, with the exception of the submental and submaxillary nodes. We treat this tumor volume to a dose of 7000 rad in seven weeks, using five fractions a week. The nodes receive a prophylactic dose of 5000 rad. Palpable nodes are given boosts using photons or electrons to bring the dose to 6500 rad in six and one-half weeks. Because the frequency of complications increases at high tumor doses, without an evident increased benefit for the patient, we do not deliver a dose higher than 7000 rad.

## Preoperative Radiotherapy

The treatment portals and techniques employed do not differ from those used for definitive radiotherapy. The only distinction made for preoperative radiotherapy is in the tumor dose, which, for different authors, varies from 2000 to 5000 rad with widely different treatment schedules. We rarely use preoperative radiotherapy. When we do, we usually choose a dose inferior to 4000 rad. Dose rates are at 1000 rad per week in five equal fractions.

## Postoperative Radiotherapy

The techniques applied to postoperative radiotherapy should be carried out with the same precision and care applied to curative radiotherapy to assure the proper immobilization and comfort of the patient. One must completely assess the real extension of the cancer as determined by the surgeon and the pathologist. After total laryngectomy the target volume may vary widely. Most important is the recognition of tumor extension in the subglottic region. The decision to include the tracheostome in the treatment fields depends on the histopathologic finding of subglottic involvement, even in a tumor macroscopically confined to the glottis. The level of the tracheostome in relation to the sternal manubrium is important. One must not shield a stoma located high in the neck, particularly at the level of the first three tracheal rings. Posteriorly, the field always includes the surgical scar.

The doses we use at IGR vary according to the pathologist's findings. If the tumor excision is complete with no nodal involvement, we give a maximum tumor dose of 5000 rad in five weeks. If the resection is inadequate, the tumor dose is 6500 rad. If there is microscopic nodal involvement and complete tumor excision, we do not deliver a dose higher than 5000 rad to the tumor bed, but we give boosts limited to the node-bearing areas, which may reach 6500 rad in cases with capsular rupture. In cases treated by partial laryngectomy, we feel that postoperative radiotherapy of the tumor bed is never indicated. On the other hand, when the pathologic examination reveals microscopic nodal involvement with capsular rupture even in the absence of macroscopic invasion, we undertake postoperative radiotherapy of the node-bearing areas. For this radiation we most frequently use an anteroposterior field with systematic midline shielding.

We practice elective postoperative radiotherapy only if there is (1) inadequate resection of tumor, (2) extensive laryngeal involvement, (3) tumor extension into the cricothyroid space or along the paratracheal space, or (4) extension to the thyroid gland. We also employ postoperative radiotherapy if pathologic examination shows involvement of the lymph nodes, especially if there is rupture of the lymph node capsule. Areas of treatment and doses are different after total or subtotal laryngectomy.

### Total Laryngectomy

If postoperative radiotherapy is indicated after total laryngectomy, we treat the tumor bed and the bilateral neck. The dose given to the tumor bed varies from 5000 rad in five weeks, if the resection is adequate, to 6500 rad in six and one-half weeks, if the resection is inadequate. The node-bearing areas receive a dose varying from 5000 rad, if there is no nodal involvement, to 6500 rad, if there is nodal involvement with capsular rupture.

### Subtotal Laryngectomy

After subtotal laryngectomy only the node-bearing areas of the neck are treated to a dose varying from 5000 to 6500 rad. Cobalt or cobalt and electrons are used.

### Definitive Radiotherapy

Certain indications for definitive radiotherapy are derived from the contraindications for the protocol we have just described, that is: (1) poor general condition, (2) extensive local tumor involvement, (3) and extensive nodal involvement with fixation to the deep muscle layers.

We have also seen that a large exophytic tumor may immobilize the cord by its mass. We feel that these patients should be managed by irradiation of the primary tumor and the node-bearing areas of the neck. The treatment is planned to deliver a tumor dose of 7000 rad. When a dose of 3000 to 3500 rad has been reached, the patient is carefully evaluated clinically and, if necessary, repeat radiologic studies and direct laryngoscopy are performed. Often the reduction in tumor volume will allow a better evaluation of the tumor extension. If the vocal cord remains fixed, we stop the radiation at this dose and perform a total laryngectomy. If the vocal cord has regained its mobility, we continue the radiation to 7000 rad.

## Patient Management during Treatment

The immediate postoperative patient course after total laryngectomy is not complicated by any special problems. Primary wound healing takes place rapidly. We always await complete wound healing, which takes about 15 days, before beginning postoperative radiotherapy. If a salivary fistula develops and if there is rupture of lymph node capsules, we begin treatment rapidly even if healing of the skin wound is not complete.

The postoperative course after subtotal laryngectomy is much longer, with two major problems of management: (1) the restoration of the natural laryngeal airway and (2) the initiation of adequate deglutition. The acquisition of adequate deglutition for solid foods requires approximately a month, whereas problems with aspiration of liquids may persist for many months. This prolonged period of inadequate deglutition, of course, sets the stage for frequent pulmonary infection. For this reason, even if an early restoration of the natural airway is possible, removal of the tracheostomy tube is delayed until aspiration of liquids is minimal.

The radiation therapist must be much more alert while irradiating a patient with a subtotal laryngectomy than one with a total laryngectomy. It is important to watch for signs of laryngeal edema, which may be present even before radiotherapy is begun, especially in the region of the remaining arytenoid. Smoking must absolutely be forbidden from the very beginning of treatment.

When definitive radiotherapy is indicated for a tumor with vocal cord fixation due to the massive exophytic nature of the tumor, the adequacy of the laryngeal airway must be assured. We do not feel, however, that elective tracheotomy should be performed before beginning treatment. If a tracheotomy becomes necessary, it may be performed during the course of treatment.

## Follow-up

Follow-up examinations should be scheduled every two months during the course of the first two posttreatment years. One must be alert to a primary, a nodal, and/or a metastatic recurrence and also to the possibility of the appearance of a second primary in the aerodigestive tract.

Follow-up after subtotal laryngectomy and postoperative radiotherapy is most difficult. The interpretation of an edema of the remaining arytenoid or of a progressive narrowing of the subglottic region poses a problem. At the slightest doubt, direct laryngoscopy should be performed.

The same diagnostic problem arises after definitive radiation. The appearance of edema or the reappearance of fixation or of diminished mobility of a cord which had regained its normal mobility after radiotherapy should be taken as a sign of recurrence. Eliminating the diagnosis of late edema or radiotherapeutic fibrosis with certainty may be impossible, even with multiple biopsies, until time lag.

Stomal or peristomal recurrence had been an important problem for a long time. Elective tracheotomy performed before definitive surgery or radiotherapy is considered a predisposing factor. We have noted 14% peristomal recurrences in laryngeal cancers when tracheotomy was performed prior to total laryngectomy, as opposed to 3% when prior tracheotomy was not performed. These last results still may be improved by systematic intraoperative diagnosis of the subglottic region by frozen section, and by elective postoperative radiation of the stoma to a dose of 6500 rad in patients with any histologic hint of subglottic extension. It is difficult to diagnose stomal and peristomal recurrence early, but it is important to keep alert to this possibility. Successful management of this problem is now possible by such means as large surgical excision with reconstruction, interstitial curietherapy, and teleradiotherapy.

## Results

Our present approach to the management of cancer of the larynx with fixation of the vocal cord is based on the careful analysis of data obtained from two distinct series of patients treated under two very different protocols, the first from 1960 to 1965, the second from 1967 to 1972.

From 1960 to 1965, T3 T4 tumors of the larynx were treated definitively by radical telecobalt therapy to a dose of 7000 rad. Salvage total laryngectomy was performed only in patients with marked destruction of the thyroid cartilage and/or in patients showing no tendency toward tumor regression after a dose of 4000 rad.

From 1967 to 1972 total laryngectomy was indicated for lesions with complete fixation of one or two vocal cords, or invasion of cartilage, or extension to the three laryngeal levels. Nodal invasion was always managed in the same surgical procedure.

An analytic comparison of these two retrospective series allows us to draw several conclusions.

In the first series, using definitive radiotherapy, the absolute five-year survival was 38% (50 of 130) for T3 tumors, 25% (6 of 24) for T4.

In the second series, using definitive surgical management, the absolute five-year survival was 47% (53 of 113) for T3 and 45% (9 of 20) for T4.

The results of treatment of T3 cancers by telecobalt were disappointing, especially considering that the survival figures take into account salvage surgery, which could be used to manage only 60% of the failures. After salvage surgery, one may expect five-year survival for only one case in four. Definitive radiotherapy alone gave a 22% cure. In addition, conservation of laryngeal function, the goal of radiation therapy, was very mediocre. Only 42% of patients with glottic lesions and 58% of patients with subglottic lesions conserved their voice.

The five-year results of definitive surgical treatment of T3 lesions (originating in the supraglottic area) are clearly superior (49%) to those obtained by radiation therapy eventually followed by salvage surgery (38%). One must also take into account that the irradiated group includes those patients for whom surgery was contraindicated. If one considers only those patients managed by definitive surgery, the five-year survival is 57%. A total laryngectomy for a fixed larynx allows one to hope for five-year survival of almost 60%.

On the other hand, the results from the treatment of large T4 lesions (8% of our cases) and N3 nodes (9% of our cases) are poor. The 18-month survival of a patient with a T4 lesion is about 40%. The 30-month survival for a patient with an N3 neck is 30%.

A study of pattern of disease spread and the causes of death helps us to evaluate the results of treatment in relation to the natural history of the disease. Cancer of the larynx is highly curable, but one must keep in mind the limits of locoregional treatment. Almost one patient out of four will show a recurrence either local (50%), nodal (20%), nodal with metastasis and tumor (20%), or isolated metastases (10%).

Analysis of the causes of death (182 cases studied) shows local and regional recurrence in 27% of the cases, metastases in 24% of the cases, and a second primary cancer in 13% of the cases. The frequency of multiple cancers is far from insignificant. In a study of 417 cases of cancer of the larynx, we have found multiple cancers in 13% of the cases, either concomitant (7 cases) or successive (43 cases). In about half of the patients these cancers were situated in the upper aerodigestive tract and about half were situated in the lung or esophagus. The five-year survival after treatment of the laryngeal cancer in those cases was only 5%.

In comparing those two historical series, we must study the functional results. The aim of the first protocol, based on definitive radiotherapy, was to preserve the larynx and its functions.

Radiotherapy of the larynx is not without side effects, which increase in importance according to tumor volume. Fibrosis, ankylosis of articulations, and chronic edema may be associated in varying degrees which at their maximum produce the syndrome of the postradiotherapy larynx. We noted 58 cases of severe postradiotherapy changes in 225 cases treated by definitive radiotherapy. In 38 cases (17%) it became necessary to perform a tracheotomy, which in some cases became permanent. Laryngeal chondronecrosis developed in five cases (2%). It was necessary to perform a total laryngectomy for the painful, severely injured larynx in which no recurrence was found.

Vocal rehabilitation after total laryngectomy as we practice it, in three weeks of intensive full-time training, gives relatively good results. We noted 15% excellent results, 75% satisfactory, and 10% complete failures, in which it was necessary to use a vibrating prosthesis.

The major problem, which is far from being resolved, remains the social rehabilitation at both the family and professional levels. A study of the patients treated in our institute showed a low level of resumption of professional activity.

The rehabilitation of the laryngectomized patient should therefore be an essential preoccupation for the therapist and should hold an important place in the surgical management.

It is the search for a surgical procedure combining both adequate excision and conservation of laryngeal functions which has led us to introduce the various methods of subtotal reconstructive laryngectomy into our protocol. Our survival results at this time are preliminary, but we are able to evaluate the functional failures at about 10%, for whom it is impossible to recover normal deglutition and who must complete the treatment by undergoing total laryngectomy.

## References

Cachin, Y., and Eschwege, F. Combination of radiotherapy and surgery in the treatment of head and neck cancer. *Cancer Treat. Rev.* 2:177–191, 1975.

Micheau, C. et al. Modes of invasion of cancer of the larynx. A statistical, histological, and radioclinical analysis of 120 cases. *Cancer* 38:346–357, 1976.

## Chapter 8

# *Current Controversies in the Management of Cancer of the Tongue and Floor of the Mouth*

# Alando J. Ballantyne

There has never been unanimity of opinion regarding the preferred means of treatment of oral cavity cancer. With the advent of newer modalities of treatment and various combinations of treatment, the confusion regarding choice of treatment has increased. Rather than present an exhaustive review of all of the literature, citing the advantages and disadvantages of various modalities of treatment, I would prefer to present a somewhat didactic and perhaps opinionated outline of the methods of treatment that I have found effective in my own practice.

Briefly stated, the current methods available for treatment are as follows:

1. Surgery.
2. Radiation therapy.
3. Electrocoagulation.
4. Cryosurgery.
5. Combinations of the above.

Electrocoagulation and cryosurgery play a minor role in most centers.

In addition to the primary modalities of treatment, one should add chemotherapy and immunotherapy. Neither of these, at present, seems curative by itself, but each has been advocated for use either pre- or postoperatively in combination with any of the primary treatment modalities. Until chemotherapy for head and neck squamous cell carcinoma becomes more efficient, its role would seem to be relatively limited. Immunotherapy, likewise, has only limited and doubtful usefulness as an adjunctive treatment. Much additional work needs to be done before deciding the place this modality of treatment will occupy in the treatment of cancer of the tongue and floor of the mouth.

Obviously, the best method of treatment would be prophylaxis. Numerous studies have demonstrated that the incidence of cancer of the tongue and floor of the mouth is higher in those who use tobacco than in those who do not. Intemperate use of alcohol may act as a promoting factor for whatever carcinogen there is in tobacco.

In some parts of the world where the use of the betel nut and lime in various forms is employed intraorally, the elimination of these forms of chemical and mechanical irritation would markedly reduce the incidence of cancer of the oral cavity. Short of educational efforts to reduce the use of known factors seeming to have an association with the genesis of oral cancer, it is unlikely that any means of prophylaxis will be forthcoming in the near future.

As with all forms of cancer, early recognition, diagnosis, and treatment provide the best opportunity for cure. Because of the comparative infrequency of oral cavity cancer and the type of patient in whom this kind of cancer is likely to develop, it is quite unlikely that mass screening efforts will be productive from an economic standpoint. The best means of promoting early diagnosis and treatment is general education of the public and specific education of the dentist and other medical professionals who are most likely to detect disease either in a symptomatic or asymptomatic form. It is distressing to find patients who have gone either to a dentist or physician for evaluation of mouth complaints or for the presence of nodes in the neck who have not received an adequate intraoral examination. The tools for an adequate intraoral examination are simple, straightforward, and available in any reasonably-equipped dentist or doctor's office. Any suspicious lesion should be biopsied, but the practice of making large biopsies or of attempting excision of suspicious intraoral lesions by one not qualified to manage the entire problem is to be discouraged. Any suspicious lesion without significant infiltration which can be adequately excised by a competent oral surgeon or general surgeon should be totally excised as a biopsy procedure. Any larger lesions should be initially treated by a small biopsy only, without the placement of sutures. The practice of making large biopsies and extending these into the adjacent normal mucosa with the introduction of sutures for closure of the defect is to be decried.

Once a diagnosis of intraoral malignancy has been made, careful examination of the cancer and the host should form the basis for the assessment as to the best mode of treatment. The manner of growth of the primary tumor, size, possible extensions, the probability of invasion of adjacent structures, and the presence or absence of nodal metastases should be carefully noted. Host factors are also of great significance. The personal habits, particularly with regard to the use of tobacco and alcohol, and the occupation and emotional performance of the patient should be assessed. In addition, the wishes of the patient regarding treatment should be determined, to some extent, by the examining physician. Of considerable importance in the total evaluation of the problem is the level of dental hygiene and the state of repair of the teeth because these influence both the decision as to mode of treatment and the need for dental prophylaxis if radiation therapy is to be elected. The age of the patient is of significance since the late effects of radiation therapy become more prominent when this form of treatment is to be administered to the younger patient.

Cancers of the anterior two-thirds of the tongue, the floor of the mouth, and the base of the tongue have different biologic behaviors, and no statement should be made categorically about the preferred means of treatment for each of these distinctive sites. Inasmuch as each of these structures contributes to the processes of speech and swallowing, it would seem that that form of treatment which would be most likely to conserve function should be the one elected. The only presumed advantage of radiation therapy is conservation of tissue and, hence, function. Radiation therapy, however, is always accompanied by undesirable sequelae which increase with the size of the dosage delivered, the volume of tissue irradiated, and the elapsed time after radiation therapy. There are two phases of the complications of radiation therapy:

1. Early complications, which occur during and immediately following the radiation treatment. These consist of mucositis, discomfort, dysphagia, and erythema of the skin, if external radiation therapy is given. The early changes tend to subside in time, and the late changes then begin to show themselves at various intervals from the time of completion of the radiation therapy.
2. Late changes consist of atrophy, fibrosis, intimal thickening of the blood vessels, xerostomia, and, on occasion, changes in the peripheral nerves and sometimes in tissue of the central nervous system. In addition, if the patient is young, the chances for development of radiation-induced cancer increase as time goes by.

The disadvantages of surgery are, of course, readily apparent. Most are acute and then become static, with the disability either remaining stationary, improving, or becoming capable of improvement by reconstructive procedures or by other means.

With the primary object of cure firmly in mind, one must then select, on the basis of personal experience, that form of treatment most likely to result in the greatest cure with the best preservation of function and the fewest undesirable early and late sequelae. Small lesions of the oral tongue, base of tongue, or floor of the mouth can be treated either by radiation therapy or surgery with an almost equal cure. As the cancers progress in size, and particularly as they become more infiltrative, the presumed advantage of radiation therapy diminishes, and when one is dealing with large, infiltrative, and destructive cancers, whether of oral tongue, floor of mouth, or base of tongue, the results with surgery are considerably better than those achieved by radiation therapy. Recent studies reported but not published by Guillamondegui, Hayden, and Oliver (1980) and by White and Byers (1980) have shown that at the M. D. Anderson Hospital, where both radiation therapy and surgery are presumably performed by experts, the larger and more infiltrative lesions are treated considerably better by surgery.

As a case in point, a small lesion of the oral tongue can be surgically excised with minimal sacrifice of tissue and little or no disturbance of function. As the lesions progress in size and surgery becomes more extensive, the disadvantages of alteration of function from extensive sacrifice of tissue increase. It is remarkable, however, the way the tongue hypertrophies and, as time goes by, the patient adjusts to the change in the conformation of the tongue and the amount of disability significantly decreases. Conversely, although the use of interstitial radiation to eradicate a small tumor and conserve function may result in an initial good result, as time goes by, the effects of radiation fibrosis and atrophy reduce the function of the remaining tongue. It is not at all unusual to find after five to ten years that an initially good result obtained by radiation therapy for an oral tongue cancer has subsequently resulted in marked radiation fibrosis and hemiatrophy, with an end result that is much less satisfactory than that obtained by simple surgical removal of the tumor with minimal initial morbidity and no late sequelae.

Surgery would seem to be the treatment of choice for those patients having multiple areas of leukoplakia, with or without multiple areas of invasive cancer, and for the alcoholic smoker who can be expected to develop multiple primary cancers. Approximately 30% of the patients with oral cavity cancer who survive can be expected at some time in their follow-up period to develop a second primary of the aerodigestive tract, and this second primary can be much better managed if it occurs in a field which has not been previously irradiated. In addition, since the morbidity from a surgical procedure is relatively small, it is apparent that an elderly patient would probably tolerate the insult of minimal surgical morbidity much better than that of the prolonged morbidity of heavy radiation.

Surgery would seem to be the treatment of choice for the majority of oral tongue cancers and cancers of the floor of the mouth, particularly in the following circumstances:

1. Infiltrative cancers, particularly when they are attached to or are immediately adjacent to the mandible.
2. Cancers occurring in patients having multiple intraoral primaries or marked areas of leukoplakia who can be expected sometime to develop other squamous cell carcinomas.
3. Cancers occurring in alcoholic smokers who will not change their habits, tolerate radiation therapy poorly, and are more likely to have undesirable sequelae in the postradiation course.
4. Cancers occurring in elderly patients.
5. Cancers occurring in psychotic or uncooperative patients who cannot be expected to undergo any prolonged course of radiation therapy.

There are a number of controversies surrounding surgical procedures for cancer of the oral tongue and floor of the mouth. These can be listed briefly as follows:

1. Feasibility of intraoral resection of cancer of oral tongue and floor of mouth.
2. Safety of surgical margins.
3. Is sacrifice of mandible necessary?
4. Role of elective neck dissection.
5. Type of surgical repair.

1. It was previously held that if a surgical procedure were to be done for an oral tongue cancer, it was necessary to do a composite resection along with resection of the primary. For some time at our institution, however, we have been doing all T1 and T2 floor of mouth and oral tongue primaries through the intraoral approach, with a neck dissection, if necessary, done discontinuously. Additionally, many T3 and some T4 lesions can be similarly approached with conservation of the functional portion of the mandible by doing a coronal or marginal resection of the mandible adjacent to the tumor. Such a surgical procedure requires adequate exposure and can only be done with adequate assistance and in the relatively bloodless field. The use of the electrosurgical unit has been found most helpful in providing such a field.

2. The adequacy of the extent of surgical margins. It has sometimes been advocated that a hemiglossectomy for a T1 lesion of the oral tongue is necessary, and it has also been held that a margin of 2 cm is necessary for all tongue cancers. A consideration of the anatomy of the tongue plus knowledge of the routes of spread would indicate that neither of these tenets is justifiable. There is no firm barrier between the two halves of the tongue, and tumors generally do not conform to a precise geometric pattern, but rather tend to spread along paths of predilection. The tongue is not a large enough organ to allow a margin of 2 cm around any primary cancer, since the total width of the tongue between the mandible, at the level of the posterior third of the oral tongue, is only about 6 cm. The most logical surgical approach to removal of a tongue or floor of mouth cancer is to perform the procedure under a relatively bloodless field using an electrosurgical unit and to remove an adequate volume of tissue around the primary cancer as determined by clinical evaluation during the surgical procedure and also with the aid of frozen section microscopic studies. It is mandatory, if surgery is to be done on intraoral cancers, that surgeons have access to competent frozen section studies, that they take the specimen to the surgical pathologist and go over the most likely areas of extension in consultation with their colleague. It is the surgeon who is most likely to be able to point out the areas likely to be suspect and to recognize the possibility that tumor can be spreading along submucosal, muscular, or neurovascular planes. If there is any question as to the adequacy of the surgical resection, additional margins of tissue should be taken and submitted for diagnostic studies, so that a controlled excision of the primary cancer is done. This results in a more certain resection of the

cancer with less sacrifice of normal tissue. In situations in which the primary cancer is accompanied by multiple areas of in situ carcinoma or leukoplakia, it is advisable to resect the mucosa at risk and, if necessary, cover the entire remaining musculature of the tongue with a skin graft. Such a resurfacing gives protection against the development of new primaries in the immediate vicinity of the original cancer, plus adequate coverage with good function of the remaining tongue.

3. The necessity for resection of the mandible. It has sometimes been held that the mandible should be resected, both to get better access to the primary and because of the possibility that lymphatic structures might be located immediately adjacent to the mandible. Although the sacrifice of the horizontal ramus of the mandible behind the mental foramen does not result in any significant cosmetic or functional deformity, the sacrifice of the anterior arch of the mandible results both in marked anatomic deformity and loss of function. It is particularly advisable, therefore, in the anterior mandible, to do a primary intraoral resection without disturbing the mandible if tumor is not immediately adjacent to the mandible. If it is close to the mandible, then a marginal resection of the mandible should be done. When the anterior mandible is grossly invaded by a cancer, resection and primary reconstruction of the mandible should be performed, if feasible. It is not necessary or advisable to split the lip in order to gain access to the intraoral cavity. The arguments for removing the mandible because of the possibility that lymphatic structures may lie adjacent to the mandible would seem to be largely specious.

4. Another point of controversy regarding the surgical treatment of floor of mouth and oral tongue cancers concerns the advisability of doing an elective neck dissection. The subject has been hotly debated over the years and cannot be satisfactorily resolved on purely statistical grounds. The incidence of nodal metastasis is considerably greater for cancers originating in the oral tongue than for those beginning in the floor of the mouth. The advisability of doing an elective neck dissection for cancers of the oral tongue would seem to be reasonable, particularly if the patient is one who cannot be followed. An upper neck dissection is not an adequate procedure for most cancers of the oral tongue—particularly for anteriorly-placed lesions—since nodal metastases may be to the lower third of the jugular chain. It is quite possible to do an adequate neck dissection removing all of the nodes at risk while at the same time preserving the spinal accessory nerve, the sternocleidomastoid muscle, and the internal jugular vein.

5. Another point of controversy concerns the manner of surgical repair of defects of the floor of the mouth and oral tongue. Small defects of the floor of the mouth or oral tongue can be either closed primarily or left open with the expectation of rapid healing and good function. Larger defects of the floor of the mouth can be satisfactorily treated by application of a split-thickness skin graft. There are those who would object to the use of split-thickness skin grafts since they maintain that they all contract and produce undesirable loss of function. If the skin graft, however, has been properly placed, is made

large enough and redundant enough, and is stented adequately, the success rate is extremely high. Defects in the tongue can be closed by primary approximation, or, if a hemiglossectomy has been done, the tip of the remaining tongue can be turned back on itself to refashion an organ which looks and functions quite normally. It would seem unnecessary to use nasolabial flaps, platysmal myocutaneous flaps, or flaps with free vascular anastomoses for many of the defects created unless one anticipates giving postoperative radiation to a patient who has had a marginal resection of the mandible. Although theoretically the full-thickness flaps would give more pliability and better function, they actually are bulky in many instances and do not give any greater function than can be achieved by a properly placed split-thickness skin graft. Free grafts with vascular anastomoses should probably be reserved for those patients who have had either preoperative radiation with resection of a large portion of tongue, floor of mouth, or mandible or in patients in whom a marginal resection of the mandible has been done and postoperative radiation is to be employed.

## Cancers of the Base of the Tongue

Previous discussion has dealt with cancers of the oral tongue and floor of the mouth. Cancers of the base of the tongue have a different biologic behavior since they have a considerably higher rate of metastasis and tend both to have bilateral nodal metastases and, occasionally, retropharyngeal nodal metastases. Because of the importance of the base of the tongue in the performance of the act of deglutition, plus the more diffuse metastases which can be expected, radiation therapy would seem to play a greater role than it does in cancers of the floor of mouth and oral tongue. It has been my experience, however, that essentially no large infiltrative base of the tongue cancers are salvaged by radiation therapy, and it would seem at the present time that all such cancers are best treated surgically. The decision as to whether or not to remove the larynx should be based on two factors: first, on the proximity of the base of tongue cancers to the hyoid bone and the necessity for including all tissue to which the base of tongue might spread and, second, on the age and physiologic state of the patient. An elderly patient with an extensive base of the tongue cancer who could not tolerate repeated bouts of aspiration should have the larynx removed along with the base of tongue cancer as the primary surgical procedure. Because of the high rate of bilateral nodal spread, a bilateral neck dissection should be done at the time of the initial surgical procedure. Such neck dissections can be modified with preservation of the sternocleidomastoid muscle, spinal accessory nerve, and internal jugular vein, provided the nodes are freely movable and do not infiltrate any of the structures in the neck. Bilateral neck dissections of this type which preserve both internal jugular veins are accompanied by a negligible morbidity and mortality.

## Controversies Regarding Radiation Therapy

Small cancers of the oral tongue or floor of the mouth can be treated either by primary interstitial radiation or by the use of intraoral cone. If the lesions are larger, however, with greater risk of metastasis to the upper neck, preliminary radiation to approximately a tumor dose of 5000 rad should be given to the neck, to be followed by radium implant. It has been found that if a radium implant alone is done for the larger lesions, the risk of implanting cancer cells into the neck is increased. There are other controversies regarding the total dose to be employed and the volume of tissue to be irradiated, but these are technical and not within the scope of this chapter. The use of other forms of radiation such as the neutron beam is being evaluated. The place of the neutron beam has yet to be determined. It would seem that neutron beam, as the sole modality of treatment, will not find great use because of the pronounced effect on normal tissue. There may be a place for this form of energy when it is combined with the more conventional radiation achieved with the cobalt teletherapy unit.

## Pre- or Postoperative Radiation

Regarding the combination of radiation therapy with surgery in an effort to achieve a greater cure, there is a continuing debate as to whether the radiation should be delivered pre- or postoperatively. The presumed advantages of preoperative radiation are:

1. The volume of tumor is reduced, and hence the surgical procedure is facilitated.
2. The tumor cells are devitalized so that the risk of implantation is less.
3. The peripheral extensions of the tumor are sterilized and only the central nidus remains.
4. The magnitude of the surgical procedure can be decreased.

The drawbacks to the employment of preoperative radiation are as follows:

1. Morbidity is increased. Four to five weeks of preoperative radiation followed by a recovery period of equal duration and then the hospitalization for the surgical procedure add up to a lengthy period of morbidity.
2. The usual anatomic and pathologic markers are absent at the time of surgery. Frequently, neither the surgeon nor the pathologist can tell whether viable tumor is present, or how it is spreading.
3. Inevitably some patients will refuse surgery after preoperative radiation has been completed. Since the radiation dose delivered has usually been less than cancerocidal, the patient is most likely to get a recurrence. Although it has been stated that the number of surgical complications following preoperative radiation is not increased, it would seem that if the radiation is given to a tumor dose of 5000 rad, to both the primary and neck, it is more difficult to secure primary wound healing and convalescence is prolonged.

A review of the literature has not shown conclusively any series in which the use of preoperative radiation has resulted in a significant rate of improvement of long-term survival. Any study performed would be difficult to randomize: a number of patients would have to be eliminated from the preoperative radiation group inasmuch as they would be unsuitable either physiologically or emotionally to undergo the combined procedure. Probably the best indication for preoperative radiation would be in those patients who have large or fixed nodes in which neck dissection is facilitated and the risk of local recurrence is reduced by delivering the radiation therapy preoperatively.

Postoperatively, radiation has been advocated as being better tolerated by the patient and as being equally effective in controlling the risk of local recurrence. Here again no study has conclusively shown that survival is significantly enhanced by postoperative radiation. Probably postoperative radiation adds but little to an excellent surgical procedure. No surgeon should be deluded by the siren song of postoperative radiation into doing a less than "adequate" surgical procedure in the hopes that gross disease left behind can be satisfactorily eradicated by the radiotherapist. Probable indications for postoperative radiation are:

1. Microscopic disease at margins.
2. The presence within the neck of multiple positive nodes at multiple levels.
3. The presence of extensive perineural lymphatic spread.
4. The presence of soft tissue metastases in the neck outside of the regional lymph nodes.

The arguments for preoperative radiation versus postoperative radiation are fairly well defined. They are as follows:

1. Preoperative radiation would seem to have the advantage of being given to an area not scarred by a surgical procedure. The surgical procedure always produces scarring with relatively anoxic areas, and the radiotherapist would prefer not to give the radiation postoperatively.
2. A delay in wound healing would postpone the time at which postoperative radiotherapy might be beneficial.
3. The reduction of tumor burden by preoperative radiation has a theoretical advantage as does also the devitalization of the tumor cells in the alteration of the tumor bed to reduce the risk of implantation of viable cancer cells.

The advantages of postoperative radiation are:

1. It is better tolerated.
2. It is performed with a better knowledge of the true extent of the tumor, both as to local routes of spread and to the extent of the cervical metastases. Such knowledge permits better planning of the radiation fields.

When one weighs the advantages and disadvantages of the two adjuvant methods of radiation therapy, they would seem to balance out. Since postoperative radiation is better tolerated, it is the procedure preferred by the majority of surgeons.

The place of chemotherapy in the treatment of cancer of the tongue and floor of the mouth is still under debate. It has been claimed that the addition of chemotherapy to radiation or surgery results in greater local control. The series reported, however, has not had long-term follow-up, and the cases selected have not been adequately randomized. It is readily apparent that the addition of chemotherapy to radiation or surgery increases the morbidity and also the expense. Initially, there was great enthusiasm for the use of the various combinations of Cis-platinum, bleomycin, methotrexate, and 5-fluorouracil, for this regimen apparently resulted in a marked shrinkage of some tumors. Some of the tumors undergoing considerable shrinkage, however, were those tumors that were largely exophytic and would be expected to respond to radiation therapy. In our experience, the use of preoperative chemotherapy, either in combination with radiotherapy or surgery, or using all three combined, has not been of significant benefit to those patients in whom we would expect poor results by conventional treatment. Since chemotherapy is available, there is a temptation to employ it in combination with radiotherapy in the hope of avoiding an extensive surgical procedure that might well be curative. In our hands, the use of this form of combined treatment for extensive infiltrative cancers of the base of the tongue has been futile.

When new and better drugs come along for the treatment of squamous cell carcinomas of the oral tongue, floor of mouth, and base of tongue, chemotherapy may have an integral place in the treatment, either by combination with radiotherapy or surgery. At the present time, the combinations of chemotherapy, radiotherapy, and surgery are best left to institutions with a sufficient volume of material and adequate numbers of skilled personnel to conduct proper clinical trials.

## Summary

In a dogmatic presentation such as this, it might seem that a set form of treatment is elected for all cancers of the floor of the mouth and tongue. In actual practice, treatment is highly individualized, with all tumor and host factors weighed in the balance and a treatment plan outlined that seems to offer the patient under consideration the greatest chance of cure with the least morbidity and disturbance of function, and with the fewest undesirable sequelae. The weighing toward surgery, radiation, or combinations will vary among institutions depending upon the skills of the specialists.

## References

Guillamondegui, O. M.; Hayden, R.; and Oliver, B. Cancer of the anterior floor of the mouth: selective choice of treatment and analysis of our failures. Submitted to *Am. J. Surg.* October 1980.

White, D., and Byers, R. M. What is the preferred initial modality of treatment for squamous carcinoma of the oral tongue? Submitted to *Am. J. Surg.* October 1980.

# Chapter 9

# *An Inquiry on the Quality of Life after Curative Treatment*

Juan V. Fayos and
François Beland

Surgery, radiation, or a combination of both modalities of treatment constitute the only alternatives available today for the cure of carcinomas of the head and neck region, as several chapters in this book will attest.

Regardless of the modality of treatment, the outcome is measured in one of two ways: by determining whether the primary or metastatic disease is cured, or by assessing the survival of the patient after treatment. The former describes efficacy of treatment; the latter, quantity of life, ordinarily measured in months or years after the beginning of treatment.

Both of these measures can be easily computed, and they are customarily reported when the results of a treatment are presented either in medical literature or at meetings, as a means of judging the superiority of one treatment over another.

With the widespread use of computers for data analysis in medicine, it is very simple to let the "machine" do the computations and generate actuarial life tables or graphs in rapid fashion.

Another way the clinician ordinarily assesses the outcome of treatment is by determining how many patients suffered a complication as a result of the treatment given. In general, complications are described by the pathologic damage produced or by the anatomic structure in which they occurred, as when describing radionecrosis of the jaw bone, dehiscence of a surgical wound, and so on. Seldom is there a quantification or a social description of the functional, psychic, or emotional damage produced in the patient as a consequence of a given treatment.

Furthermore, when an individual with a carcinoma of the oral tongue, for example, is treated with a mutilating procedure such as hemiglossectomy, hemimandibulectomy, or radical neck dissection, the outcome of treatment with the ensuing defect is considered as the new "normal state" for the patient and not as a complication of treatment. This "normal state" is assumed in spite of the speech and swallowing disabilities the patient might experience which could cause him severe social disturbances.

It is becoming imperative, therefore, that a new dimension be considered in evaluating the outcome of treatment, in addition to the current determination of treatment efficacy and quantity of life following treatment. This new dimension measures outcome by determining the quality of life a patient enjoys after treatment. To be sure, one of the difficulties in determining quality is the lack of a developed methodology to make the information relevant, reliable, and systematically applicable by a treating physician.

## The Quality of Life: Concept and Value

Unfortunately, there is no straightforward manner in which "quality of life" can be defined. The concept of quality of life is rather impervious. Our understanding of that concept is still intuitive and is based on some normative notion of well-being, often defined according to the values and biases of the researcher (Andrews and Withey 1976; Bunge 1975; Donabedian 1973; Harwood 1976; McPeek, Gilbert, and Mosteller 1977; U.S. Department of Health, Education, and Welfare 1969).

The notion of quality of life is thus value-laden. Consequently, it is important that in any study of quality of life the values and normative orientations of the researcher be displayed. We have chosen to define quality of life as the ability of patients to manage their lives as they evaluate it.

In the case of patients with cancer of the head and neck, how will the treatment they must endure modify the quality of their lives? When patients come to a radiotherapist or surgeon, they might know they are suffering from a life-threatening disease. They have probably gone through anguishing moments and presumably their quality of life has already been lowered. There is no point, however, in trying to ascertain how much it has been altered. Rather, we want to know if the treatment process will improve it, diminish it, or not affect it at all.

There are at least two prevailing opinions regarding the importance of assessing the patient's quality of life in the treatment process. The first contends that enhancing the quality of life of patients can be conceived of as a part of the treatment process. The second opinion maintains that the proper goal of medical activity is the cure of the disease, not the betterment of the patient's quality of life. Of course, if there is a relationship between cure and quality of life, so much the better, but this is not the main objective of the treatment. The main objective, the second opinion concludes, is to cure the patient. Consequently, in order to do research on the quality of life of patients one must choose between these two positions.

Whatever the opinion of the medical team, however, the fact remains that patients under treatment will bear further disruptions from their usual way of life. As a consequence of their illness, they will have to adapt to a different schedule for the period of treatment and perhaps afterwards. They will live through periods of anguish, uncertainty, hope, and lack of confidence. After the treatment period, patients will either resume or relinquish all or part of their former activities, but the state of their illness and the consequences of a setback cannot be ignored.

Research on the quality of life, therefore, should focus on the patients' own evaluation of their lives in the domains affected by the disease and the treatment process. The patient suffering from cancer and being treated by some means must deal not only with physical disabilities and functional limitations of disease and treatment, but also with major social and psychological problems of varying degrees, depending upon the impact of disease and treatment. These additional problems involve social isolation, relationships with family and friends, working disabilities, and so on. The patient still has to mobilize resources and take part in different social contexts (Gerson 1976). We emphasize that selecting activities as determinants of the quality of life is a normative choice, but one we believe to be in general agreement with the prevailing value system (Parson 1964).

## The Measurement of Quality of Life

Our intuitive conception of quality of life as the ability of patients to manage their lives links itself with the notion of health used in health surveys, which is defined as the capacity of individuals to sustain their usual roles in society (Moriyama 1968; Sigemann and Elieson 1977). We will thus distinguish impairment from disability (Haber 1967). Patients may suffer impairment of their habitual functions. This becomes a condition that varies to some extent according to the social context. The social context either enhances or impairs the ability of individuals to manage their lives. A disability, on the other hand, is a physical or mental condition defined by a clinical diagnosis (Ruesch and Brodsky 1968). Impaired individuals are never fully capable of managing their own lives, whereas disabled individuals can be free from impairments and can therefore continue to manage their own lives.

Having patients evaluate their own capacity to sustain activity is one way to conceptualize their well-being. It also indicates something about the measurement of well-being. The literature describes several indexes of health that measure many aspects of the problem. One of them is the Sickness Impact Profile (SIP) developed by the Department of Health Services, University of Washington (Gibson 1975). This index appears to fit the clinical situation of patients with cancers of the head and neck. The SIP index coincides with our assumptions and conceptual framework, and also conforms to the rules of scaling and interviewing techniques.

SIP was developed to provide an appropriate outcome measure for use in assessing health care services (Carter et al. 1976). It is a behavior-based measure of sickness-related dysfunction. It is comprised of 136 items covering the broad activities involved in carrying on one's life (Gibson 1975). These statements are divided into 12 categories, each representing a specific area of activity. The main aspects evaluated are those corresponding to physical dimensions, psychosocial dimensions, and the feeling of well-being (University of Washington 1978). The items it explores are shown in table 9.1. The patient receives a questionnaire covering each of the items in table 9.1. Each of the questions is weighed. Partial or total scales of the physical and psychosocial dimensions could be obtained if necessary, but the test is designed to be evaluated in its entirety.

Since the SIP measures the ability of patients to manage their lives at one moment in time and since the treatment of a cancer patient is also a process requiring time, the measurement process should be longitudinal; that is, many measurements should be made on the same patient. The most significant periods would be before treatment, at the end of treatment (whether surgical or with radiation), and at convenient times in the immediate post-treatment period. Because patients are bound to resume their usual activities two or three months after the treatment concludes, while still under the real threat of recurrence of the disease (75% of recurrences occur within one year), it is desirable to measure the health indexes at least once during the first year after treatment at the most appropriate time selected by the investigator.

The application of indexes of health to patients is in its infancy. We have initiated a pilot program to test the concept of quality of care in patients with cancer of the head and neck who are undergoing radiation therapy. It is still too soon to determine whether the SIP index will be sufficiently sensitive or an appropriate test to validate and measure quality of life in patients after treatment, although our initial impression is that it will be.

**Table 9.1**
The Dimensions of the SIP Index

| |
|---|
| A. Social interaction |
| B. Ambulation |
| C. Sleep and rest |
| D. Taking nutrition |
| E. Usual daily work |
| F. Household management |
| G. Mobility and confinement |
| H. Communication activity |
| I. Leisure and recreation |
| J. Emotion, feelings, and sensations |
| K. Body care and movement |
| L. Alertness behavior |

It is even more difficult to assign risk values to the given treatment based upon the quality of life remaining after treatment. If there were such a measure, it would be of considerable value to the physician. Prescription of treatment will not be made on the basis of a referral pattern when patients are irradiated because they have been referred to a radiation therapy facility, nor will it be made when they have surgery because they have been referred to a surgeon. Treatment should be based upon a global concept. Control of the neoplasm, quality of life, and maximum quantity of life all depend upon the stage and type of the neoplasm from which the patient is suffering. The result of all the measurements on a patient will be a picture of the patient's quality of health during a given period of time.

The following two cases illustrate the need for measuring quality of care and integrating it into the therapeutic decision-making process.

1. The patient was a 65-year-old man who was found to have a large tumor of the oropharynx, most likely arising from the right tonsil. Biopsies were obtained showing moderately well-differentiated squamous cell carcinoma. He was admitted to the University of Michigan Hospital, where in May 1978 he had a supraglottic laryngectomy and right radical neck dissection. The specimen showed a large fungating partially-exophytic tumor involving the supraglottic portion of the larynx and extending to the pyriform recesses on both sides. It was an infiltrating squamous cell carcinoma. Sections showed the neoplasm extending into the preepiglottic space. Mucosal margins were free of tumor. The radical neck dissection specimen showed a large tumor in its middle third. The mass was in the soft tissues and presumably represented a replaced lymph node by metastatic squamous cell carcinoma. The carcinoma invaded to within 1 mm of the wall of the jugular vein.

Postoperatively, the patient had difficulty swallowing. Instructions given to help him overcome his disability failed, and he was discharged in July with a nasogastric tube so nutritional status could be maintained. Weight loss during his hospitalization was approximately 30 pounds.

In October 1978 the patient was admitted again into the hospital because of inability to swallow, right-sided headache, weight loss, and hypercalcemia. His work-up at this time centered around the latter. Subsequently, because of the hypercalcemia he underwent a neck exploration with biopsies of parathyroid glands and excision of the right lobe of the thyroid. There was no evidence of any pathologic abnormality in either the thyroid or parathyroid glands.

Because of continued difficulty swallowing, a total laryngectomy was contemplated. This was not done, however, because of the detection of an enlarging mass in the right upper cervical region at the level of the angle of the mandible. A biopsy of an ulcerated area on the right pharyngeal wall showed recurrent squamous cell carcinoma. The patient began a course of radiation therapy because of the definite recurrence of the primary lesion and neck metastasis. Treatment began on November 27, 1978 and terminated on January 12, 1979. He was treated using cobalt 60 radiation at a source-skin distance of 80 cm through two opposing lateral fields that cross-fired the primary and the metastatic nodes in the neck. A midplane dose of 6000 rad was given for 47 days in 30 fractions. The lower neck was treated through an anterior bilateral neck field measuring 8×21 cm. An incident dose of 5000 rad at 0.5 cm beneath the surface of the skin was also given for 47 days.

During the middle of treatment, radiation had to be interrupted because the patient could not lie flat for treatment due to excessive coughing. This made him refuse treatment for a period of four days. After that, treatment was resumed until termination, but at no time was there any significant change in the size of the tumor either at the primary or metastatic sites. He was discharged from the hospital on January 19, 1979, and died at home five days later.

During this second admission to the hospital, the patient became very depressed and withdrawn. Questions to him would be met by a shrug of his shoulders or a blank stare. He refused to communicate, although occasionally he would pound on his bedside stand to gain attention. The nurses caring for him charted almost daily his depression and continued withdrawal, but no mention of this was ever made in the daily physician's notes.

The approximate cost of his first hospitalization was $13,000, and the second, $25,000, both covered by Medicare. This did not include professional fees, which were billed separately. Radiation therapy fees were $1216, about equally divided between professional and hospital components. The patient had also been followed by urology, medical oncology, otology, and general surgery, and none of these can be documented. It is estimated that the cost of this illness was higher than $40,000 and the outcome was death after a prolonged period of suffering.

At no time was there any measure of the psychosocial disturbance that the treatment, either by surgery or radiation, might have caused. Even though he had a supraglottic laryngectomy, the patient was unable to express himself after initial surgery either in English or in Spanish. This may have been due to functional disability or to a marked withdrawal resulting from the disturbance of his psychosomatic condition.

2. This patient was a 48-year-old man with a six-week history of daily elevated temperature and bilateral enlarging masses in his upper neck. He was first treated by his family physician with antibiotics. When there was no improvement in his symptoms, a biopsy of a left neck lymph node was performed elsewhere and reported as lymphosarcoma. He was referred to the hematology service of University Hospital, where initial evaluation in July included a gallium scan, liver/spleen scan, and bone marrow aspirate. When the patient was presented to lymphoma conference, the pathologic slides were reviewed and showed a diffusely, moderately well-differentiated squamous cell carcinoma. A direct laryngoscopy was performed, and a biopsy of the base of the tongue showed poorly-differentiated squamous cell carcinoma.

The patient was evaluated by the radiation therapy department, and treatment was advised with good probability of controlling the primary tumor, but with a considerably less chance of controlling the metastatic adenopathy. The patient, however, was placed on a chemotherapy regimen to be followed by a surgical procedure. His first surgery was performed on September 28, 1978 and consisted of a left composite resection and left radical neck dissection, with removal of a segment of the mandible and base of the tongue. The pathologic diagnosis was infiltrating poorly-differentiated squamous cell carcinoma. Large metastatic lymph nodes were present in the upper and middle cervical regions. On October 17, 1978, the patient had a right radical neck dissection which also showed infiltrating moderately well-differentiated squamous cell carcinoma within soft tissue and lymph nodes. After surgery, the patient began to sleep in a sitting position. Because he had difficulty eating, he was placed on nasogastric feedings.

One month after the right radical neck dissection was done, the patient was again referred to radiation therapy for consideration of radiation treatment. Upon examination, he was found to have marked torticollis and two nodules in the skin of the right neck (fig. 9.1). Motion of the neck was very limited, associated with difficulties in swallowing and speech. Needle aspirate biopsies of the nodules were done, and they showed recurrent carcinoma. Because of the presence of rapidly growing recurrence in the neck and the deterioration of his general status, the patient was admitted to the hospital in December 1978. He had increasing difficulty breathing, pain, dysphagia, right facial swelling, and decreased ability to speak. An emergency tracheostomy was performed the day after admission. The patient's general condition declined rapidly until his death on January 10, 1979. No radiation therapy was given to this patient at any time.

The patient had four admissions to this hospital. The cost per admission was: August, \$7000; September, \$2000; October, \$10,000; and January, \$19,000. Added to these costs were the professional fees, which could not be documented. As in the previous case, the total cost was estimated to be higher than \$40,000, with a fatal outcome after repeated therapeutic attempts.

These two cases raise numerous questions and provide few answers. Would these two patients have been better off receiving treatment other than initial surgery? Should a more conservative treatment (for example, radiation therapy) have been instituted initially, reserving surgery for the event of recurrence only? It is obvious that subsequent events in these patients' histories militate against having used surgery initially, particularly in the second case, where the patient had a poorly-differentiated lesion, which is known to respond fairly well to radiation. Moreover, the second patient had an open biopsy of the adenopathy prior to surgery, a poor prognostic risk in patients who are to undergo surgery.

These two patients had in common advanced disease of the primary when initially evaluated. From the prognostic point of view, neither patient had but a small probability of local control by any therapeutic means. Both were treated surgically, with grave psychosomatic disturbances resulting.

**Figure 9.1**

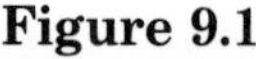

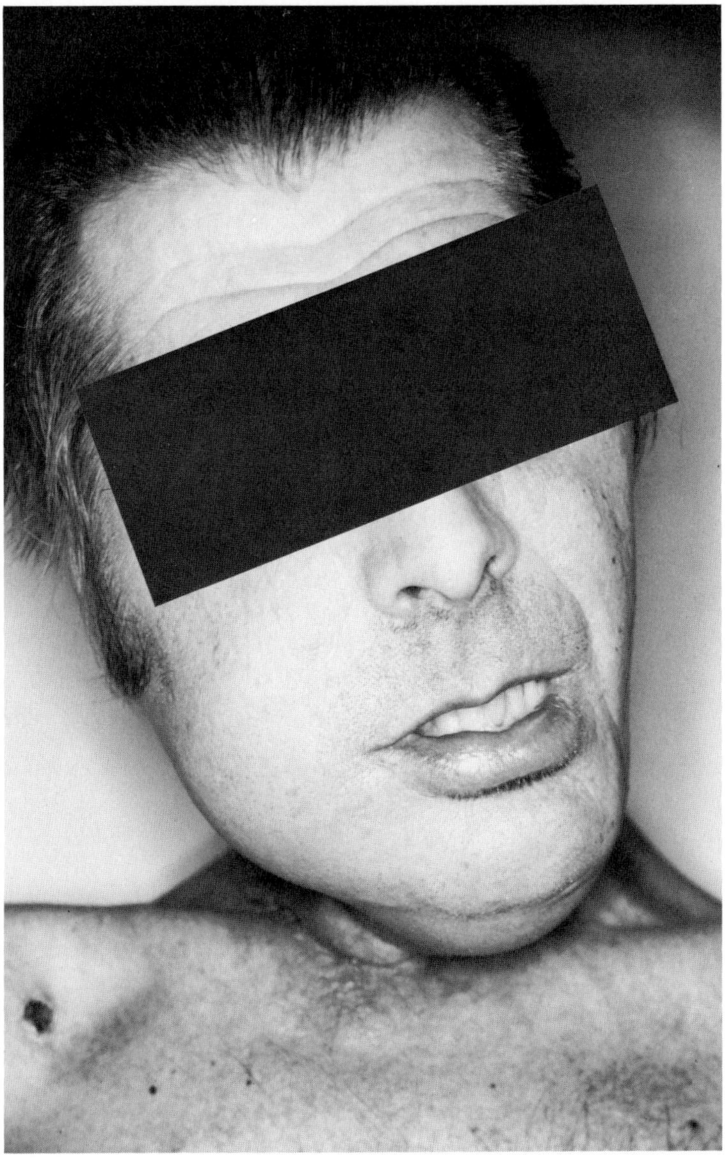

A

*Photographs of patient described as case 2, showing torticollis and recurrent cancer after surgery and chemotherapy.* ***A,*** *facial view;* ***B,*** *lateral view.*

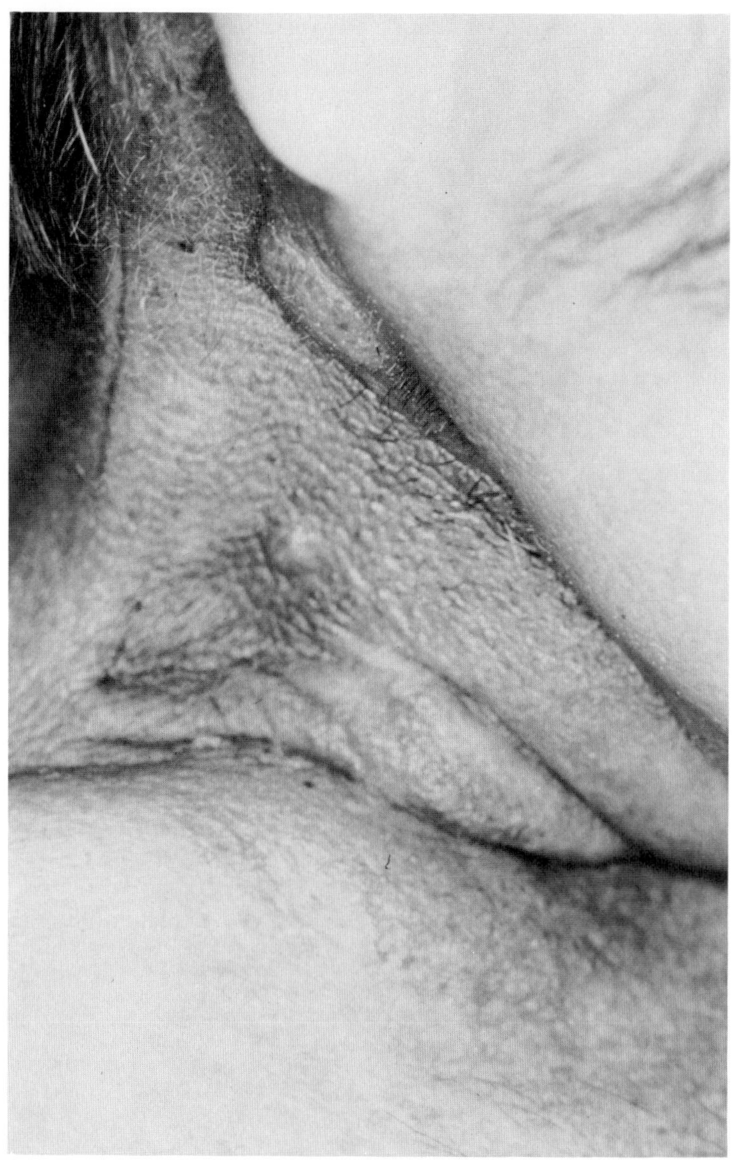

B

Death followed rapidly after treatment. We postulate that the treatment decision-making in either case would have been greatly helped if measures of the quality of life after treatment existed. In this way, the patients would have been able to make a more intelligent decision concerning risks and disabilities before acceptance of treatment. With more enlightening information, the patients could have made a deliberate decision to maximize their wishes and life-styles and to trade the disability resulting from treatment for potential survival. This, in effect, is what the proper informed consent of the patient should entail.

We began this discussion with a very general concern about quality of life. We were then able to define our area of interest as the quantification of the ability of patients to manage their lives (manageability being conceived, in this case, as resource mobilization, social context participation, and negotiation actions of the patients). Without attempting explicitly to define these areas of actions, it appeared to us that the ability of patients to engage in a significant number of activities and tasks was to be the concept that would direct our choice of a concrete index of quality of life. We found that the SIP, with its implicit assumptions and goals and its basic dimensions, is a proper index of quality of life, for the SIP is a measure of the behavior capacities of individuals as they are affected by their health or by any modifications in their clinically-defined condition induced by a treatment.

The two cases illustrated potential benefits that could accrue from the development of a methodology that would measure quality of life after treatment. By informing patients of the total outlook of the disease and the impairments resulting from treatment, they would be able to maximize their decision-making and trade potential lengthening of life against disabilities that could follow from disease and therapy (McNeil, Weichselbaum, and Pauker 1978).

In an era of soaring medical care expenses, how heavily should cost weigh in a therapeutic decision? In the above instances the cost of hospitalization, surgery, and so on, exceeded $40,000 for each patient.

The two patients derived little benefit from the treatments. In fact, the treatments may have had deleterious effects. Although cost considerations could become a factor in altering treatment decision-making (Abt 1975, 1977; Green 1977; Neuhauser 1977; Pliskin and Taylor 1977), cost alone does not play a significant part in therapeutic decisions for the present.

## References


Abt, C. C. The social costs of cancer. *Soc. Indicators Res.* 2:175–190, 1975.

Abt, C. C. The issue of social costs in cost-benefit analysis of surgery. In *Costs, risks, and benefits of surgery,* eds. J. Bunker, B. Barnes, and F. Mosteller. New York: Oxford University Press, 1977.

Andrews, R. W., and Withey, S. B. *Social indicators of well-being: American perceptions of life quality.* New York: Plenum Press, 1976.

Bunge, M. What is quality of life indication? *Soc. Indicators Res.* 2:65–79, 1975.

Carter, W. B. et al. Validation of an internal scaling: the sickness impact profile. *Health Serv. Res.* 11:516–528, 1976.

Donabedian, A. *Aspects of medical care administration: specifying requirements for health care.* Cambridge, Mass.: Harvard University Press, 1973.

Gerson, E. M. On quality of life. *Am. Sociol. Rev.* 41:473–806, 1976.

Gibson, B. S. et al. The sickness impact profile: development of an outcome measure of health care. *Am. J. Public Health* 65:1304–1310, 1975.

Green, J. R. Cost-benefit analysis of surgery: some additional caveats and interpretations. In *Costs, risks, and benefits of surgery,* eds. J. Bunker, B. Barnes, and F. Mosteller. New York: Oxford University Press, 1977.

Haber, L. P. Identifying the disabled: concepts and methods in the measurement of disability. *Soc. Secur. Bull.,* 1967, pp. 17–34.

Harwood, P. de L. Quality of life: ascriptive and testimonial conceptualizations. *Soc. Indicators Res.* 3:471–497, 1976.

McNeil, B. J.; Weichselbaum, R.; and Pauker, S. G. Fallacy of the five-year survival in lung cancer. *N. Engl. J. Med.* 299:1397–1401, 1978.

McPeek, B.; Gilbert, J. P.; and Mosteller, F. The end result: quality of life. In *Costs, risks, and benefits of surgery,* eds. J. Bunker, B. Barnes, and F. Mosteller. New York: Oxford University Press, 1977.

Moriyama, T. M. Problems in the measurement of health status. In *Indicators of social change,* eds. E. Sheldon and W. Movie. New York: Russell Sage Foundation, 1968.

Neuhauser, D. Cost-effective clinical decision-making: implications for the delivery of health services. In *Costs, risks, and benefits of surgery,* eds. J. Bunker, B. Barnes, and F. Mosteller. New York: Oxford University Press, 1977.

Parson, T. Definitions of health and illness in the light of American values and social structure. In *Patients, physicians, and illness,* ed. E. Jaco. New York: Free Press, 1964.

Pliskin, N., and Taylor, A. K. General principles: cost-benefit and decision analysis. In *Costs, risks, and benefits of surgery,* eds. J. Bunker, B. Barnes, and F. Mosteller. New York: Oxford University Press, 1977.

Ruesch, J., and Brodsky, G. M. The concept of social disability. *Arch. Gen. Psychiatry* 19:394–403, 1968.

Sigemann, A. T., and Elieson, J. Newer socio-medical health indicators: implication for evaluation of health services. *Med. Care* 15(suppl.):84–91, 1977.

University of Washington, Department of Health Services. *The sickness impact profile: a brief summary of its purpose, uses, and administration.* Seattle: University of Washington, 1978.

U.S. Department of Health, Education, and Welfare. *Toward a social report.* Washington, D.C.: U.S. Government Printing Office, 1969.

# Chapter 10

## *Ineffectiveness of Combined Therapy (Radiation and Surgery) in the Management of Malignancies of the Oral Cavity, Larynx, and Pharynx*

Jose J. Terz and
Walter Lawrence, Jr.

The role of radiation therapy as a preoperative adjuvant to surgical resection in the management of head and neck cancer has remained a controversial subject. Enthusiasm for this approach arose from a series of reports of clinical experience with selected patient populations wherein the authors have generally concluded that radiation therapy has a beneficial role when administered prior to surgical resection. This is still an assumption by many, but the validity of this approach is accepted by a large number of head and neck surgeons, in spite of the lack of clearcut, scientifically acceptable evidence to support this approach. We believe that a critical analysis of the published information on the results of preoperative radiation therapy not only may dispel some misconceptions but also may provide a basis for the planning of more fruitful prospective studies of adjuvant radiotherapy in the management of head and neck cancer.

## Material Reviewed

With the above purpose in mind, we reviewed all literature reporting the results of clinical experience with preoperative radiation for head and neck cancer published between 1969 and 1979. Because of the heterogeneity of these reports, we considered only those wherein each treated population was well identified by primary site and/or stage of disease and was followed for no less than two years after the primary treatment. Twenty-two published papers met these minimal criteria; 19 reported the results by retrospective analysis of selected patient populations treated with preoperative radiation therapy followed by standard resections (Biller, Davis, and Powers 1969; Bryce and Ryder 1971; Constable et al. 1972; Flynn, Mullins, and Moore

1973; Fu et al. 1977; Goffinet et al. 1973; Goldman et al. 1972; Hendrickson and Liebner 1968; Hirata et al. 1975; Inoue, Shigematsu, and Sato 1973; Kazem 1974; Krause, Lee, and McCabe 1973; Levitt et al. 1971; Lord et al. 1973; Marks et al. 1978; Perez, Marks, and Powers 1977; Roswit et al. 1972; Skolnik et al. 1975; Wang, Schulz, and Miller 1972). Only three reports communicated the results of prospective randomized studies exploring the role of preoperative radiation (Hintz et al. 1979; Strong et al. 1978; Terz, King, and Lawrence 1980), and only two of these three reports gave survival data more than two years after primary treatment. Because a significant number of these published papers use the results of primary radiation therapy or primary surgery for comparative purposes, we included in our tabulation 12 additional papers reporting results with surgery alone, and/or radiation therapy alone (Daly and Strong 1975; Fayos and Lampe 1971; Hendrickson

**Table 10.1**
Profile of the 34 Papers Used in this Review

| | Number of Retrospective Reports | Number of Prospective Reports |
|---|---|---|
| Treatment Method(s) | | |
| Preoperative radiation therapy only | 8 | — |
| Preoperative radiation therapy vs surgery alone | 7 | 2 |
| Preoperative radiation therapy vs surgery alone vs radiation therapy alone | 4 | 1 |
| Preoperative radiation therapy vs radiation therapy alone | 1 | — |
| Surgery vs radiation therapy | 1 | 1 |
| Surgery alone | 4 | — |
| Radiation therapy alone | 5 | — |
| Clinical Categories Specified | | |
| Primary sites only | 15 | 1 |
| Primary sites and stage of disease | 15 | 3 |
| Maximum Follow-up Intervals (in years) | | |
| Two | 4 | 2 |
| Two–three | 1 | — |
| Two–five | 1 | — |
| Three | 7 | 1 |
| Three–five | 8 | 1 |
| Five | 9 | — |

and Liebner 1968; Hintz et al. 1979; Lees 1976; Razack 1977; Shah and Tollefsen 1974; Shah et al. 1976; Snow et al. 1977; Wang 1971, 1972, 1974). These were included in an attempt to balance a number of patients treated with each modality in the overall comparative assessment attempted, thereby bringing the total number of publications analyzed to 34. The differing types of studies in the papers included in this review are summarized in table 10.1.

## Methods of Analysis

All pertinent clinical information on the individual primary sites, the clinical stage of disease, the dose of radiation, the specific mode of treatment(s), and the follow-up interval employed (in years) was entered into a computer, an IBM 370/158 operating under OS/VS2 using the statistical analysis system (Brown and Benetti 1976; Goodman and Kruskal 1954, 1959, 1963, 1967). All patients were pooled in groups depending on the follow-up interval used in the reports and the initial treatment given (preoperative radiation, surgery only, radiation therapy only). Survival was analyzed at two, three, or five years, depending on the follow-up intervals reported and according to the primary site (oral cavity, pharynx, or larynx), stage of disease (I to IV), and dose of preoperative radiation (less or more than 4000 rad). Frequency tables were generated with this information and the differences among various groups were tested by the chi-square method. The results of the preoperative radiation and the surgery only groups reported in the retrospective studies were compared with results for corresponding groups undergoing similar management in the randomized trials.

This study was undertaken only to establish if there is evidence that preoperative radiation therapy followed by surgery is better than standard single modalities of treatment. The results of radiation therapy alone and surgery alone that are quoted in the analysis are used for comparative purposes only. It is not within the scope of this review to analyze the relative value of primary surgery versus primary radiation therapy in the management of head and neck cancer.

## Results: Combined Analysis of Retrospective and Randomized Prospective Reports

### Two-Year Survival Data

Table 10.2 includes a comparative summary of data from reports using two-year survival data only (Flynn, Mullins, and Moore 1973; Fu et al. 1977; Hendrickson and Liebner 1968; Hintz et al. 1979a, 1979b; Kazem et al. 1974;

**Table 10.2**
Combined Analysis of All Reports Using Two-Year Survival Data, according to Primary Sites

| Treatment | All Cases (No./%) | Primary Site: Oral Cavity (No./%) | Pharynx (No./%) | Larynx (No./%) |
|---|---|---|---|---|
| Preoperative radiation | 336/57 | 138/51 | 22/40 | 162/66 |
| Surgery only | 203/65 | 29/65 | 66/66 | 95/68 |
| Radiation only | 215/51 | 62/58 | 8/50 | 128/51 |

Levitt et al. 1971; Perez, Marks, and Powers 1977). In general, these data demonstrate survival figures for patients receiving preoperative radiation followed by surgery similar to those obtained by either surgery alone or radiation therapy alone. Actually, there was a tendency for the patients treated only by surgery to have a better survival experience than the preoperative radiation group in this particular analysis. Consideration of the dose range of preoperative radiation administered did not alter these results in this group of reports (table 10.3). The lack of sufficient information on the stage of disease treated in these reports using two-year survival information precludes further analysis of these data, but there is nothing to support the hypothesis that preoperative radiation therapy is beneficial.

## Three-Year Survival According to Primary Site and Stage of Disease

Table 10.4 includes a comparative summary of those reports (Biller, Davis, and Powers 1969; Bryce and Rider 1971; Goldman et al. 1972; Healy et al. 1976; Inoue, Shigematsu, and Sato 1973; Krause, Lee, and McCabe 1973; Lord et al. 1973; Snow et al. 1977; Strong et al. 1978; Terz, King, and Lawrence 1980; Wang 1971, 1972, 1974; Wang, Schulz, and Miller 1972) using

**Table 10.3**
Combined Analysis of All Reports Using Two-Year Survival Data, according to Dose of Preoperative Radiation

| Treatment Dose | All Cases (No./%) |
|---|---|
| (< 4000 rad) | 163/58 |
| (> 4000 rad) | 173/57 |

**Table 10.4**
Combined Analysis of All Reports Using Three-Year Survival Data, according to Primary Site and Stage

| Treatment | All Cases (No./%) | Primary Site: Oral Cavity (No./%) | Pharynx (No./%) | Larynx (No./%) |
|---|---|---|---|---|
| Stage I | | | | |
| Preoperative radiation | 31/80 | 17/64 | | 14/100 |
| Surgery only | 7/85 | 7/85 | | |
| Radiation only | 409/87 | 5/40 | | 404/88 |
| Stage II | | | | |
| Preoperative radiation | 176/62 | 61/54 | 9/44 | 106/68 |
| Surgery only | 80/56 | 53/56 | 10/60 | 17/52 |
| Radiation only | 83/73 | 18/27 | | 65/86 |
| Stage III | | | | |
| Preoperative radiation | 345/41 | 33/41 | 14/42 | 252/41 |
| Surgery only | 85/30 | 15/32 | 12/25 | 27/29 |
| Radiation only | 72/20 | 16/12 | | 56/23 |
| Stage IV | | | | |
| Preoperative radiation | 108/33 | 30/26 | 20/20 | |
| Surgery only | 35/20 | 18/22 | 17/23 | |
| Radiation only | 15/— | 14/— | | |

NOTE: No difference statistically significant between preoperative radiation and surgery-only groups.

three-year survival data and indicating both the primary site and stage. The combined group of patients with stage II and stage III cancers receiving preoperative radiation therapy did show a higher survival than those treated by either surgery or radiation alone, but this survival advantage did not prove to be statistically significant. When all reports using three-year survival data are examined (both those with and without staging), absolutely no advantage is seen with preoperative radiation over surgical resection alone by primary site or in toto (table 10.5).

Despite our inability to demonstrate value from preoperative radiation therapy in these reports using three-year survival data, survival was examined in terms of the dose of preoperative radiation administered to the patients included in these reports (table 10.6). Those patients with primary tumors arising in the oral cavity that received more than 4000 rad preoperatively did show a significantly higher survival ($P = 0.01$) when compared with those receiving less than 4000 rad. This could not be demonstrated in patient groups with pharyngeal or laryngeal lesions. When broken down by stage, those patients receiving the higher dose level had a significantly better survival than those receiving low-dose radiation for all stages other than

**Table 10.5**
Combined Analysis of All Reports Using Three-Year Survival Data, All Stages Combined

| Treatment | All Sites (No./%) | Primary Site: Oral Cavity (No./%) | Pharynx (No./%) | Larynx (No./%) |
|---|---|---|---|---|
| Preoperative radiation | 1090/44 | 247/47 | 238/30 | 605/49 |
| Surgery only | 477/45 | 248/46 | 119/35 | 87/51 |
| Radiation only | 1207/54* | 370/35† | 214/26 | 623/74‡ |

*"Radiation only" group superior to surgery (with or without radiation); $P = 0.0005$.
†"Radiation only" group inferior; $P = 0.001$ (all other differences not significant).
‡Includes a high proportion of stage I cancer (see table 10.4).

stage III (table 10.7). Nevertheless, preoperative radiation at either dose failed to yield overall survival data superior to those achieved by surgery alone, thereby making these data on radiation dose less compelling than they otherwise would be.

## Five-Year Survival According to Stage and Primary Site of Disease

Table 10.8 includes a comparison of those reports (Constable et al. 1972; Goffinet et al. 1973; Goodman and Kruskal 1959; Hirata et al. 1975; Inoue, Shigematsu, and Sato 1973; Krause, Lee, and McCabe 1973; Lees 1976; Marks et al. 1978; Perez, Marks, and Powers 1977; Razack et al. 1977; Roswit et al. 1972; Shah et al. 1974, 1976; Snow et al. 1977; Skolnik et al. 1975; Terz, King, and Lawrence 1980; Wang 1971, 1972, 1974) using five-year survival data and indicating both primary site and stage of patients treated. Patients with stage IV lesions who received preoperative radiation did show a signif-

**Table 10.6**
Combined Analysis of All Reports Using Three-Year Survival Data, according to Dose of Preoperative Radiation and Site of Primary Tumor

| Treatment | Primary Site: Oral Cavity (No./%) | Pharynx (No./%) | Larynx (No./%) |
|---|---|---|---|
| (<4000 rad) | 117/42* | 199/31 | 132/45 |
| (>4000 rad) | 70/60* | 39/23 | 473/50 |

*$P = 0.01$ (other differences not significant).

**Table 10.7**
Combined Analysis of All Reports Using Three-Year Survival Data, according to Dose of Preoperative Radiation and Stage of Disease

| | **Stage** | | | | |
|---|---|---|---|---|---|
| **Treatment** | **I (No./%)** | **II (No./%)** | **III (No./%)** | **IV (No./%)** | **All (No./%)** |
| (<4000 rad) | 17/64 | 90/52 | 115/40 | 50/35 | 508/38 |
| (>4000 rad) | 14/100 | 86/73 | 230/42 | 58/41 | 582/49 |
| $P=$ | 0.01 | 0.004 | NS | 0.05 | 0.005 |

icantly higher survival than those who had surgery only ($P=0.0005$), but no statistically significant difference could be demonstrated between these two groups when broken down by primary site and stage. When all reports using five-year survival data (table 10.9) are examined (both those with and without staging), the group undergoing surgery alone did better than those receiving preoperative radiation. The trend for surgery to be superior over combined therapy holds for the entire group as well as for specific regions such as oral or laryngeal lesions. On the other hand, the pharyngeal lesions in the preoperative radiation group appeared to do better than those undergoing either surgery or radiation alone. Another observation of interest was the higher survival following radiation alone for the group of patients with laryngeal lesions. Examination of table 10.8, however, demonstrates a disproportionate concentration of stage I lesions in this radiation-only group.

When dose levels were examined in the reports employing five-year survival statistics, there was a statistically significant superior result ($P=0.01$) with the higher dosage (> 4000 rad) than with a low dose (< 4000 rad), but there was no overall advantage demonstrated for preoperative radiation over surgery or radiation alone.

## Combined Assessment of Two- , Three- , and Five-Year Survival

It is clear that pooling data from these reports with data presented in varying detail and with patients being followed for differing periods failed to produce data suggesting a survival advantage from preoperative radiation therapy. A few selected comparisons, in terms of primary site or stage, showed a significant advantage for one group or the other, but these few individual differences favored "surgery only" as often as they did the preoperative radiation group. The failure to discover a convincing difference between the preoperative radiation groups and surgery-only groups in this combined analysis occurred despite the claim in many of the individual reports that preoperative radiation produced major survival benefits.

## Analysis of Randomized Trials

Of the three reports of randomized clinical trials included in this analysis, one contained limited data in terms of patient numbers and staging information, as well as having follow-up intervals of only two years (Hintz et al. 1979b). The other two randomized clinical trials, comparing surgery alone with preoperative radiation and surgical resection, had follow-up intervals of three years (Strong et al. 1978) and three to five years (Terz, King, and Lawrence 1981) after low-dose preoperative radiation therapy. These data are combined for analysis in table 10.10. There was no statistically significant advantage to preoperative radiation (over surgery alone) for any primary site, stage of disease, or primary site and stage combined. These results confirmed the conclusions of the authors of these individual reports when they were analyzed separately.

**Table 10.8**
Combined Analysis of All Reports Using Five-Year Survival Data, according to Primary Site and Stage

| | | Primary Site | | |
|---|---|---|---|---|
| Treatment | All Cases (No./%) | Oral Cavity (No./%) | Pharynx (No./%) | Larynx (No./%) |
| Stage I | | | | |
| Preoperative radiation | 6/83 | 6/83 | | |
| Surgery only | 382/83 | 73/82 | | 272/89 |
| Radiation only | 535/79 | 132/65 | | 403/84 |
| Stage II | | | | |
| Preoperative radiation | 59/60 | 34/76 | 9/11 | 16/56 |
| Surgery only | 296/63 | 20/70 | 110/38 | 116/78 |
| Radiation only | 185/58 | 119/50 | | 66/74 |
| Stage III | | | | |
| Preoperative radiation | 88/45 | 65/47 | 12/16 | 11/63 |
| Surgery only | 593/35 | 37/48 | 254/18 | 302/47 |
| Radiation only | 275/27 | 183/27 | | 92/26 |
| Stage IV | | | | |
| Preoperative radiation | 58/36* | 20/20 | 18/11 | |
| Surgery only | 74/6* | 4/25 | 64/6 | |
| Radiation only | 67/5 | 67/5 | | |

NOTE: All other differences regarding preoperative radiation not significant.
*$P = 0.0005$.

**Table 10.9**
Combined Analysis of All Reports Using Five-Year Survival Data, according to Primary Sites

| Treatment | All Cases (No./%) | Primary Site: Oral Cavity (No./%) | Pharynx (No./%) | Larynx (No./%) |
|---|---|---|---|---|
| Preoperative radiation | 737/40 | 217/43 | 280/30 | 240/47 |
| Surgery only | 1662/50 | 232/54 | 533/24 | 897/64 |
| Radiation only | 1576/47 | 879/35 | 136/19 | 561/73* |
| $P$ = (preoperative radiation vs surgery only) | 0.0005 | 0.025 | 0.05 | 0.0005 |

*Includes a high proportion of stage I cancer (see table 10.8).

### Comparison between Survival Data and Retrospective Studies and Randomized Trials

Since many reports of retrospective trials of preoperative radiation therapy claim benefit for this approach, while the authors of the two randomized trials analyzing data at three years do not, a comparison of survival data between these two categories of studies was carried out (table 10.11). Preoperative radiation groups have similar survival data in the retrospective and the randomized studies except for a slightly better survival experience with stage II lesions in the retrospective studies. Surgical results in the randomized trials were somewhat inferior to those reported in retrospective evaluations, but this was only significant in the analysis of the entire group. The data certainly show no selective bias favoring the surgery-only group in the randomized, and more meaningful, assessments of preoperative radiation therapy for head and neck cancer.

## Discussion

Although there are many problems associated with pooling data from different retrospective reports, it did seem possible that trends might be observed that would be meaningful. There were a few specific stages or primary sites that inconsistently showed significant survival differences, but there were no convincing trends favoring preoperative radiation over treatment by surgery alone. Actually, those few comparisons suggesting the possibility of an advantage from preoperative radiation proved spurious because of marked disproportions in the number of cases analyzed in each category. Other comparisons with larger groups showing no advantage from preoperative radiation confirmed the lack of improvement in results despite the frequent

**Table 10.10**
Three-Year Survival, Combination of Two Randomized Trials

| Primary Site | Stage II (No./%) | Stage III (No./%) | Stage IV (No./%) | Total (No./%) |
|---|---|---|---|---|
| Oral Cavity | | | | |
| Preoperative radiation | 39/56 | 37/40 | 13/38 | 89/47 |
| Surgery only | 35/51 | 40/30 | 16/16 | 91/34 |
| Pharynx | | | | |
| Preoperative radiation | 9/44 | 14/42 | 20/20 | 43/32 |
| Surgery only | 10/60 | 12/25 | 17/23 | 37/31 |
| Larynx | | | | |
| Preoperative radiation | 20/50 | 22/31 | | 42/40 |
| Surgery only | 17/52 | 27/29 | | 44/34 |
| All Sites | | | | |
| Preoperative radiation | 68/52 | 28/38 | 33/27 | 174/41 |
| Surgery only | 62/53 | 79/29 | 33/21 | 172/34 |

SOURCE: Strong et al. 1978; Terz, King, and Lawrence, 1981.
NOTE: No differences were statistically significant.

claim of some authors that it is beneficial. In fact, there were a number of comparisons in these data demonstrating a small statistically significant survival advantage for those patients treated by surgery alone. Viewed as a whole, the patient data from both retrospective and randomized trials fail to show significant benefits from preoperative radiation therapy when survival figures are examined in this admittedly crude fashion.

It is a well-established fact that the therapeutic effectiveness of radiation is directly related to the dose employed. Despite our inability to demonstrate an advantage from preoperative radiation, it was of interest that survival data appeared better for patient groups receiving more than 4000 rad preoperatively than for those treated with a lower dose. This was not a consistent finding, however. At three years, significant benefit was seen in the analysis of the overall group of patients at stage II and IV and patients with tumors arising in the oral cavity. In the five-year analysis, the only apparent benefit from the higher dose level was seen in the evaluation of the total group and in the group with carcinoma of the larynx. We must assume from this analysis that we have failed to establish that a higher dose of preoperative radiation will produce benefits, but the lack of prospective randomized trials employing a high dose of radiation leaves open the question regarding a possible therapeutic advantage from high-dose preoperative radiation.

Although all retrospective studies tend to report a higher survival than do randomized trials, this difference is only significant when the groups undergoing surgery alone are compared in the two types of studies, and it certainly does not invalidate the negative conclusions of the authors of the randomized trials of low-dose preoperative radiation whose studies were reviewed.

The lack of benefit from preoperative radiation shown in this analysis contrasts with the favorable conclusions of most of the authors of these same retrospective reports. If one assumed that the data in some of these retrospective studies actually did demonstrate benefit from preoperative radiation, the validity of such a finding would be in question for a host of reasons. These include:

1. Patient selection on the basis of physician bias in terms of optimal therapy for this group of diseases. This cannot be eliminated without randomization.
2. The frequent retrospective staging procedure in these studies is grossly inaccurate and very dependent on the accuracy of the medical report.
3. A single mode of therapy employed in a population of patients is frequently compared with so-called historic controls receiving another type of management and often treated at an earlier time than the study group, a time when the technology of the treatment method might not be so well developed.
4. Lack of uniformity of dosage of preoperative radiation and/or the subsequent surgical procedure for individual patients adds another variable which is difficult fully to assess.
5. Trends in the results are often reported without evidence of statistical significance of the observations.

It is clear that there are multiple problems in assessing retrospective studies or prospective studies that fail randomly to assign patients to treatment groups with a single or limited number of variables. Despite our feeling that all such studies usually fail to yield the information we need, this anal-

**Table 10.11**
Comparison of Data from Retrospective and Randomized Studies Using Three-Year Survival Data (All Sites)

| Treatment | Type of Study | Stage II (No./%) | Stage III (No./%) | Stage IV (No./%) | Stage Total (No./%) |
|---|---|---|---|---|---|
| Preoperative radiation | Retrospective | 108/68 | 272/40 | 25/36 | 916/45 |
| | Randomized trials | 68/52 | 28/38 | 33/27 | 174/41 |
| *P* = | | 0.03 | NS | NS | NS |
| Surgery only | Retrospective | 18/66 | 6/50 | 2/50 | 305/51 |
| | Randomized trials | 62/53 | 79/29 | 33/21 | 172/34 |
| *P* = | | NS | NS | NS | 0.0003 |

ysis was carried out to discover leads that might stimulate a more refined attempt to answer the important questions involved. Our analysis failed to demonstrate strong evidence in favor of preoperative radiation.

The randomized prospective clinical trials summarized in this report were designed to eliminate most of the objections described above. Analysis of these studies shows a good balance in each arm of the study in each instance from the standpoint of age, sex, stage of disease, and sites of primary tumor as well as subsequent analysis of the incidence of lymph node metastases and morbidity and mortality. The results of these studies when analyzed alone or in combination failed to demonstrate any higher survival for those patients receiving preoperative radiation when compared with control groups treated by surgical resection alone. Analysis by stage and primary site further substantiates the results obtained.

There were two discrepancies noted in the results obtained in the two randomized prospective clinical trials that were evaluated for three or more years. Analysis of the incidence of distant metastases in the two groups in the study reported by Strong and associates (1978) showed a lower incidence of such metastases in those patients receiving preoperative radiation than in those treated by surgery alone, while this was not observed in our own randomized trial (Terz, King, and Lawrence 1981). In our study, there was a lower incidence of local recurrence following preoperative radiation, despite the lack of any survival benefits, but this finding was not observed in the other randomized trials.

The randomized trials summarized here might appear finally to have answered the question regarding the role of preoperative radiation in the management of head and neck cancer in a negative sense, but an objection to this conclusion might well be the fact that using a low dose (less than 4000 rad) might not be as effective in this setting as a higher dose schedule given over a longer period of time. This may be a valid point, and it is a legitimate basis for additional trials of preoperative radiation therapy using radiation in this dose range. It is clear that it is essential that such an assessment be carried out using prospective randomized trials.

## Conclusions

The careful statistical review of current data on the role of preoperative radiation therapy in the management of head and neck cancer fails to establish the often-described benefits of this approach. These negative conclusions regarding low-dose preoperative radiation are already demonstrated by the randomized trials reviewed here. Observations suggest, however, that adjuvant radiation therapy might play a role in the management of head and neck cancer, particularly with selected high-risk populations (such as the presence of lymph node metastases). A randomized clinical trial using a higher radiation dose with a fractioned schedule (5000 to 6000 rad in five to six weeks), either preoperatively or postoperatively, may well provide an answer to this incompletely resolved controversy in the management of head and neck cancer.

The higher incidence of postoperative complications associated with a full course of radiation may well preclude the feasibility of a preoperative radiation approach. A reasonable alternative would be a similar clinical trial using postoperative radiation. Such a study would offer the advantage that the high-risk group most likely to benefit from such an approach would be clearly identified from the pathologic analysis of the cervical lymph nodes in the operative specimen. Randomized assignment of these patients to a postoperative course versus no radiation would yield data of great interest and potential importance.

## References

Biller, H. F.; Davis, W. H.; and Powers, W. E. Planned preoperative irradiation for carcinoma of the larynx and laryngopharynx treated by total and partial laryngectomy. *Laryngoscope* 79:1387–1395, 1969.

Brown, M. B., and Benetti, J. K. Asymptotic standard errors and their sampling behavior for measures of associations and correlation in a two-way contingency table. Technical report #23, Health Science Computer Facility, University of California, Los Angeles, 1976.

Bryce, D. P., and Rider, W. D. Preoperative irradiation in the treatment of advanced laryngeal carcinoma. *Laryngoscope* 81: 1481–1490, 1971.

Constable, W. C. et al. High dose preoperative radiotherapy and surgery for cancer of the larynx. *Laryngoscope* 82:1861–1868, 1972.

Daly, C. J., and Strong, E. W. Carcinoma of the glottic larynx. *Am. J. Surg.* 130:489–492, 1975.

Fayos, J. V., and Lampe, I. Radiation therapy of carcinoma of the tonsillar region. *Am. J. Roentgenol.* 3:85–94, 1971.

Flynn, M. B.; Mullins, F. X.; and Moore, C. Selection of treatment in squamous carcinoma of the floor of the mouth. *Am. J. Surg.* 126:477–481, 1973.

Fu, K. K. et al. Results of integrated management of supraglottic carcinoma. *Cancer* 40:2874–2881, 1977.

Goffinet, D. R. et al. Carcinoma of the larynx. *Am. J. Roentgenol.* 117:553–564, 1973.

Goldman, J. L. et al. High dosage preoperative radiation and surgery for carcinoma of the larynx and laryngopharynx—a 14-year program. *Laryngoscope* 82:1869–1881, 1972.

Goodman, L. A., and Kruskal, W. H. Measures of association for cross-classification I. *J. Am. Stat. Assoc.* 49:732–764, 1954.

Goodman, L. A., and Kruskal, W. H. Measures of association for cross-classification II. *J. Am. Stat. Assoc.* 54:123–163, 1959.

Goodman, L. A., and Kruskal, W. H. Measures of association for cross-classification III. *J. Am. Stat. Assoc.* 58:310–364, 1963.

Goodman, L. A., and Kruskal, W. H. Measures of association for cross-classification IV. *J. Am. Stat. Assoc.* 62:415–421, 1967.

Healy, G. B. et al. Carcinoma of the palatine arch. *Am. J. Surg.* 132:498–503, 1976.

Hendrickson, F. R., and Liebner, E. Results of preoperative radiotherapy for supraglottic larynx cancer. *Ann. Otol. Rhinol. Laryngol.* 77:222–229, 1968.

Hintz, B. et al. Randomized study of local control and survival following radical surgery or radiation therapy in oral and laryngeal carcinoma. *J. Surg. Oncol.* 12:61–74, 1979a.

Hintz, B. et al. Randomized study of control of the primary tumor and survival using preoperative radiation, radiation alone, or surgery alone in head and neck carcinomas. *J. Surg. Oncol.* 12:75–85, 1979b.

Hirata, R. M. et al. Carcinoma of the oral cavity. *Am. J. Surg.* 182:98–103, 1975.

Inoue, T.; Shigematsu, Y.; and Sato, T. L. Treatment of carcinoma of the hypopharynx. *Cancer* 31:649–655, 1973.

Kazem, I. et al. Preoperative short intensive radiation therapy of $T_3$-$T_4$ laryngeal carcinoma. *Acta Radiol.* 14:524–528, 1974.

Krause, C. J.; Lee, J. G.; and McCabe, F. F. Carcinoma of the oral cavity. *Arch. Otolaryngol.* 97:354–358, 1973.

Lees, A. W. The treatment of carcinoma of the anterior two-thirds of the tongue by radiotherapy. *Int. J. Radiat. Oncol. Biol. Phys.* 1:849–858, 1976.

Levitt, S. H. et al. Combination of preoperative irradiation and surgery in the treatment of cancer of the oropharynx, hypopharynx, and larynx. *Cancer* 27:759–767, 1971.

Lord, I. J. et al. A comparison of preoperative and primary radiotherapy in the treatment of carcinoma of the hypopharynx. *Br. J. Radiol.* 46:175–197, 1973.

Marks, J. E. et al. Carcinoma of the pyriform sinus. *Cancer* 41:1008–1015, 1978.

Perez, C. A.; Marks, J.; and Powers, W. E. Preoperative irradiation in head and neck cancer. *Oncology* 4:387–397, 1977.

Razack, M. S. et al. Carcinoma of the hypopharynx: success and failure. *Am. J. Surg.* 134:489–491, 1977.

Roswit, B. et al. Planned preoperative irradiation and surgery for advanced cancer of the oral cavity, pharynx, and larynx. *Am. J. Roentgenol.* 114:59–62, 1972.

Shah, J. P. et al. Carcinoma of the hypopharynx. *Am. J. Surg.* 132:439–443, 1976.

Shah, J. P., and Tollefsen, H. R. Epidermoid carcinoma of the supraglottic larynx. *Am. J. Surg.* 128:494–499, 1974.

Skolnik, E. M. et al. Combined therapy in the management of laryngeal carcinoma. *Cancer J. Otolaryngol.* 4:236–245, 1975.

Snow, G. B. et al. Squamous carcinoma of the oropharynx. *Clin. Otolaryngol.* 2:93–103, 1977.

Strong, M. S. et al. A randomized trial of preoperative radiotherapy in cancer of the oropharynx and hypopharynx. *Am. J. Surg.* 136:494–500, 1978.

Terz, J. J.; King, E. R.; and Lawrence, W. Preoperative irradiation for head and neck cancer: results of a prospective study. *Surgery,* 4:449, 1981.

Wang, C. C. Radiotherapeutic management of carcinoma of the posterior pharyngeal wall. *Cancer* 27:894–896, 1971.

Wang, C. C. Management and prognosis of squamous cell carcinoma of the tonsillar region. *Radiology* 104:667–671, 1972.

Wang, C. C. Treatment of glottic carcinoma by megavoltage radiation therapy and results. *Am. J. Roentgenol.* 120:157–163, 1974.

Wang, C. C.; Schulz, M. D.; and Miller, D. Combined radiation therapy and surgery for carcinoma of the supraglottis and pyriform sinus. *Am. J. Surg.* 124:551–554, 1972.

# Chapter 11

# *The Value of Lymphadenectomy in Melanomas of the Head and Neck*

F. Kristian Storm and
Frederick R. Eilber

Cutaneous malignant melanoma is occurring more frequently, with an incidence now equal to that of primary brain tumors and Hodgkin's disease. Primary melanoma of the head and neck accounts for 20% to 35% of all newly diagnosed melanomas, and while significant advancements in primary tumor microstaging have helped clarify the natural history of this disease in general, little data are available to aid the clinician in the treatment of melanoma arising in the head and neck.

When compared to that of other parts of the body, the skin of the head and neck is unusual in several respects. It is constantly exposed to the sun and other elements, and is unique in the character of its epidermis and dermis, as well as its proximity to regional lymph nodes. Thus several questions arise when treating diseases of this area. Is the natural history of melanoma of the head and neck similar to that of melanoma arising in other sites? Is similar therapy applicable? Is clinical staging reliable? What is the incidence of lymph node metastases based upon primary tumor microstage? Are certain sites of head and neck melanoma more apt to have lymph node metastases, and do these locations bear upon survival? Which parameter, primary tumor microstage, or status of regional lymph nodes is of greater predictive value in determining prognosis? Finally, what is the role of regional lymphadenectomy in melanoma of the head and neck?

## Clinical Trials

In an effort to answer these fundamental questions, 92 patients with primary cutaneous melanoma arising in the head and neck were prospectively evalu-

This investigation was supported by U.S. Public Health Service grant CA-12582 from the National Institutes of Health and contract CB-64076 awarded by the National Cancer Institute, Department of Health, Education, and Welfare, and Surgical Services of the Sepulveda Veterans Administration Hospital.

ated from 1973 to 1979. Follow-up ranged from one month to six years. Ages ranged from 12 to 80 years, with a median age of 51 years. There were 60 males and 32 females (ratio of 2:1). Primary lesions were located in the eyelid, nose, and lip (4 patients), forehead or temple (10 patients), ear (16 patients), cheek (17 patients), scalp (18 patients), and neck (27 patients).

Sixty-one patients had no evidence of disease spread beyond the primary and were classified as clinical stage I, and 25 who had palpable parotid or cervical adenopathy were classified as clinical stage II. Primary tumor microstaging for level of invasion (Clark, From, and Bernardino 1969) and more recently for depth of invasion (Breslow 1970) was obtained on all but 10 lesions. Of the clinical stage I patients, 9 were at level II or III, with less than 0.65 mm depth of invasion; 16 were at level III, with invasion greater than or equal to 0.65 mm; 19 were at level IV; 9 were at level V; and 6 were at an indeterminate level because of an earlier shave biopsy and cauterization of the base of the lesion before referral to UCLA. Of the 25 patients with palpable regional lymph node disease, 4 were at level II or thin level III; 4 were at deep level III; 14, level IV; 7, level V; and 4 were at an indeterminate level.

In this prospective study, all patients underwent a radical wide excision of their primary lesion with at least 2.5 cm margins, and 5 cm where anatomically feasible (namely, scalp and neck). Using this technique, 3 out of 92 (3%) patients had localized disease recurrence at the primary tumor site at the 11-month median. Those with level III lesions greater than or equal to 0.65 mm depth of invasion, and all those with level IV, V, and level indeterminate also underwent a radical neck dissection, whether or not the lymph nodes were clinically suspicious (83 patients). Patients with primary tumors of the eyelid, cheek, forehead, temple, and anterior ear also underwent resection of the superficial parotid lymph nodes, as this has been shown to be the first-echelon drainage site of tumors of this location (Storm et al. 1977). Nine patients who had level II or thin level III melanoma underwent lymphadenectomy only when adenopathy became manifest.

This prospective trial showed that the clinical stage of the patient's disease at initial presentation was related to prognosis. Of the 58 patients followed from 1 to 78 months (18-month median) who initially had disease clinically confined to the site of the primary, 9 (16%) died at 3 to 59 months (20-month median). Of 25 patients with obvious regional lymph node metastases followed from 2 to 114 months (30-month median), 13 (52%) died at 7 to 51 months (24-month median).

After clinical staging, 83 patients with deeply invasive melanoma underwent histopathologic staging of their regional lymph nodes. Of 58 patients at clinical stage I, 8 (14%) had occult microscopic lymph node metastases. All 25 patients at clinical stage II had pathologically proved regional disease. The prognosis based upon surgical staging showed a projected five-year survival of 75% for patients with histopathologically uninvolved nodes, and only 25% for those with regional node metastases (fig. 11.1).

**Figure 11.1**

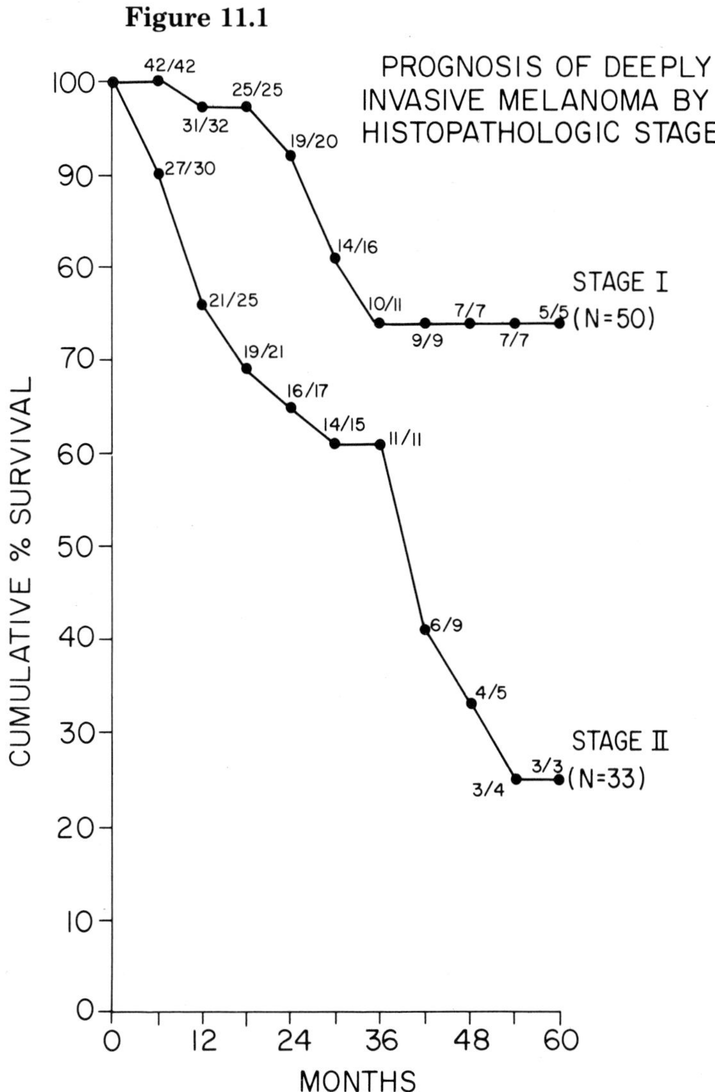


*Influence of histologic stage on survival.*

**Figure 11.2**

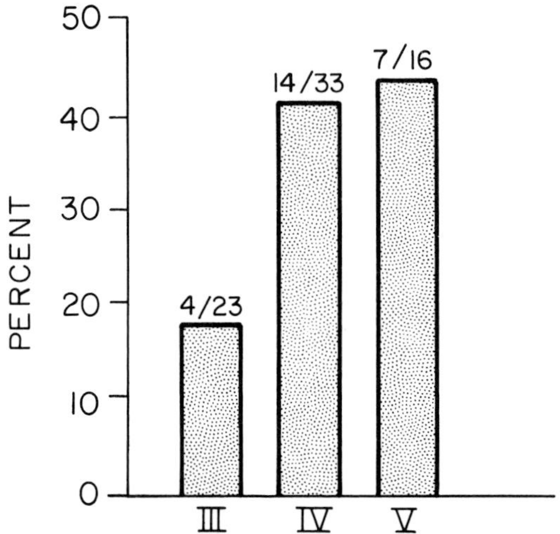


*Incidence of lymph node metastases and micróstage.*

Histopathologic evaluation of the primary tumor microstage for level and depth of invasion also correlated with the incidence of regional lymph node metastases and survival. Patients with level III melanoma greater than or equal to 0.65 mm depth of invasion had 17% incidence of regional metastases; level IV, 42%; and level V, 44% (fig. 11.2). The projected five-year survival by microstage was 91% for melanoma of level II and III less than 0.65 mm invasion, 62% for level III greater than or equal to 0.65 mm, 32% for level IV, and 36% for level V (fig. 11.3).

The prognostic significance for clinically palpable regional lymph node metastases was compared to that for clinically occult but histopathologically positive nodes. In each group, the number of lymph node metastases was approximately equivalent, and recurrence rates were similar during the same interval of follow-up. Projected five-year survival suggests that clinically palpable regional disease may have a worse prognosis than micrometastases (fig. 11.4).

To determine which of the two variables was of greater value for predicting outcome—the microstage of the primary tumor or pathologic involve-

**Figure 11.3**

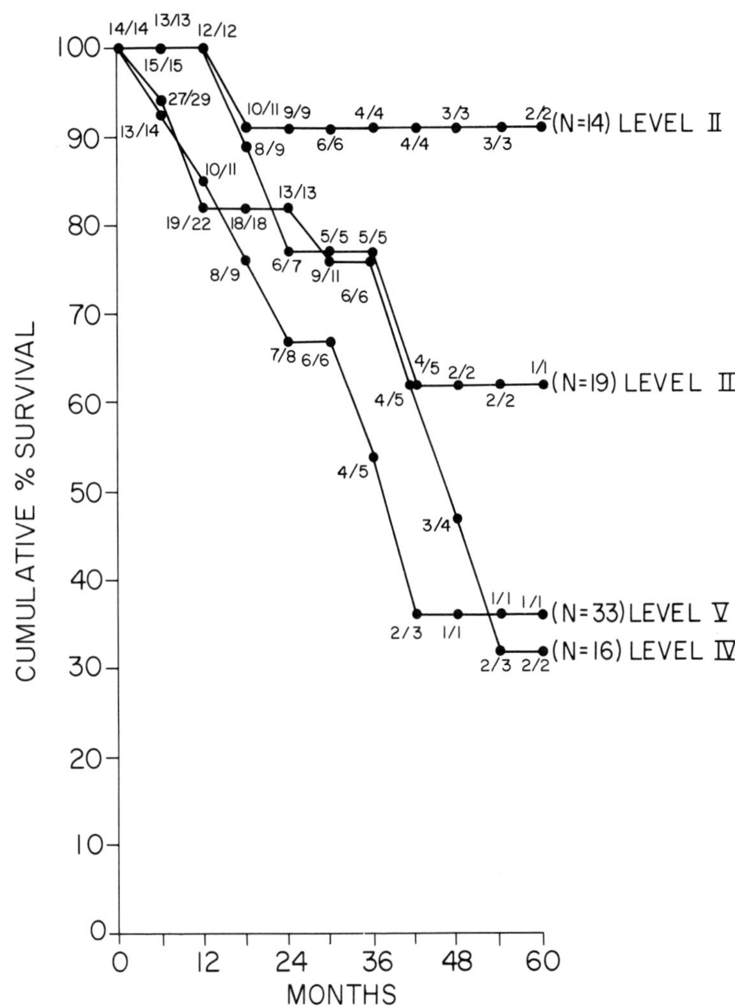


*Influence of microstage on survival.*

ment of the regional lymph nodes—the level of primary tumor invasion, with and without regional lymph node metastases, was compared to survival during the same period of follow-up (fig. 11.5). Patients with level III and IV melanoma had survival greater than or equal to 95% if lymph nodes were

**Figure 11.4**

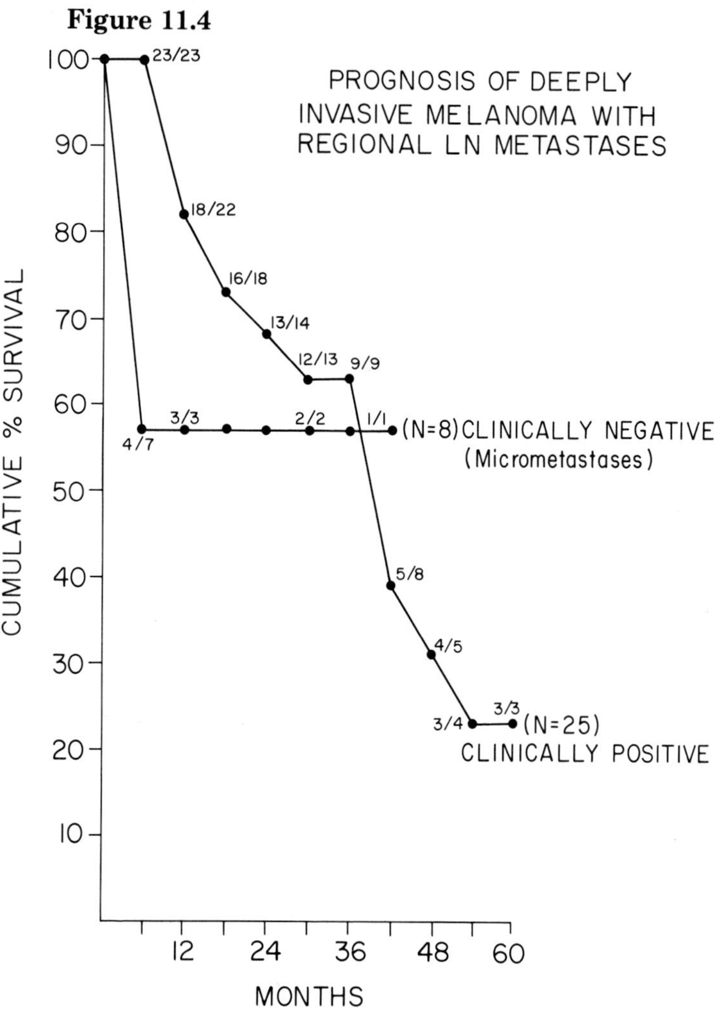


*Influence of occult and gross lymph node metastases on survival.*

histologically negative, while patients at level V had only 66% survival. In the presence of lymph node metastases, prognosis was poor regardless of level. These data suggest that the presence of regional metastases is the most significant indicator of prognosis.

The anatomic location of the primary tumor was compared to the incidence of regional lymph node metastases and prognosis (fig. 11.6). The data suggest that lesions arising in the scalp have the highest incidence of regional disease and the poorest prognosis.

**Figure 11.5**

% SURVIVAL BY PRIMARY TUMOR MICROSTAGE IN THE PRESENCE OR ABSENCE OF REGIONAL LN METASTASES

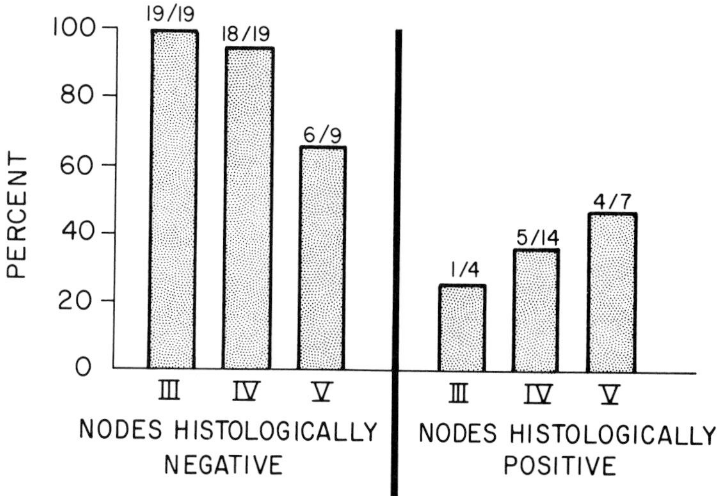


*Influence of histologically negative and positive nodes on survival.*

# Conclusions

## Incidence and Etiology

The results of our prospective clinical trial suggest that cutaneous melanoma arising in the head and neck region is not significantly different from melanoma arising in other anatomic sites. Primary tumor microstaging that was possible in 82 patients revealed the incidence of superficially and deeply invasive melanoma to be similar to the incidence of melanomas in other locations. Interestingly, 69 out of 82 (85%) of these tumors were classified as deep level III, level IV, or level V at the time of initial presentation. Thus any benefits based upon earlier detection of head and neck melanoma are doubtful.

In this study of head and neck melanoma patients, males were predominant by a factor of 2:1. This is contrary to what is found in melanoma series in general, where prevalence favors women, because of an increasing incidence of melanoma of the lower extremity attributed to increased sun exposure and contemporary clothing fashions. If this logic is valid, it may be that the incidence of head and neck melanoma is higher in men because of increased occupation-related sun exposure.

**Figure 11.6**

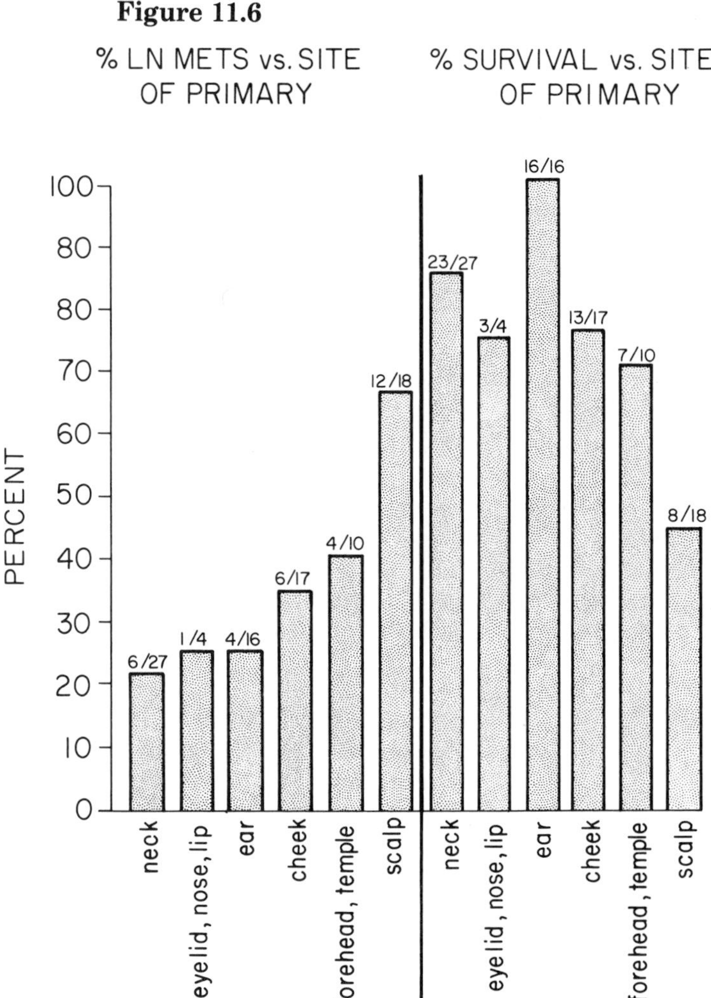


*Influence of incidence of positive lymph node metastases and survival with primary site.*

## Treatment of the Primary Tumor

Radical wide excision of the primary tumor is generally advocated for melanomas of the trunk and extremities, but it is our impression that some surgeons tend to reduce surgical margins for head and neck melanomas, probably for cosmetic considerations. In our clinical trial, strict adherence to at least 2.5 cm margins, and 5 cm margins where anatomically feasible (namely, neck and scalp), resulted in only 3% locally recurrent disease at the site of original resection during the interval of follow-up. In our previous review of 15 patients with locally recurrent disease referred for treatment after initial therapy elsewhere, all had had wide excisions with less than 2.5 cm margins and had disease recurrence at an eight-month median (Storm et al. 1978). These data suggest that radical wide excision of the primary, as practiced in other parts of the body, is also applicable to melanomas of the head and neck region and should result in a lowered incidence of locally recurrent disease.

Lesions of the ear present a vexing problem. In our experience, these tumors may be treated by a wide V excision, rather than auriculectomy (Storm et al. 1978). This technique provides a better functional and cosmetic result and does not appear to compromise local disease control.

## Clinical and Histopathologic Disease Staging

Clinical stage was related to prognosis. At a similar interval of follow-up, 84% of patients with disease clinically confined to the site of the primary at the time of initial presentation were alive, while only 48% of those with evident regional lymph node metastases survived. Moreover, patients with clinical stage II disease seemed to die somewhat earlier (24 months) than those with clinical stage I disease (30 months).

Histopathologic disease staging of all patients with deeply invasive melanoma revealed a 14% incidence of occult micrometastases in those patients with clinically uninvolved regional lymph nodes. Thus clinical staging for the presence of lymph node metastases may be in error in nearly one-sixth of patients with head and neck melanoma.

A study of five-year survival based upon histopathologic disease stage revealed a 75% survival for patients with uninvolved lymph nodes, and 25% for those with regional node metastases (fig. 11.1). These statistics are somewhat worse than those for melanoma arising in other parts of the body, particularly for stage I disease, and suggest that head and neck melanoma may carry a graver prognosis.

## Primary Tumor Microstaging

Histopathologic evaluation of the primary tumor for level and, more recently, depth of invasion was related to the status of the regional lymph nodes and survival. Patients with deeply invasive melanoma had a 17% to 44% incidence of regional disease (fig. 11.2). A study of five-year survival by microstage revealed 91% of patients with level II melanoma alive, 62% of those with level III, 32% of those with level IV, and 36% of those with level V (fig. 11.3). These data indicate that increasing depth of primary tumor invasion bears heavily on the overall prognosis for head and neck melanoma, as is true with melanoma of other sites.

## Prognostic Predictors

It is clear that both the pathologic involvement of the regional lymph nodes and the primary tumor microstage influence survival. To determine which of these two variables was of greater value for predicting outcome, however, the level of primary tumor invasion—with and without regional lymph node metastases—was compared to survival over the period of follow-up (fig. 11.5). The absence of regional disease was better for prognosis overall than with nodal spread, which appeared to be independent of level. These data indicate that the status of the regional lymph nodes is the most significant indicator of prognosis. It is not known why patients with level V melanoma apparently confined to the site of the primary fare worse, but these patients may have earlier blood-borne spread of disease.

## Anatomic Location

Primary tumor sites were nearly equally distributed throughout the head and neck region, although lip lesions were distinctly uncommon. To determine if a particular site of primary tumor influenced outcome, each location was compared to the incidence of regional metastases and survival (fig. 11.6). The data suggest that lesions arising in the scalp had the highest incidence of regional disease spread and the gravest prognosis.

## Role of Regional Lymphadenectomy

Regional lymphadenectomy is clearly indicated for the treatment of clinically evident lymph node metastases and also for accurate disease staging.

Of 25 patients at clinical stage II in our study, all had histologically confirmed lymph node metastases. This suggests that patients with clinically suspicious regional nodes should undergo resection rather than biopsy, which has the attendant risk of field contamination. While the overall prognosis for patients with palpable disease spread is poor, adequate resectional therapy (standard Martin neck dissection) may achieve a 25% five-year survival (fig. 11.1). This is far superior to the results for chemotherapy or radiation therapy (Storm and Morton 1979).

To determine the accuracy of clinical disease staging, 58 patients at clinical stage I with deeply invasive melanoma underwent elective regional lymphadenectomy. In nine patients with level II and thin level III (< 0.65 mm) the staging lymphadenectomy was not performed because of the extremely low incidence of regional disease spread in these superficial lesions. Staging lymphadenectomy consisted of a modified neck dissection (with preservation of jugular vein, eleventh nerve, and sternocleidomastoid muscle) and, while providing complete lymph node removal, also resulted in satisfactory cosmesis (Eilber and Storm 1981). Patients with primary tumors of the forehead, temple, eyelid, cheek, and anterior ear also underwent superficial parotidectomy, a procedure confirmed by earlier studies which showed that the superficial parotid nodes are first-echelon drainage sites of lesions arising in these areas (Storm et al. 1977). Elective regional lymphadenectomy has not been shown to increase the risk of late in-transit metastases in extremity melanomas (Storm, Sparks, and Morton 1979), and, on review, did not increase local recurrences in this trial.

Histopathologic lymph node staging revealed a 14% incidence of occult micrometastases in patients at clinical stage I. Thus clinical staging is falsely negative in nearly one-sixth of patients with deeply invasive melanoma at initial presentation. As was mentioned earlier, regional lymph node status—rather than primary tumor microstage—is the most significant predictor of outcome and may be an independent variable bearing on prognosis. Histopathologic staging definitely revealed a poorer prognosis for patients with melanoma of the head and neck (fig. 11.1) than that generally reported for melanoma arising in other sites of the body, and which had not been adequately defined in earlier trials using clinical staging alone.

Histopathologic lymph node staging is certainly mandatory in judging the adequacy of comparative adjuvant treatment trials. Elective lymphadenectomy in the absence of palpable disease will reveal a significant number of patients with occult micrometastases who remain at high risk for recurrence (Holmes, Moseley, and Morton 1977). In our prospective evaluation of patients with melanoma of the head and neck, histopathologic staging of clinically uninvolved lymph nodes revealed a 14% incidence of occult regional disease spread. In adjuvant trials where the presence of residual metastases may have significant bearing on results, clinical staging is totally inadequate (Eilber, Townsend, and Morton 1976). This finding appears to be as true for melanoma arising in the head and neck as for melanoma arising in other parts of the body.

Elective regional lymphadenectomy also has a therapeutic role in selected patients with head and neck melanoma. In the absence of prospective randomized trials to evaluate scientifically the efficacy of elective lymph node dissection in melanoma arising in the head and neck region, philosophical bias must intervene in the interpretation of available data. The extremely low yield of lymph node metastases and excellent prognosis of patients with level II and thin level III lesions suggests lymphadenectomy is not warranted unless nodes become clinically suspicious. In our prospective clinical trial all patients with lesions at deep level III, IV, V, and indeterminate level underwent lymphadenectomy, whether or not the nodes were clinically positive. When one compares prognoses, the survival trend suggests that patients with micrometastases fared significantly better than those with palpable disease at three years (fig. 11.4), as has been seen with melanoma arising in other parts of the body (Das Gupta 1977). A longer follow-up will be necessary to determine if, in fact, the patients who had surgical resection of clinically unsuspected microscopic regional lymph node metastases will have a longer ultimate survival than those with palpable regional metastases. Whether or not these patients with micrometastases would have fared as well without lymphadenectomy will remain unknown; however, resection was associated with an encouraging prognosis. Since the morbidity and cosmetic impairment from elective regional lymph node resection (particularly modified neck dissection) are extremely low when the patient is in skilled hands, and since the prognosis for patients who develop manifest regional disease is so low, it appears to be a worthwhile procedure.

## References

Breslow, A. Thickness, cross-sectional areas, and depth of invasion in the prognosis of cutaneous melanoma. *Ann. Surg.* 172:902–908, 1970.

Clark, W. H.; From, L.; and Bernardino, E. A. The histogenesis and biologic behavior of primary human malignant melanomas of the skin. *Cancer Res.* 29:705–726, 1969.

Das Gupta, T. K. Results of treatment of 269 patients with primary cutaneous melanoma: a five year prospective study. *Ann. Surg.* 186:201–209, 1977.

Eilber, F. R., and Storm, F. K. Surgical procedures for diseases of the neck. In *Reconstruction of the head and neck,* ed. M. A. Lesavoy. Baltimore: Williams and Wilkins, 1981.

Eilber, F. R.; Townsend, C. M.; and Morton, D. L. Results of BCG adjuvant immunotherapy for melanoma of the head and neck. *Am. J. Surg.* 132:476–479, 1976.

Holmes, E. C., Moseley, H. S.; and Morton, D. L. A rational approach to the surgical management of melanoma. *Ann. Surg.* 186:481–490, 1977.

Storm, F. K. et al. A prospective study of parotid metastases from head and neck cancer. *Am. J. Surg.* 134:115–119, 1977.

Storm, F. K. et al. Malignant melanoma of the head and neck. *Head Neck Surg.* 1:123–128, 1978.

Storm, F. K., and Morton, D. L. Treatment of metastatic disease. In *Advances in surgery,* vol. 13, eds. G. L. Jordan et al. Chicago: Year Book Medical Publishers, 1979.

Storm, F. K.; Sparks, F. C.; and Morton, D. L. Treatment for melanoma of the lower extremity with intralesional BCG and hyperthermic perfusion. *Surg. Gynecol. Obstet.* 149:17–21, 1979.

# Chapter 12

# *Treatment of Melanoma*

Samuel L. Perzik

## Definition

The term melanoma implies a malignant lesion. The use of the adjective malignant, as in malignant melanoma, is superfluous. The benign counterpart is a pigmented nevus. To modify the latter by adding the term benign is redundant. Due to the confused use of these terms, most pathologists and clinicians use the names malignant melanoma and benign nevus in order to avoid any misinterpretation which might result in grave therapeutic misadventures.

## Location

Melanoma originates in a single primary site, most frequently in a preexisting pigmented nevus or de novo. Premonitory manifestations of impending or already developed malignancy may be suggested when a pigmented nevus begins to itch, becomes painful, hyperpigmented, or depigmented, or enlarges by superficial spreading or topographical nodulation. The malignant evolution may occur without clinical evidence of alteration, in which case the time of transition from the benign to the malignant state is indeterminable. Surface melanomas may occur on the skin or mucosal surfaces, in the latter from the hyoid-hypopharyngeal level outward to the mucocutaneous junction. Exceptions, as reported in other primary sites, should be looked upon with suspicion (Pack, Perzik, and Scharnagel 1946; Perzik and Baum 1969; Perzik 1979; Moore and Martin 1955; Catlin 1967; Robinson and Hukill 1970; Principato, Sika, and Sandler 1965; Walker and Snow 1969).

Melanomas that are subsurface or in viscerae are to be considered as metastatic lesions. Those that appear as presumed primary lesions in other mucosal surfaces, as in the gut or bronchial tree, will often reveal a submucosal origin without junctional changes but with secondary ulceration into the lumen by direct invasion indicating their metastatic status.

The choroid melanoma must be considered separately and is not included in this discussion.

## Pathology

The pathogenesis, on microscopic study, reveals that the primary lesion progresses from its junctional location by direct cellular infiltration, centrifugally, up through the epidermis and down into the dermis and beyond (Fitzpatrick, Brown, and Reid 1972; Fisher 1977; Handley 1907). The cells invade the subepidermal (papillary) and deeper dermal lymphatics down to and including the lymphatic plexuses of the deep fascia. Within the lymphatic channels the tumor cells grow by progressive local permeation, blocking the tributary orifices, thereby facilitating retrograde tumor growth, resulting in the production of local subepithelial satellitosis. Concomitantly tumor emboli flowing freely through the lymphatic channels may be trapped and grow in the first group of regional lymph nodes draining the area. The extent of these developments depends upon the biologic potential of a specific primary lesion and is not necessarily directly proportional to the temporal duration or size of the primary lesion (figs. 12.1 and 12.2).

Distant metastases result from invasion of contiguous capillary vessels paralleling the papillary lymphatics in the primary lesion. There is no evidence that such vascular invasion normally originates by way of lymphatic-capillary crossover in the involved lymph nodes. The exception would be a rupture of a well-developed metastatic lesion into an adherent vascular channel through direct tumor invasion of its wall. The latter seldom occurs and can readily be anticipated in the presence of such an advanced clinical picture. Metastases in melanoma are the result of two simultaneous or asynchronous mechanisms, both originating in the primary site. After total removal of the primary lesion, the subsequent clinical appearance of any metastases, whether immediate or delayed, arises from occult sites that were seeded before the primary lesion was completely excised.

When melanoma proves fatal, it is the result of involvement of a distal vital organ such as the brain, liver, lungs, adrenals, kidneys, heart, or spinal cord. The latter presumes a vascular spread which could only have originated in the primary site before it was totally excised. Death does not occur as a result of progressive disease still confined to the primary site or regional lymph nodes, except in the rare cases of far-advanced, nonresponding, ulcerated, bleeding, infected local and regional tumor masses.

**Figure 12.1**

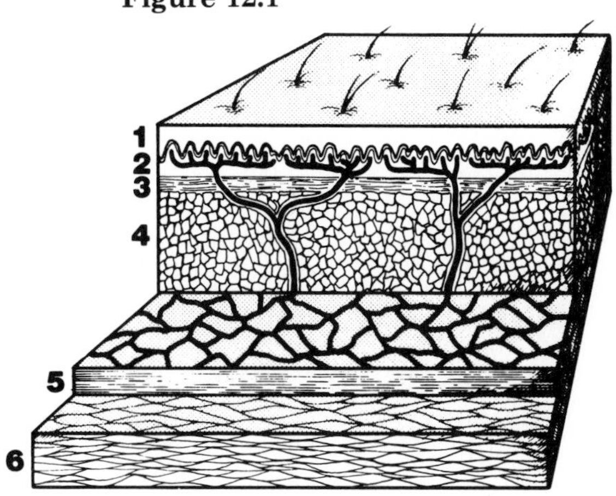


(1) *Epidermis.* (2) *Junctional interphase with papillary dermis and lymphatic and vascular channels arising in the papillae (subepidermal lymphatics). Site of origin of permeating lymphatic and embolic vascular metastases.* (3) *Reticular (deep) dermis with oblique collecting lymphatic channels; source of blockage of lymphatic channels resulting in retrograde growth and satellitosis.* (4) *Subcutaneous fat with major vertical dermal lymphatics.* (5) *Deep fascial surface complex of network of lymphatic channels draining toward regional lymph nodes.* (6) *Muscle.*

# Treatment

With the rare exception as noted, surgical cure in melanoma can only be attained by complete removal of the primary lesion before it has metastasized. Any additional treatment, whether elective or therapeutic, is palliative, which by definition should only be instituted when indicated by an existing or obviously anticipated disability. The discussion of treatment is based upon the preceding premise.

## Biopsy

Depending on circumstances of location and size, a biopsy may be either incisional or excisional. In the past there has been an aversion to cut into a pigmented lesion on the presumption that this might result in spreading of the melanoma, if present (Pitt 1977). This presumption is based upon the misinterpreted observation that after an incisional biopsy on an apparently

**Figure 12.2**

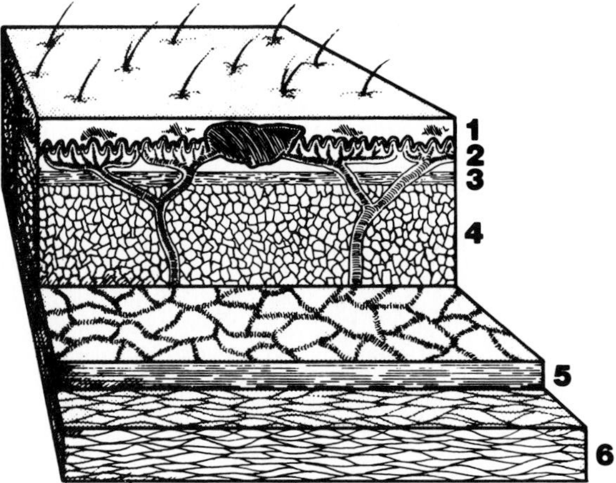


*Melanoma developing at junctional interphase* (2) *permeates the subepidermal lymphatics in the superficial (papillary) layer of the dermis* (2). *By retrograde (permeation) extension the overlying intraepithelial layer is involved (satellitosis)* (1). *Progressive permeation of the second and third echelons of collecting lymphatics extends the disease into the reticular (deep) dermis* (3), *resulting in additional centrifugal retrograde satellitosis. Continued deep extension through the subcutaneous fat* (4) *connects with the deep fascial lymphatics* (5), *which drain toward the regional lymph nodes (by permeation or tumor emboli or both).*

quiescent pigmented lesion, satellitosis or regional or distant metastases frequently appear within several weeks or months, whereupon it is assumed that this must have been caused by the procedure (Perzik 1979; Ballantyne 1970). What most likely occurred was that a very subtle pathologic change, developing in the primary lesion in the months preceding biopsy, escaped the casual or inexperienced examination by the patient, or the patient may have consciously rejected the likelihood that such a threatening alteration was possibly occurring. The clinical manifestation may only have been a slight sensation of local itching, or a nonrecognizable increase in size or alteration in topography or coloration of the lesion. The presence of such subtle clinical signals may have crystallized a hesitant recognition of the existence of the lesion. Nonchalantly the lesion would be called to the attention of the attending physician without any extenuating associations. These subtle changes were simply the prodromal manifestations of the more obvious signs and symptoms soon destined to appear as a result of the increasing local infiltrative and metastasizing activity now taking place. A biopsy performed at this time would relatedly be followed in a few weeks or months by these clinical manifestations, all of which were destined to appear whether a biopsy was or was not performed. To the unsophisticated observer, the sequence of events following the biopsy suggests that the subsequent manifestations of local growth and metastatic spread were the result of the surgical invasion of a presumably quiescent primary malignant lesion of long standing.

There is no documented, unequivocal clinical evidence that an incisional biopsy of a melanoma is an etiologic factor in its local or distant spread.

If a pigmented lesion is of small size in a favorable location, it can be managed by an excisional biopsy, which, in many instances, will be definitive treatment whether it is a benign nevus or a malignant melanoma.

## Primary

Initial management of melanoma is accomplished by total removal of the primary lesion, with not over 1 cm of apparently uninvolved tissue in all directions (Perzik and Baum 1969; Perzik 1979; Catlin 1966; Hansen and McCarten 1974). The extent of removal circumferentially is apparent; the depth will include the full thickness of the lesion plus the uninvolved subcutaneous fat. If the subcutaneous fat has not been invaded and is less than 1 cm thick, only that which is present need be excised. Only if the lesion is in contact with the deep fascia need the latter be excised. The specimen will have a cylindrical shape. There is no theoretical or practical advantage in beveling the excision outward, as has been frequently recommended (Pack, Perzik, and Scharnagel 1946; Pitt 1977). If satellite lesions are already present either in the epidermis, dermis, or subcutaneous fat then the excision will be more extensive, including the same 1 cm of apparently uninvolved tissue in all directions. If operators are concerned with respect to their ability to delineate the extent of the lesion, then it behooves them to remove as much apparently uninvolved tissue as their personal judgment dictates. *The amount removed under these conditions will be in inverse proportion to the experience of the operator.* Once the deep fascia is organically involved, a wider excision of this layer and the underlying muscle is warranted, since the deep fascial lymphatics parallel this layer as they extend toward the most proximal draining lymph nodes. Under the latter circumstances, operators must accept the fact that they are now faced with more than just a local primary lesion. The situation now requires management as for a metastasizing lesion.

In the presence of postoperative local recurrence, the primary site must be managed by totally removing the recurrent tumor plus all of the prior operative site. Such a recurrence suggests that the residual of the incompletely removed tumor may have been seeded in all the tissue layers exposed during the initial operation. In such a situation the deep fascia almost invariably must be taken, whether grossly involved or not.

## Lymphatics

The management of the lymphatic drainage basin should be considered in three categories: (1) in the presence of clinically negative nodes; (2) in the face of clinically positive nodes; (3) in the presumed situation of the existence of possibly involved lymphatic channels between the primary lesion and the first group of regional lymph nodes.

Based on the natural history of this disease, patients who succumb to melanoma do so as a result of involvement of distal vital organs and not from the disease in the primary site or regional lymph nodes. *Such distal involvement results from vascular spread from the primary site and not from secondary lymphatic disease.* The rare exception is the situation in which a neglected large ulcerated primary or lymph node mass inadvertently and by direct infiltration bursts into a contiguous vascular channel. Accepting this pathogenesis, treatment of the lymph nodes is a palliative procedure, adding nothing to the curative objective. There is no indication, therefore, for elective lymphadenectomy (Perzik and Baum 1969; Perzik 1979; Catlin 1966; Ballantyne 1970; Polk and Linn 1971; Veronesi et al. 1977; Conrad 1972; Cohen et al. 1977; Sim et al. 1978). Contrary opinions abound in the literature (Pack, Scharnagel, and Morfit 1945; Conley and Pack 1963; Simmons 1968; Fortner et al. 1977; Goldsmith 1979; Gumport and Harris 1974).

In the presence of clinically positive nodes, the therapeutic lymphadenectomy should be categorized as a palliative procedure and only performed with the definition of that term in mind. Since positive nodes may become locally disabling, they should be removed for anticipated palliation if there is no contraindication to the operation. Such nodal disability may be due to local functional restriction, pain, or ulceration, with bleeding and infection. Node removal will, however, not enhance the patients' chance of survival if metastases are present in a distant vital organ. In most instances, when lymphatic metastases are present, the chances are that distant metastases, by way of the vascular channels, have also occurred. Metastases usually originate simultaneously from the primary site through the contiguous papillary lymphatic and vascular channels and not secondarily from the lymphatics into the blood stream. The rare exceptions occur when infiltrative advanced nodal disease ruptures into an adherent vein or from a permeated and blocked thoracic duct.

When the removal of a primary lesion results in an extensive operative invasion of an underlying lymph node area, then an elective node dissection may be considered. This is advised in order to render a later indicated palliative therapeutic node dissection less hazardous by avoiding the fibrosis and adhesions that would ordinarily develop subsequent to the removal of a primary lesion so located.

There is no specific indication for an elective dissection-in-continuity. Therapeutically it may be more convenient and possibly of greater palliative effect, with a primary very close to a positive node-bearing area, to include the intervening skin to fascia soft parts. A bit more occult disease may thus be removed. The resulting added morbidity must be neutralized by the increased palliation anticipated from the dissection-in-continuity.

### Distant Metastases

With very few and extremely rare exceptions the management of distant vascular metastases is palliative (Gilchrist et al. 1977; Cahan 1973). By simple definition this implies doing more good than harm. Yet in some enthusiastic quarters there has been a tendency to apply modalities, mostly still experimental, that presumably yield a so-called favorable response, a nonmeasurable and objective regression of limited degree, often for periods of only days or weeks. At best, this therapeutic meddling only delays temporarily the inevitable progression of the disease. The price in morbidity, paid by the patient for these chemo- and immunotherapeutic attacks, has been well documented by the referring physicians and more seasoned medical oncologists. Certainly these modalities should continue to be used—but only in an experimental framework with due regard for the associated complications and sequelae. Further reduction in the patients' quality of remaining life by the disabling results of palliative procedures is not justified. To propose these agents as substitutes for available proved modalities such as surgery or radiation or medicinal hospice care which offer true palliation, when indicated, is unacceptable.

## Host Resistance

Melanoma, like many malignant tumors, often remains occult and dormant for years before late recurrence becomes manifest. Medical oncologists should devote all of their efforts in determining what the host factors are that keep such occult disease in check. They would then possess a modus operandi that could be used in managing either occult or obvious distant metastases. Until such a fortuitous time arrives, currently acceptable surgical and radiation palliatives, when properly selected, may prove useful.

When recurrent melanoma appears as a safely resectable lesion, an operative procedure should be performed, regardless of the anticipated prognosis. Such recurrent disease has been locally excised from node-bearing areas—the breast, the small bowel, the brain, and other locations—often in the same patient, over a period of several years following the initial treatment, and in turn to be followed by a clinically disease-free interval of many years, without benefit of chemo- or immunotherapy. In some instances, after intraabdominal extirpations, nonresectable, retroperitoneal melanoma has remained in situ without treatment and symptomless for a period of years. This points to the patient's intrinsic resistance, which for shorter or longer periods keeps the residual disease in check. This may also explain the reported instances of so-called spontaneous cure. All of the preceding have been observed without benefit of adjunctive, prophylactic, or therapeutic chemo- and immunotherapy, as now available (Perzik 1979; Barr, Gartside, and Goldman 1979; see also Appendix).

## Prognosis

The prognosis is determined by the inherent biologic potential of the disease modified by occult host resistance factors. Theoretically, the only certain curative procedure, regardless of the type of lesion or the host resistance, is the fortuitous total elimination of the primary lesion before it has metastasized.

A study of the natural history of melanoma reveals its very protean nature. As is true of all malignant tumors, the more undifferentiated the cell, the greater will be the tendency to locally and expansively infiltrate and metastasize by way of the lymphatics and blood stream.

The nodular lesion carries the gravest prognosis, followed, in order, by the superficial spreading melanoma and the lentigo maligna melanoma (Hutchinson's freckle).

Microscopically, the seriousness of the lesion is determined primarily by its degree of local infiltration in depth. When strictly confined to an intraepithelial location, it is often designated as melanoma in situ and carries an excellent prognosis. As the lesion infiltrates the deeper layers of the skin, the prognosis becomes more threatening in the following order: junctional interface, papillary dermis, reticular dermis, and subcutaneous fat (Clark et al. 1979). Breslow (1976) suggests an excellent prognosis if the lesion measures less than 0.75 mm in thickness, fair between 0.75 mm and 1.5 mm, and poor when thicker than 1.5 mm. Although no mention is made of an active junctional nevus, this diagnosis, after minimal local excision, has been followed by the subsequent appearance of involved regional lymph nodes and distant metastases. After a review of the microscopic slides in one such case the diagnosis was finally changed to possible in situ melanoma (Perzik and Baum 1969). The finding of disease at the primary site permeating the local lymphatic and vascular channels determines the outlook for survival regardless of the gross aspects of size, ulceration, depth, or topography of the lesion. Reference has been made to the correlation of prognosis with the parameters of cellular undifferentiation; number of mitoses; size, topography, ulceration, and extent of the area of infiltration and involvement of local lymphatic and vascular channels; and the presence of positive regional lymph nodes and distant metastases. There is nothing unique to melanoma in using these parameters in prognosticating end results. These parameters are used in prognosticating end results in all malignant tumors on an individual basis (Fitzpatrick, Brown, and Reid 1972; Clark 1969; Breslow 1976; Kapelanski, Block, and Kaufman 1979.)

The thickness of the primary lesion always has been and still is a good prognostic indicator, but its use as a parameter for selection of prophylactic (elective) treatment for the purpose of favorably influencing the prognosis has not been proved (Veronesi et al. 1977).

When cure is the objective, the protean clinical nature of melanoma warrants a therapeutic approach by the accepted modalities of surgery and, to a lesser extent, radiation to the primary site. Treatment of metastases is palliative and is to be applied with an understanding of the inherent factors of host resistance that may influence the course of the disease in any individual case.

## Material

In 1946, Pack, Perzik, and Scharnagel reported on 862 cases of melanoma treated in the prior 20 years. With constant changes in regimens, it was concluded that a very radical operative approach might yield better end results than the more minimal therapeutic measures used in the early years of the study. The recommended operation consisted of very wide and deep removal of the primary lesion, including the deep fascia, which almost invariably required some type of plastic closure plus a radical dissection of the regional lymph nodes, electively or therapeutically, preferably in-continuity if it was anatomically indicated.

Further observation by the author over a period of about 20 years led to a reevaluation of this thesis suggesting that it was probably too radical, resulting in marked and often disabling morbidity without compensating improvement in end results. A regimen of very limited local excision of the primary lesion with the elimination of elective (clinically negative) node dissection was instituted. Rarely was radiation therapy used, and then only in a palliative situation. Adjunctive, elective, or therapeutic chemo- and/or immunotherapy were not used.

The results in 164 consecutive cases of melanoma so managed were published in 1969 by Perzik and Baum. The five-year salvage for all cases was 52.7% (table 12.1). As might be expected, the more advanced the stage of the disease, the poorer was the result. With positive nodes the salvage rate was 24.6%. If these nodes were positive on entrance the five-year salvage was reduced to 20.5%.

The data as obtained in a correlation of specific gross clinical and histologic findings with respect to prognosis in this series of 164 cases were as follows.

The five-year salvage was 62.5% for women versus 43.4% for men (table 12.2), probably because women were more sensitive to the presence of pigmented lesions of the skin, as a result of which their lesions were managed at an earlier stage. The same might account for the 45.2% survival in the over-45-year group versus the 60% survival in the under-45-year group (table 12.3). Parents, because of their concern, more frequently detected pigmented

**Table 12.1**
Five-Year End Results in All Cases

| Cases | Percentage | Number of Cases |
|---|---|---|
| All Cases | 52.7 | 148 |
| Primary only on entrance | 66.3 | 104 |
| Positive nodes, all cases | 24.6 | 69 |
| Positive nodes on entrance | 20.5 | 44 |
| Positive nodes, elective | 16.6 | 6 |
| Negative nodes, elective | 74.3 | 39 |
| Negative nodes, all cases | 66.6 | 45 |

lesions in the younger age group, whereas the seniors and aged had a tendency to vacillate and ignore such pigmented lesions for prolonged periods of time.

If the primary lesion was under 1.5 cm in diameter, the five-year salvage was 62.5%; if over 1.5 cm, it decreased to 45.6% (table 12.4). This is explainable on the basis that, as a rule, the larger lesions have been present longer and have had more time to infiltrate the local lymphatic and vascular channels with a resulting increase in metastases.

With ulceration the five-year salvage was reduced to 45.9%, as compared to 75.4% for the nonulcerated lesions (table 12.5). As a rule ulceration is a manifestation of a more active infiltrating type of lesion, one with a greater propensity to metastasize.

On the basis of thickness and depth of invasion this study revealed that the so-called intraepithelial, active junctional nevus, or in situ melanoma had a 100% five-year salvage; the papillary-dermal invader (superficial melanoma) yielded an 87% salvage; the reticular-dermal invader (deep dermal), 56%; but, with involvement of subcutaneous fat there was no five-year salvage (table 12.6). These observations were made before Clark and associates (1969) enunciated their parameters of microscopic levels, or Breslow (1976) reported the use of the ocular micrometer. Also no patient received adjunc-

**Table 12.2**
Five-Year End Results versus Sex

| Sex | Percentage | Number of Cases |
|---|---|---|
| Male | 43.4 | 76 |
| Female | 62.5 | 72 |

**Table 12.3**
Five-Year End Results versus Age

| Age | Percentage | Number of Cases |
|---|---|---|
| Over 45 years | 45.2 | 73 |
| Under 45 years | 60.0 | 75 |

tive, elective, or therapeutic chemo- or immunotherapy. Management was solely surgical except for a few instances of added palliative radiation therapy.

## Discussion

The basis for the use of the current therapeutic regimen is a better appreciation of the natural history of melanoma. Whereas the radical onslaught on this disease was almost universal up to about 10 years ago, practitioners running scared, as it were, when presently faced with melanoma are now looking back over their shoulders, minimizing their panic, and developing a more reasonable evaluation based upon their personal observations. The current literature bears this out (Perzik 1979; Pitt 1977; Polk and Linn 1971; Veronesi et al. 1977).

During the period when radical and wide extirpative excision was the almost universally accepted method of management of the primary melanoma, reports appeared in the literature suggesting that a more limited operation on primary melanoma of the skin of the head and neck was equally effective (Perzik and Baum 1969; Catlin 1966; Ballantyne 1970). Many of these advocates nevertheless continued to recommend the wider, more radical excisions on the trunk and extremities. It would appear that this revelation was the result of serendipity: the more horrendous cosmetic and functional disability resulting from the application of the then-accepted rad-

**Table 12.4**
Five-Year End Results versus Size of Primary Lesion

| Size of Lesion | Percentage | Number of Cases |
|---|---|---|
| Primary over 1.5 cm | 45.6 | 46 |
| Primary under 1.5 cm | 62.5 | 88 |

**Table 12.5**
Five-Year End Results versus Ulceration of Primary Lesion

| Lesion | Percentage | Number of Cases |
|---|---|---|
| Ulcerated primary | 45.9 | 57 |
| Nonulcerated primary | 75.4 | 61 |

ical management of the primary melanoma forced the head and neck operator to limit markedly, either consciously or subconsciously, the extent of the excision. The surgeon's misgivings after long periods of follow-up were replaced with the happy clinical discovery that in spite of such very limited excisions, cure without local recurrences was equal to that obtained with the mutilating and unnecessary wider excisions which previously were thought to be necessary. The precept of limited excision of a primary melanoma of the skin of the head and neck was thus established. What was developed in the head and neck by force of circumstances was then applied gradually by many surgeons to primary melanoma of the trunk and extremities, with surprisingly good results.

Veronesi and associates (1977), reporting on a randomized prospective study by the WHO melanoma group, showed that there was no difference in survival time between two groups of patients, one receiving and the other not receiving elective regional node dissection for clinically uninvolved nodes. This also held true when compared for sex, site of origin, size of the lesion, or its depth by the criteria of both Clark and Breslow.

Cohen and colleagues (1977), from the National Cancer Institute, stated that after five years "there is no difference in survival between patients with lower extremity melanoma randomly allocated to receive either prophylactic lymph node dissection or not, even among patients with large or deeply invasive melanomas." They concluded that the factors of depth of invasion of

**Table 12.6**
Five-Year End Results versus Pathology

| Pathology | Percentage | Number of Cases |
|---|---|---|
| Active junctional nevus | 100 | 3 |
| Superficial melanoma | 87 | 16 |
| Dermal involvement | 56 | 39 |
| Fat invasion | none | 10 |
| Local satellitosis | 27 | 11 |

the primary melanoma were of prognostic value "rather than for identification of patients that would benefit from a prophylactic node dissection."

Polk and Linn (1971) conclude that there is no evidence that routine prophylactic (elective) regional node dissection in the presence of clinically negative nodes is of any value in favorably influencing the end result in the management of melanoma, especially when consideration is given to the morbidity and mortality associated with such routine operations. They suggest that when signs and symptoms indicating the presence of occult disease in clinically negative nodes are available, then consideration can be given to the usefulness of such an operation. Peer pressure and medicolegal implications should have no place in influencing the attending surgeons' judgment based on their individualization of a specific case.

## Conclusions

Malignant melanoma is a surgical disease. Radiation in a few selected situations may be used palliatively.

Incisional biopsy may be safely performed.

The only curative operation in malignant melanoma is the total excision of the primary lesion before it has metastasized.

The primary lesion need only be excised with a margin of 1 to 2 cm of apparently uninvolved tissue; the limits of the excision will be determined by the extent of the lesion and the experience and judgment of the operator.

The cosmetic stimulus limiting the extent of local excision and elective radical neck dissections in the management of melanoma of the skin of the head and neck, serendipitously led to the use of these principles in the treatment of melanoma of the skin of the rest of the body.

Plastic reconstruction or excision of the deep fascia is warranted only if the size of the primary lesion necessitates such extensive excision of specific tumor-involved tissue.

Recurrent primary site lesions will require the total elimination of the prior exposed operative field, regardless of the size of the recurrence.

The factors of size, depth, ulceration, and nodular topography are directly related to the biologic threat of the disease with respect to more extensive development of metastases. This in turn is modified by the effectiveness of the individual's inherent protective host factors. Eventual mortality will not be influenced by performing elective (prophylactic) regional node dissection on the basis of the earlier excision of presumably present occult disease.

Elective (prophylactic) node dissection is not indicated except when the node-bearing area is extensively invaded during the removal of the primary lesion.

Mortality in melanoma, with rare exceptions, is due to fatal involvement of vital organs and not to the disease still present in the primary site or regional lymph nodes.

Distant metastases to vital organs have their genesis in vascular spread from the primary site and not from secondary lymph system involvement. The rare exception is an obviously well-advanced metastatic lesion which, due to uncontrolled local infiltrative growth, ruptures into a contiguous blood vessel.

Host resistance may be associated with the individual's hormone and/or immune apparatus, which will require further study for its delineation. Such a successful study will reveal the host factors determining spontaneous regression, the different rates and variability of growth, and the long intervals of quiescence in the existing symptomless and occult metastases preceding their subsequent objective reappearance, often after many years. Their discovery and therapeutic utilization hold out the promise of future control in malignant melanoma.

After a primary melanoma has metastasized, the patient will eventually succumb to the disease if he or she lives long enough and does not expire from an unrelated cause.

Elimination of metastases, by any modality, is only for palliation. The aggressive use of palliative procedures is based upon the protean nature of malignant melanoma. By definition, such a palliative procedure should not result in greater morbidity or earlier mortality than would be associated with nontreatment.

Adjunctive, prophylactic, or therapeutic chemo- and/or immunotherapy are not indicated as primary modalities; they should be used only in experimental situations.

# Appendix: Case Histories Depicting Protean Nature of Malignant Melanoma

Every physician involved with the management of malignant melanoma has experienced the extensive manifestations of its protean nature. An attempt to categorize the disease on the basis of a common denominator has revealed a maximum of exceptions, leading to frustration in this vain endeavor. Recognition of the many variables has led to a routine of individualizing the management of each case on the basis of a few accepted generalities.

An analysis of the following case histories will exemplify some of the variables emanating from apparently similar clinical starting points.

These variables include various degrees of host resistance, multiple asynchronous primaries, and massive or minimal primary disease with or without regional and/or distant vascular involvement.

Certain tentative common phenomena are revealed: death from melanoma results from distant vital organ involvement by vascular spread unrelated to prior regional node metastases; prognosis correlates with the depth of invasion by the primary lesion and the presence of metastases; the reliability of limited excision of the primary lesion; the ineffectiveness of elective (prophylactic) node dissection; the absence of any evidence of cure through the medium of chemo- or immunotherapy, at this time; the value of palliative persistent excision of resectable recurrences; and the tendency to overtreat with elective radical extensive surgery when cure is the objective.

## Case I: Woman, 29

This patient had a 1.5-cm superficial melanoma widely excised from mid-forearm in June 1947; the 8-cm defect was repaired with a split-thickness graft. The following sequence of events occurred:

**August 1950.** Therapeutic right axillary dissection with black striae in the axillary fat.

**February 1951.** Therapeutic right supraclavicular neck dissection.

**April 1951.** Therapeutic right upper neck dissection.

**May 1951.** Local excision of recurrence in subcutaneous fat of right breast.

**June 1951.** Excision of recurrent lesions of posterior triangle of right neck over trapezius muscle.

**September 1951.** Completion of right neck dissection for recurrences.

**October 1951.** Pregnant.

**June 1952.** Delivered normal child.

**June 1979.** No evidence of recurrent disease since June 1951 (28 years).

### Discussion

It is reasonable to assume that occult disease was still present at the time of the last operation. Yet, in a period of 28 years, since June 1951, there has been no clinical manifestation of recurrent melanoma, in spite of the fact that no other treatment, including chemo- or immunotherapy, was used in this case.

This case exemplifies host resistance.

It also shows the value of palliative extirpation of recurrences whenever and wherever they appear, regardless of the presumed poor prognosis signified by their appearance.

## Case II: Woman, 43

**October 1957.** A 0.8-cm enlarging pigmented skin lesion of six months' duration excised under local anesthesia from back of left upper neck below the hair line. The 1-cm defect was primarily closed. Diagnosis was an active junctional nevus.

**April 1959.** Left radical neck dissection for an infraparotid node with metastatic melanoma.

**October 1959.** A 1.5-cm subcutaneous recurrence of the right upper abdominal wall excised under local anesthesia.

**February 1960.** Right axillary dissection for recurrent nodal involvement.

**March 1961.** Segmental ilium resection with partial resection of melanoma-involved retroperitoneal nodes. Residual disease remaining.

**June 1979.** No recurrence or abdominal symptoms since March 1961 (18 years).

### Discussion

In this case gross recurrent disease was left in the retroperitoneal nodes. The recurrences kept appearing over a period of three and one-half years following the initial treatment. There has been no clinical evidence of further symptomatic recurrence for 18 years. No additional treatment, including chemo- or immunotherapy, was used in this case at any time. This case exemplifies spontaneous regression and host resistance.

This is an example of widespread metastases resulting from a borderline primary lesion, first diagnosed as an active junctional nevus and later, reluctantly, changed to melanoma in situ.

This case shows the value of persistent palliative excision in spite of the obvious poor prognosis.

It also verifies the efficacy of a very limited excision of a primary malignant lesion, since no local recurrence occurred.

Furthermore, it is an example of the localization of metastatic nodal involvement to the paraparotid area when drainage is through this region. In retrospect, a limited excision of the paraparotid nodes would have been adequate. Since the procedure was palliative, any subsequently appearing neck nodes could have been locally excised.

## Case III: Woman, 46

**Prior History.** In 1948 a birthmark was excised from the right posterior neck. From September 1951 through February 1952, three separate excisions were performed for what were presumably metastatic lymph nodes, posterior left neck.

**September 1952.** A 10 × 10 × 5 cm recurrence at the back of the left upper neck extending to the right side in the hairline was widely excised, including skin and underlying trapezius muscle. The 15 × 18 cm deep defect was repaired with a split-thickness skin graft. The specimen consisted of positive matted lymph nodes with infiltration of the involved trapezius muscle and subcutaneous fat.

**June 1979.** No evidence of recurrence since September 1952 (27 years).

## Discussion

There have been no further clinical recurrences for the 27 years since the last treatment. No chemo- or immunotherapy was used in this case at any time.

This case exemplifies host resistance and the value of repeated palliative excisions of recurrent disease in spite of a presumably poor prognosis.

There was never any recurrence at the primary site in spite of a very limited excision of a 46-year-old birthmark which became clinically malignant.

Control of the recurring neck nodes was accomplished by piecemeal excision of the positive nodes when and where they appeared. Of interest, the recurrences have not appeared as yet outside the retrograde lymphatic drainage basin of the back of the neck. Any elective node dissection would have directed the operator to the right axilla, which is still negative.

# Case IV: Man, 28

**Prior History.** In June 1953 a 1.5-cm itching and enlarged pigmented lesion of 15 months' duration excised under local anesthesia from the skin of the right supraspinatus area.

**July 1953.** Right therapeutic axillary dissection (nodes positive).

**August 1954.** In-continuity excision of recurrence near primary site plus a right radical neck dissection for positive nodes.

**December 1954.** Local excision of recurrence of left submental node.

**June 1979.** No evidence of recurrence since December 1954 (25 years).

## Discussion

There has been no clinical recurrence since the last treatment 25 years ago, in spite of repeated recurrences over a period of about three years, all confined to the right neck and right axilla. No chemo- or immunotherapy was used in this case at any time.

This is an example of host resistance and the value of repeated palliative excisions of recurrent disease in the face of a poor prognosis. There has never been any further recurrence at the primary site in spite of its removal by a very limited excision and primary closure. Although metastatic disease by way of the blood stream most likely occurred, it has either been held in check or has been eliminated by the patient's (host) resistance.

## Case V: Man, 61

**Prior History.** A lifelong pigmented lesion of left temple began to enlarge and ulcerate in February 1954.

**March 1954.** A 1.5-cm ulcerated melanoma excised widely from left temple in-continuity with an elective left parotidectomy and radical neck dissection; the temple defect was covered with a split-thickness graft; the nodes were negative; facial nerve was preserved.

**July 1959.** A second primary melanoma, 1 cm in diameter, was excised from the right perianal skin, along with a separate therapeutic right radical groin dissection.

**October 1961.** Died of widespread metastatic disease to liver and lungs.

### Discussion

The first primary could have been treated by a limited local excision alone. Apparently this lesion was removed before it had metastasized.

The second primary had regional positive nodes on entrance and, in spite of radical local and node excisions, the patient died of distant metastases which undoubtedly occurred synchronously by way of the capillary vessels in the primary site. The second primary exemplifies (1) the palliative situation associated with a melanoma that has metastasized before the primary is removed and (2) the uselessness of curative surgical intervention. The latter also points to a lack of host resistance and the tendency toward multiple primaries in such patients.

## Case VI: Man, 42

**Prior History.** A 2.5-cm birthmark below tip of right mastoid bone, enlarged slightly in the prior three years.

**January 1951.** Incision biopsy revealed superficial spreading melanoma.

**February 1951.** Wide local excision with split-thickness skin graft, in-continuity with right radical neck dissection, elective (nodes negative).

**1979.** No recurrence to date.

### Discussion

There has been no recurrence in the 28 years since the last treatment. No chemo- or immunotherapy was ever used.

This is an example of overtreatment by current criteria. A limited local excision with primary closure would have sufficed. An incisional biopsy was performed without complications.

## Case VII: Man, 66

**Prior History.** An untreated pigmented right cheek nodular lesion was first noted in 1948. Currently lesion is 10 cm in diameter and elevated 2.5 cm. Clinically positive nodes occupy entire right jugular chain. In past three months growth has been rapid, becoming ulcerated and infected. No clinical evidence of distant metastases.

**October 1954.** Palliative extensive wide excision of right cheek plus therapeutic right radical neck dissection and extensive plastic closure.

**January 1957.** Died of generalized distant metastases.

### Discussion

Host controlled primary growth for six years, ending in three months of very rapid local and cervical metastatic activity and a further lapse of three years before death from distant metastases. Illustrates that death is due to vascular spread to vital organs and not to a lesion in the primary site or regional nodes.

## Case VIII: Man, 77

**August 1964.** Black pigmented lesion noted on the skin of left cheek.

**August 1965.** Lesion became larger (1.5 cm), darker, and nodular.

**September 1965.** Widely removed by a $4 \times 3 \times 0.8$ cm excision, plastic closure. Diagnosed superficial/nodular melanoma with very little free margin in depth.

**March 1966.** Local nodular subcutaneous recurrence; complete clinical regression by external radiation.

**August 1967.** Died of liver metastases. No other clinical evidence of recurrence.

### Discussion

Example of local regression by radiation. No cervical nodes or further local recurrence appeared. Died of vascular distant metastases, not from local disease. No evidence of host resistance. Elective node dissection would have contributed nothing in this case.

## Case IX: Woman, 68

**June 1955.** A 1.5-cm melanoma of three months' duration of skin of posterior left upper neck treated by wide local excision and elective left radical neck dissection in-continuity (nodes negative).

**June 1960.** Superficial melanoma (1.5 cm) of middle of left cheek treated by limited local excision.

**July 1964.** Cardiac death; no melanoma recurrences.

### Discussion

Case of multiple primaries; first one overtreated; second one treated by current protocol.

No recurrences. Died from unrelated cause.

## Case X: Woman, 66

**1952.** Hutchinson's freckle, 4 cm in diameter, with focal area of superficial melanoma of left cheek, of several years' duration, minimally excised and skin-grafted.

**1963.** Local recurrence, 1.5 cm, involving lateral end of skin of eyelids; observation only.

**July 1964.** Partial excision of melanoma in situ, $1.5 \times 0.5$ cm of clinically suspicious area with primary closure.

**January 1973.** A suspicious enlargement $1 \times 0.5$ cm near external canthus excised and primarily closed with diagnosis of melanoma in situ.

**1974.** Died of other causes; superficially growing and rather extensive pigmented flat lesion still present on skin of outer halves of both eyelids and centrifugally around periphery of skin graft.

### Discussion

Indicates that the limited approach to melanoma in situ in Hutchinson's freckle, with palliative intent, is treatment of choice. Present 22 years without clinical evidence of metastases. No sacrifice of orbital content.

## Case XI: Man, 69

**July 1965.** Limited local excision of a 1-cm pigmented lesion of helix of right auricle of six months' duration. Differential diagnosis included pigmented epidermoid cancer.

**December 1965.** Right therapeutic neck dissection revealed unequivocal metastatic melanoma.

**1972.** Died with brain metastases.

### Discussion

Reveals difficulty in diagnosing primary lesion; effectiveness of minimal local excision; palliative nature of therapeutic neck dissection; death caused by vascular metastases to a vital organ (brain).

## References

Ballantyne, A. J. Malignant melanoma of skin of head and neck. *Am. J. Surg.* 120:425–443, 1970.

Barr, L. H.; Gartside, R. L.; and Goldman, L. I. The biology of human malignant melanoma. *Arch. Surg.* 114:221–230, 1979.

Breslow, A. Tumor thickness, level of invasion, and node dissection in Stage I cutaneous melanoma. *Ann. Surg.* 182:572–575, 1976.

Cahan, W. G. Excision melanoma metastases to lungs. *Ann. Surg.* 178: 703–710, 1973.

Catlin, D. Cutaneous melanoma of head and neck. *Am. J. Surg.* 112: 512–515, 1966.

Catlin, D. Mucosal melanomas of head and neck. *Am. J. Roentgenol.* 99:809–815, 1967.

Clark, W. H. et al. The histogenesis and biologic behavior of primary human and malignant melanomas of the skin. *Cancer Res.* 29:705–710, 1969.

Cohen, M. H. et al. Prognostic factors in patients undergoing lymphadenectomy for malignant melanoma. *Ann. Surg.* 186:635–650, 1977.

Conley, J. J., and Pack, G. T. Melanoma of the head and neck. *Surg. Gynecol. Obstet.* 116:15–30, 1963.

Conrad, F. G. Treatment of malignant melanoma. *Arch. Surg.* 104:582–587, 1972.

Fisher, B. Important surgical implications in cancer. *Oncology News* 3:7–11, 1977.

Fitzpatrick, P. J.; Brown, T. C.; and Reid, M. A. Malignant melanoma of the head and neck. *Can. J. Surg.* 15:90–101, 1972.

Fortner, J. G. et al. Biostatistical basis of elective node dissection for malignant melanoma. *Ann. Surg.* 186:101–115, 1977.

Gilchrist, K. W. et al. Importance of microscopic vascular invasion in primary cutaneous malignant melanoma. *Surg. Gynecol. Obstet.* 145:559–570, 1977.

Goldsmith, H. S. The debate over immediate lymph node dissection in melanoma. *Surg. Gynecol. Obstet.* 148:403–411, 1979.

Gumport, S. L., and Harris, M. N. Results of regional lymph node dissection for melanoma. *Ann. Surg.* 179:105–115, 1974.

Handley, W. S. Pathology of melanotic growths in relation to their operative treatment. *Lancet* 1:927–935, 1907.

Hansen, M. G., and McCarten, A. B. Tumor thickness and lymphocytic infiltration in malignant melanoma of the head and neck. *Am. J. Surg.* 128:557–570, 1974.

Kapelanski, D. P.; Block, G. E.; and Kaufman, M. Characteristics of the primary lesion of malignant melanoma as a guide to prognosis and therapy. *Ann. Surg.* 189:225–240, 1979.

Moore, E. S., and Martin, H. Melanoma of the upper respiratory tract and oral cavity. *Cancer* 8:1167–1170, 1955.

Pack, G. T.; Perzik, S. L.; and Scharnagel, I. M. The treatment of malignant melanoma. *Calif. Med.* 66:351–370, 1946.

Pack, G. T.; Scharnagel, I. M.; and Morfit, M. The principle of excision and dissection in-continuity for primary and metastatic melanomas of the skin. *Surgery* 17:849–859, 1945.

Perzik, S. L. The management of melanoma. *Cutis* 23:104–110, 1979.

Perzik, S. L., and Baum, R. K. Individualization in the management of melanoma. *Am. Surg.* 35:177–190, 1969.

Pitt, T. T. E. Aspects of surgical treatment for malignant melanoma; the place of biopsy and wide excision. *N.Z. J. Surg.* 47:757–782, 1977.

Polk, H. C., Jr., and Linn, B. S. Selective regional lymphadenectomy for melanoma: a mathematical aid to clinical judgment. *Ann. Surg.* 174: 402–415, 1971.

Principato, J. J.; Sika, J. V.; and Sandler, H. C. Primary malignant melanoma of tongue. *Cancer* 18:1641–1655, 1965.

Robinson, J. C. Risks of BCG intralesional therapy: an experience with melanoma. *J. Surg. Oncol.* 9:587–595, 1977.

Robinson, L., and Hukill, P. B. Hutchinson's melanotic freckle in oral mucous membrane. *Cancer* 26:297–315, 1970.

Sim, F. H. et al. Randomized study of the efficacy of routine elective lymphadenectomy in management of malignant melanoma. *Cancer* 41:948–1000, 1978.

Simmons, J. N. Malignant melanoma of head and neck. *Am. J. Surg.* 116:494–499, 1968.

Veronesi, V. et al. Inefficacy of immediate node dissection in stage I melanoma of the limbs. *N. Engl. J. Med.* 297:627, 1977.

Walker, E. A., and Snow, J. B. Management of melanoma of the nose and paranasal sinuses. *Arch. Otolaryngol.* 89:652–670, 1969.

# Chapter 13

# *Mandibular Reconstruction*

Harry C. Schwartz

Changing attitudes about reconstruction following radical tumor surgery and changing concepts about what constitutes an adequate tumor resection have become evident in recent years. Although such changes are perhaps most obvious in the case of breast cancer, they also play a role in the current management of head and neck cancer.

The basic principles of head and neck cancer surgery evolved at the turn of the century; however, widespread application was delayed until the advent of modern anesthetic techniques, blood transfusion, and antibiotics. Today, virtually no part of the head and neck is inaccessible to the cancer surgeon. Nevertheless, extensive, debilitating resections may be neither justifiable nor feasible unless reconstructive measures are available to repair the massive wounds that are created and ultimately to rehabilitate the patient.

The integrity of the mandible and its associated soft tissues is necessary for normal mastication, speech, and swallowing. The appearance of this important part of the face may be essential to the maintenance of a normal self-image and will thus influence social behavior and psychological well-being (Constable and Bernstein 1979).

The sequelae of radical resection of the mandible and associated soft tissues are quite varied. At one extreme, there are the individuals whose major postoperative difficulty is loss of the ability to chew their favorite cut of meat. At the opposite extreme, there are the recluses, shunned by family and friends, drooling uncontrollably into a handful of tissues, speaking unintelligibly, and nourished by tube feedings. We must not confuse the gratitude that these latter patients have for being alive with satisfaction in their lot. Such patients deserve consideration for reconstruction.

# Conservative Surgery versus Mandibular Resection

Improved surgical techniques and better understanding of how cancer spreads in the head and neck have changed the indications for the classical hemimandibulectomy. Traditionally the mandible was resected in any of the following situations:

1. The tumor has spread to the mandible itself.
2. The tumor abuts so closely upon the mandible that resection is necessary to obtain adequate tumor-free margins.
3. Resection facilitates access to the tumor.
4. Resection permits closure of a large soft tissue defect by direct approximation.

Recent studies have clarified the first two situations. Modern reconstructive surgery has all but eliminated the last two situations: the mandible should not be resected solely to obtain either surgical access or simple wound closure.

## Pathophysiology

The mandible becomes involved by tumor through direct spread from the oral cavity. Invasion occurs through the periosteum. The outer bony cortex is eroded relatively slowly. When tumor reaches the spongiosa, however, it can spread quite rapidly. Once tumor has entered the inferior alveolar neurovascular canal, it is free to spread quickly via perineural lymphatics (Ballantyne, McCarten, and Ibanez 1963). This mode of spread is of particular

**Figure 13.1**

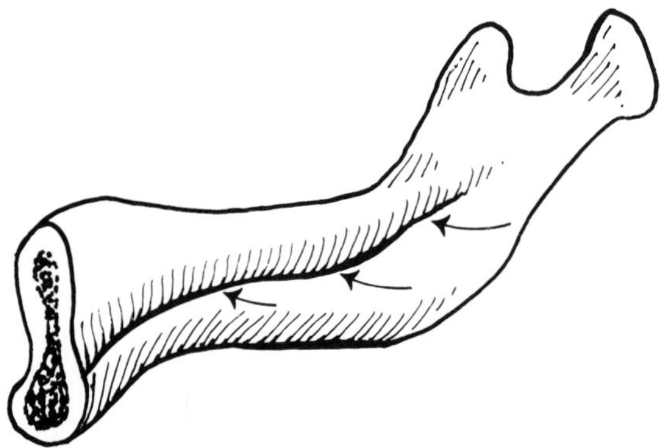

*The mylohyoid line (*arrows*). Oral mucosa contacts the mandible only above this line. If tumor has not invaded the mandible, a marginal resection may be performed at this line.*

importance in edentulous patients, whose neurovascular canals may lie just beneath the mucosa because of atrophy of the alveolar bone.

It was once felt that lymphatics from the oral cavity traverse the mandibular periosteum on their way to the cervical lymph nodes. The presence of tumor between the primary site and the lymph nodes, however, has never been convincingly demonstrated (McGregor 1977). The success of the pull-through operation further attests to this. Careful pathologic studies have shown that regardless of the size of the primary tumor and the status of the cervical nodes, tumors that do not involve the periosteum by direct extension do not spread to the mandible, even when tumor can be demonstrated within a few millimeters of the mandible (Marchetta, Sako, and Murphy 1971).

## Mandibular Resections

Equipped with modern high-speed drills and micro saws for precision bone cutting, the surgeon is capable of managing the mandible in a more conservative manner. Clearly the overall result is optimal if continuity of the mandible, from condyle to condyle, can be maintained.

Certain anatomic considerations are important in evaluating the relationship between the tumor and the mandible and in planning the resection. The floor of the mouth is formed by the mylohyoid muscle. Thus mucosa only comes into direct contact with the mandible above the mylohyoid line (fig. 13.1). Close to the angle of the mandible, the greater portion of the bone lies between the mylohyoid line and the lower border. The line runs

**Figure 13.2**

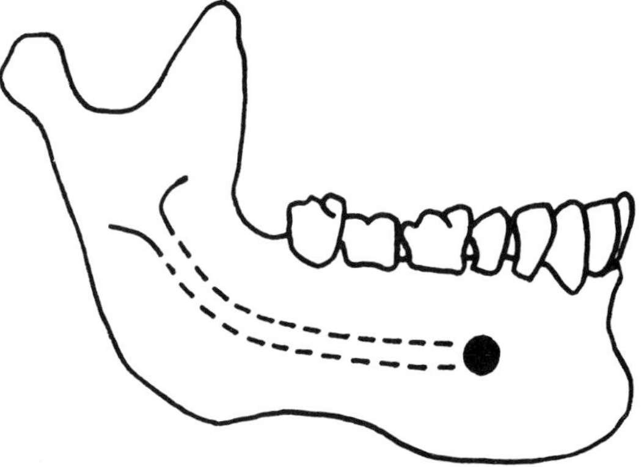

*The inferior alveolar neurovascular canal occupies most of each hemimandible. It runs from the lingula on the medial aspect of the ramus to the mental foramen on the lateral aspect of the body. If perineural tumor invasion is suspected, the entire canal should be resected.*

obliquely downward and forward, reaching the symphysis in the region of the genial tubercles. While the distance between the genial tubercles and the lower border is short, the width of the mandible is greatest at the symphysis, affording considerable support. The inferior alveolar neurovascular canal (fig. 13.2) must also be taken into account. Any suspected involvement of the canal demands its total removal. This can generally be done without disarticulating the condyle (fig. 13.3).

It is impossible to anticipate all clinical situations. The surgeon must retain sufficient flexibility to assure control of the primary tumor. Several general guidelines, however, may be useful:

1. Tumor-free margins of 2 to 3 cm, depending on the site and the extent of the primary lesion, are desirable. The margins should be confirmed by frozen section before being accepted as adequate. Because the mandible is only involved by direct invasion through the periosteum, mandibular resection is not necessarily required to obtain adequate margins.
2. When the tumor is close to the mandible, but does not directly involve the periosteum, marginal resection may be performed.
3. Where the mandible has sufficient width, as in the region of the symphysis, it may be sectioned in the sagittal plane. Thus the cortical plate adjacent to the tumor (generally the lingual plate) may be removed in lieu of, or in conjunction with, a marginal resection.
4. When the tumor involves only the periosteum or the most superficial aspect of the underlying cortex, marginal resection or a local segmental resection may be performed.
5. When the tumor invades the spongiosa or the inferior alveolar canal, a segment extending from the mental foramen to the lingula (where the neurovascular bundle enters the mandible) should be resected. The transected neurovascular bundle should be checked by frozen section. It is rarely necessary to disarticulate the condyle. Furthermore, an intact condyle is invaluable for later reconstruction.

In all resections, it is desirable to leave a cuff of normal mucosa to cover the remaining bony margins. Various soft tissue defects will be created, depending upon the size and location of the primary tumor. Most of these defects will require closure with either local or distant flaps. Osteotomy cuts should be beveled lingually and inferiorly, and all sharp margins should be smoothed to prevent soft tissue dehiscence.

## Marginal Resection

Marginal resection (fig. 13.4) may be performed by either of two methods. The tumor and the underlying bone may be excised en bloc, leaving the remaining strut of mandible and its soft tissues undisturbed. This method offers the advantage of maintaining the periosteal blood supply to the mandible. Alternatively, the soft tissues may be stripped from the strut of bone that is to be preserved. This method offers the advantage of allowing the periosteum and the surface of the retained bone to be inspected for tumor (McGregor 1977). Normal periosteum strips easily, leaving a smooth bony surface. When there is tumor involvement, the periosteum is difficult to strip, and an irregular bony surface is left behind. The disadvantage of this method is that when the inferior alveolar blood vessels have been resected, loss of the periosteal blood supply can lead to aseptic necrosis of the retained strut of bone. Preoperative radiotherapy increases the likelihood of this complication.

## Mandibular Osteotomy

While the pull-through procedure permits removal of tumors that do not involve the mandible, in continuity with the neck contents, it has been criti-

**Figure 13.3**

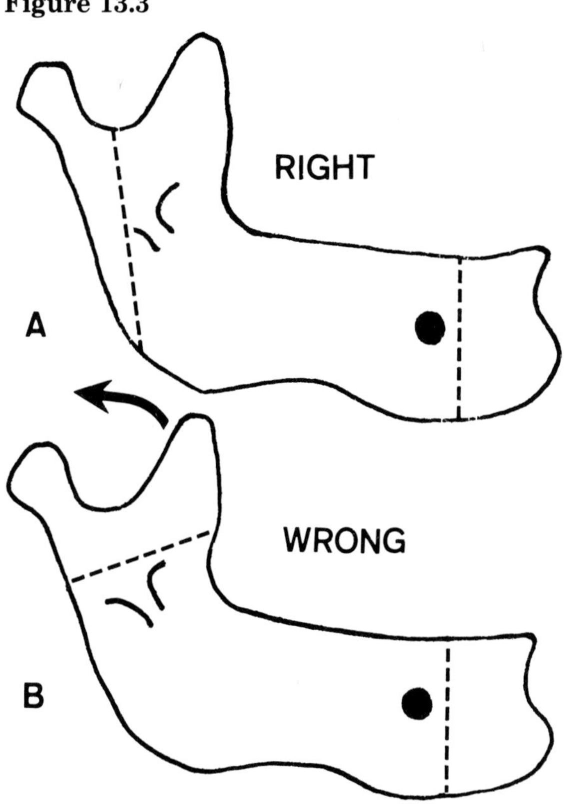


*Most mandibular resections can be done without disarticulating the condyle. Even when tumor has entered the inferior alveolar neurovascular canal, a segment running from the condyle to the angle is often safely retained. The line of resection should run vertically* (A) *so that the coronoid process is removed (see fig. 13.25). If a horizontal line of resection is used* (B), *the posterior fibers of the temporalis will pull the coronoid process up beneath the zygomatic arch (see fig. 13.7).*

**Figure 13.4**

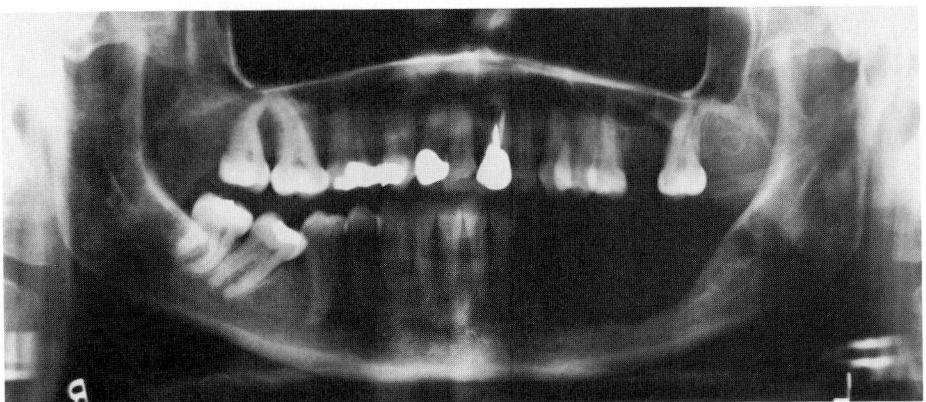

*Marginal mandibular resection gives adequate margins when tumor does not invade the periosteum. Mandibular continuity is maintained. If only a thin strut of the lower border is retained, bone grafting may be necessary to prevent stress fracture (see fig. 13.26).*

cized because of the poor surgical exposure it may afford (Conley 1967). Resection of a portion of the mandible need not be done solely for exposure, however, because of the ease with which an osteotomy can be performed.

The site of the osteotomy is governed by the location of the tumor and any remaining teeth. Lesions of the tongue and the floor of the mouth are best approached with an osteotomy at the symphysis. Lesions of the retromolar trigone, tonsil, or pharynx may require an osteotomy at the body or angle for optimal visualization. When there is a full complement of teeth, an extraction will be needed at the osteotomy site. Otherwise, edentulous areas may be used.

Mucosal incisions should be placed so that the final suture lines will not overlie the osteotomy. Mucosal flaps should be broadly based distal to the osteotomy site to insure an adequate blood supply.

The osteotomy is best given a step configuration, which aids in accurate repair and provides a broader surface area for healing. Posterior osteotomies should be given a "favorable" configuration so that the pull of the muscles of mastication tends to approximate the fragments rather than to distract them (fig. 13.5).

Posterior osteotomies will disrupt the inferior alveolar neurovascular bundle, resulting in numbness of the ipsilateral lower lip. If a thin saw blade is used with copious saline irrigation, sensation generally returns within a year.

The osteotomy should be repaired with stainless steel wire sutures. In the edentulous patient, this is all that is required. Patients with teeth should be placed in intermaxillary fixation from four to six weeks.

**Figure 13.5**

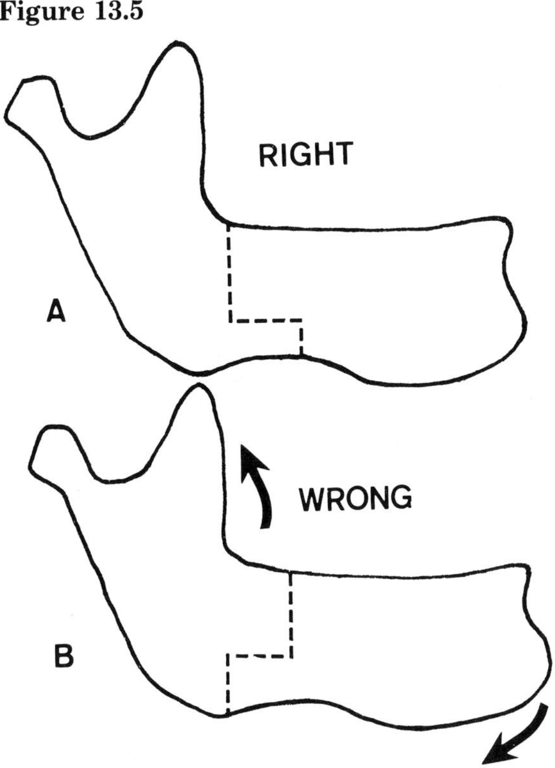


*A mandibular osteotomy improves surgical access in tumors of the posterior tongue, floor of mouth, tonsil, and retromolar trigone. The osteotomy should be stepped to insure an accurate repair. The step should be designed so that the pull of the muscles of mastication will tend to approximate the fragments* (A) *rather than distract them* (B).

## Controlling versus Disregarding Mandibular Fragments Following Resection

When a segment of the mandible has been resected, scar contracture and the unopposed pull of the muscles of mastication produce displacement of the remaining fragment(s). Such displacement serves to magnify the facial distortion and functional disability that are produced by the resection (fig. 13.6). Subsequent shortening and fibrosis of the mandibular musculature may severely limit the degree to which later reconstructive efforts can correct the deformity.

The anatomic relationships of the mandible are best maintained with a bone graft. Primary bone grafts can be hazardous, however, especially when there has been extensive soft tissue resection or preoperative radiotherapy.

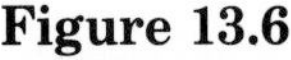

**Figure 13.6**

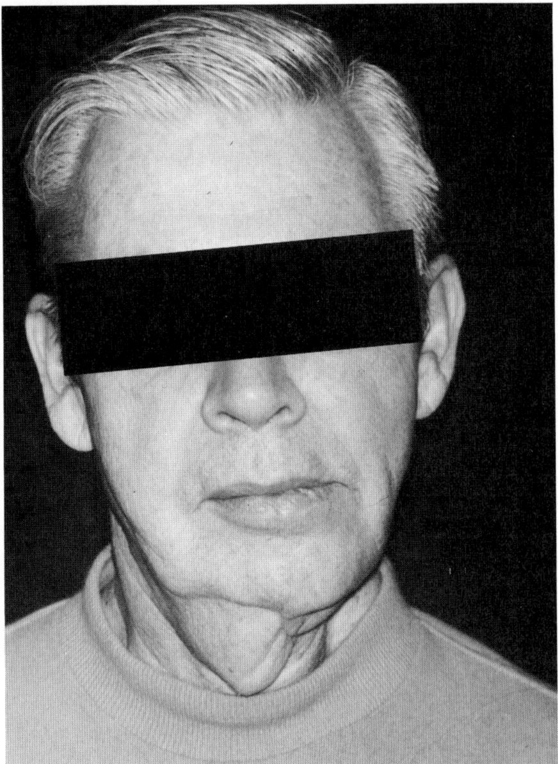

*Following resection of part of the left mandible, the major remaining fragment is displaced towards the defect. There is almost a full compliment of teeth, but they cannot come into occlusion (see fig. 13.30 for the reconstruction).*

This subject will be discussed later in more detail. More commonly, a prosthetic device is used to control the remaining mandibular fragment(s).

In a segmental resection where teeth are present on either side of the defect, either intermaxillary fixation or a dental splint may be used to maintain the proper relationship between the fragments. A splint is generally preferred, since it will permit function. Splints must be fabricated preoperatively and must allow the surgeon flexibility in performing the resection. They should not impinge upon mucosal surfaces or interfere with soft tissue flaps. A variety of cast cap splints, cast arch bars, cast metal or acrylic lingual splints, and orthodontic appliances have been used for this purpose.

When teeth are present on only one side of the defect, controlling the fragments is more difficult. If the occlusion of the remaining teeth is to be preserved, then their relationship with the maxillary teeth and with the temporomandibular joints must be precisely maintained. Various dental splints have been used for this purpose, but they have frequently been unsuccessful in stabilizing the edentulous fragment. The flange that fits upon the edentulous ridge may produce pressure necrosis of the underlying mucosa and may interfere with soft tissue flaps. Circummandibular wiring will increase stability, but at the expense of increasing pressure on the soft tissues and salivary contamination of the resection bed. Ideally, a rigid internal or external strut should be applied while the remaining teeth are in intermaxillary fixation. Such a strut can be created from a prosthetic implant or from an external pin fixation device. Both methods will be discussed later.

When the smaller mandibular fragment consists of only the condyle, attachment of a prosthetic strut is technically difficult, although occasionally possible. External pins generally cannot be placed. Often this fragment must be ignored (fig. 13.7), and only the major fragment is dealt with prior to reconstruction.

**Figure 13.7**

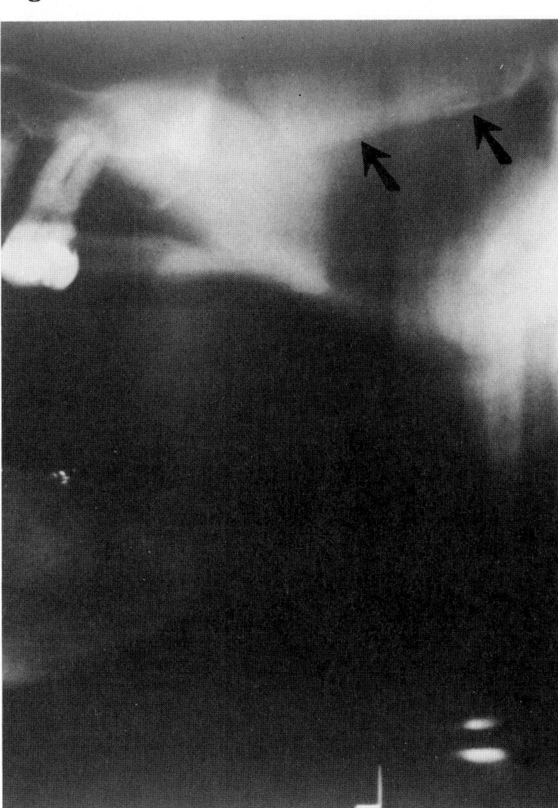

*Radiograph of the patient shown in figure 13.6. The condylar fragment* (arrows) *has been drawn up beneath the zygomatic arch because the coronoid process was not removed (see fig. 13.3).*

**Figure 13.8**

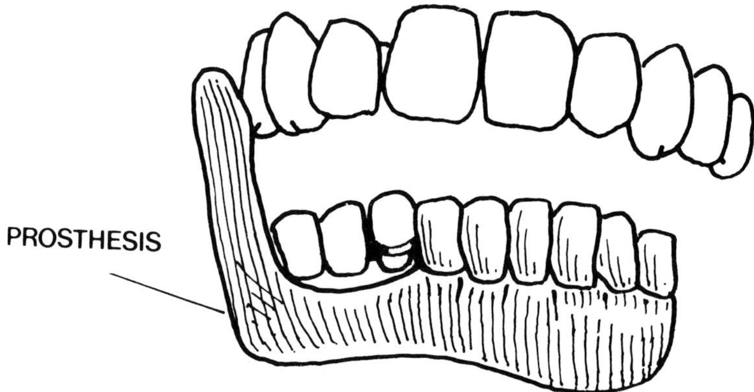


*Mandibular guide flange prosthesis. The left mandible has been resected. The vertical flange prevents medial deviation of the right mandible by maintaining contact with the buccal surfaces of the maxillary teeth.*

**Figure 13.9**

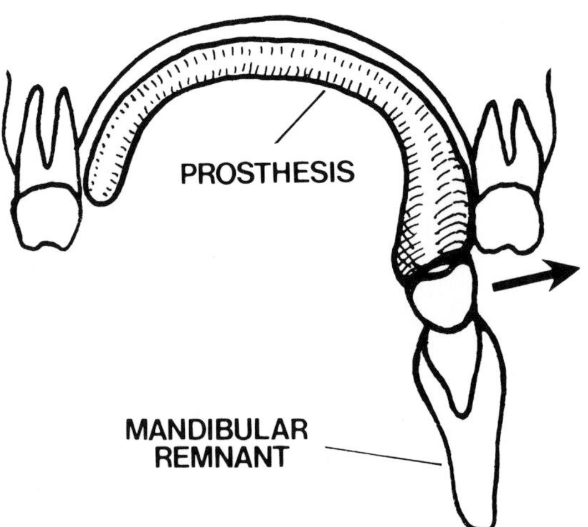


*Maxillary inclined plane prosthesis. The prosthesis is worn on the palatal aspect of the maxillary teeth. The remaining fragment of mandible is drawn medially by unbalanced muscular forces. As it is closed onto the inclined plane, a lateral component of force is generated* (arrow) *which brings it back into occlusion.*

In the case of "terminal" resections, where there has been disarticulation of one of the mandibular condyles, the presence of teeth on the remaining fragment is very helpful in controlling that fragment. Intermaxillary fixation is the simplest method of preventing distraction of the mandibular remnant. A guide flange prosthesis (fig. 13.8) permits the remnant to continue to function. The flange is attached to the buccal aspect of the mandibular teeth, and it extends vertically into the buccal sulcus alongside the maxillary teeth. As the mouth is opened, contact between the flange and the buccal surfaces of the maxillary teeth prevents deviation of the mandible. Finally, a maxillary inclined plane prosthesis (fig. 13.9) may be useful in encouraging the mandibular remnant to maintain occlusal contact. The occlusal incline runs from the palatal aspect of the maxillary teeth to their occlusal surfaces. As the medially-deviated mandibular remnant is closed, the principle of the inclined

**Figure 13.10**

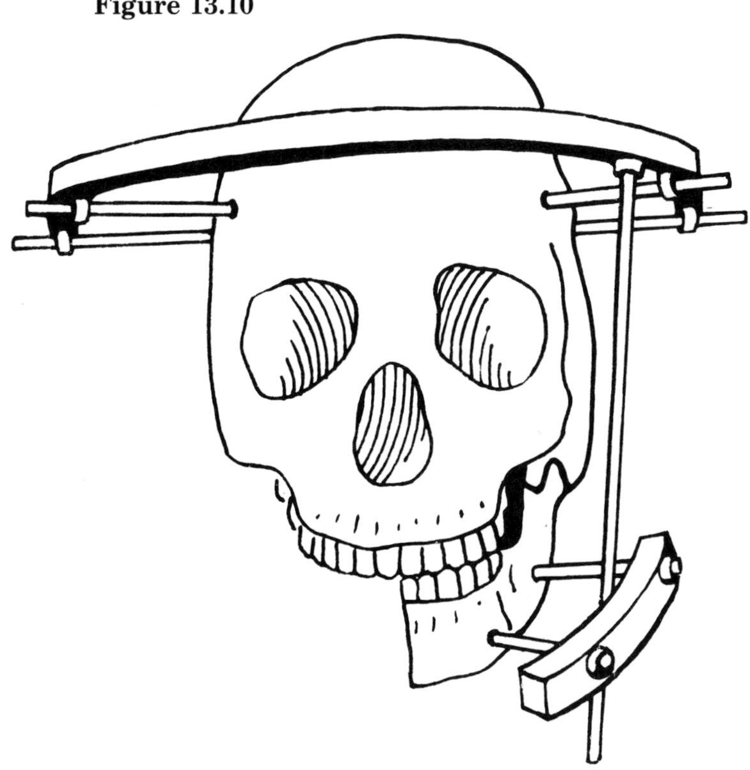

*Deviation of the mandibular remnant can be prevented by an external skeletal device. A vertical rod is attached to the head frame. During function, the rod contacts the inner surface of an acrylic bar that connects two mandibular pins. This technique is particularly useful in edentulous patients.*

plane produces a laterally-directed component of force that brings the teeth into contact.

Edentulous terminal resections are the most difficult to control. The only really effective method uses external skeletal pins in both the skull and the mandibular remnant (fig. 13.10). A vertical rod connected to the cranial pins is placed on the inner surface of a horizontal rod connected to the mandibular pins. This prevents medial displacement of the mandible when the mouth is opened.

## Prosthetic Implants

Biocompatible implants have long appealed to surgeons desiring to reconstruct the mandible. Despite numerous favorable preliminary reports, time and the stress of function have brought to light the same serious disadvan-

**Figure 13.11**

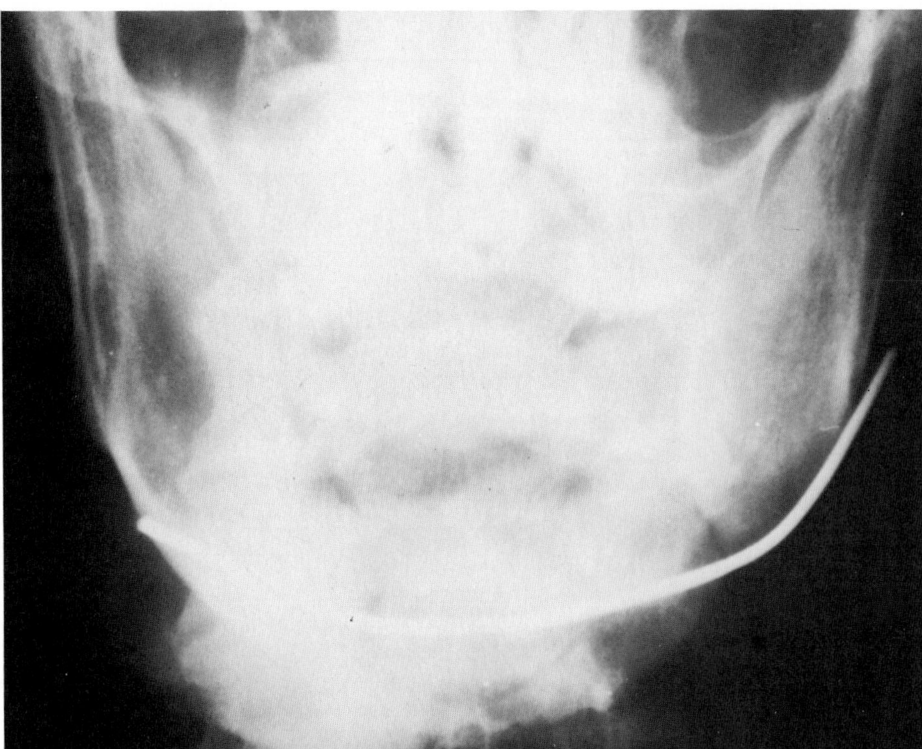

*A stainless steel wire is easily inserted, contoured, and removed. It adequately maintains the anatomic relationships of the mandibular fragments prior to definitive reconstruction with a bone graft.*

tage in all of them: they do not become incorporated by the host tissues, and they are, therefore, subject to failure at the biologic-prosthetic interface. This leads to loosening and extrusion. The best results reported in several large series (Benoist 1978; Bowerman 1974; Terz et al. 1978; Towers and Wilson 1974) are no better than the results of primary bone grafting (Millard et al. 1969). Implants should thus be reserved for use as temporary space-maintainers in most instances.

Prosthetic implants range from simple stainless steel wires, plates, or mesh to more sophisticated customized devices fabricated from titanium, Vitallium, tantalum, ticonium, Silastic, Teflon, polymethyl methacrylate, and metallo-plastic composites. When the purpose of the implant is to act as a temporary spacer that will ultimately be replaced by a bone graft, simplicity is of some advantage. It should be easily altered at surgery to fit the needs of the individual patient, and it should be easily inserted and removed using a minimum of specialized equipment. In most instances, threaded wires and small bone plates fulfill these criteria adequately (fig. 13.11) and are preferred over more complex prostheses.

**Figure 13.12**

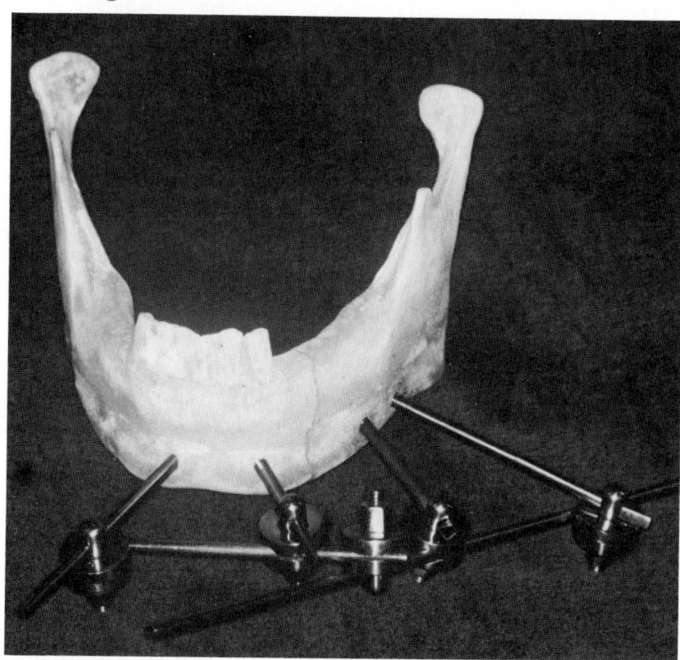

*Modified Roger Anderson appliance for mandibular fixation. The apparatus is unwieldy. The projecting ends of connecting rods may catch in clothing or strike objects or people in the environment. The universal joints must be tightened at intervals.*

## External Skeletal Fixation

Rigid external skeletal fixation devices, making use of pins or bone screws in the major fragments, have been used in the treatment of fractures of the long bones since the end of the nineteenth century (Parkhill 1897). The method attained popularity after Anderson (1936) standardized the technique and the armamentarium in the 1930s (fig. 13.12).

Further development of the method by Morris (1949) eliminated the bulk and unwieldiness and greatly increased the versatility by replacing the joints and connecting bars with a smooth, lightweight bar of cold-cure acrylic (fig. 13.13). Patients accept this device readily and have no difficulty in caring for it at home. Its use in treating avulsive injuries of the mandible led directly to application in the management of mandibular resections (fig. 13.14) (Fleming and Morris 1969).

**Figure 13.13**

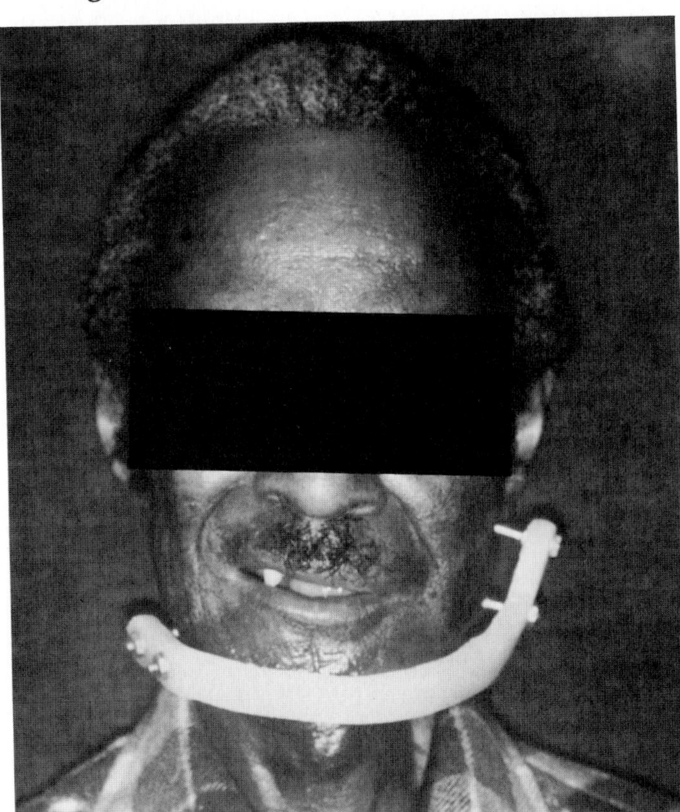

*Morris mandibular splint. The four bone screws are connected by a rigid, lightweight acrylic bar. The contour is smooth, and there are no sharp projections.*

**Figure 13.14**

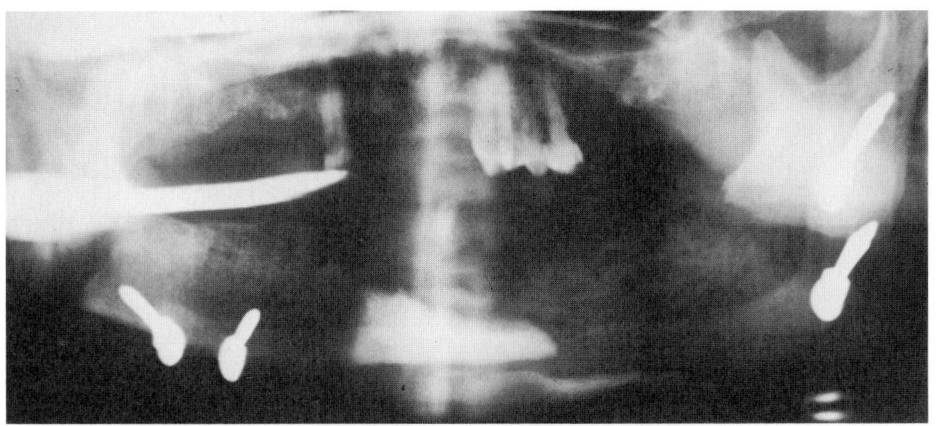

*X-ray of patient shown in figure 13.13. Most of the left mandible has been resected. Anatomic relationships and facial form have been maintained. The long radiopacity on the patient's right is a technical artifact.*

Placement of the Morris appliance is simple. Two bone screws are placed in each mandibular fragment through small incisions. It is important to tap to the minor diameter of the screws so that the bone between the turns is not subject to pressure necrosis. With viable bone between the turns, the screws can remain in place for many months without loosening. If the resection has been performed already, universal joints and connecting rods are attached to the screws temporarily to hold the mandibular fragments in the proper position. The acrylic bar is then prepared and adapted to the screws while it is still pliable. After the heat of polymerization has dissipated, the temporary mechanical splint is removed. If the limits of resection can be reliably determined prior to surgery, the splint may be placed before the resection is performed. This eliminates the need for the temporary mechanical splint and allows the mandibular fragments to remain precisely in their preoperative relationship. It may, however, limit surgical access and impede retraction. Morris has designed a kit (Walter Lorenz Surgical Instruments, Inc., Jacksonville, Florida), which greatly facilitates use of this method of fixation.

While certain clinical situations clearly call for external skeletal fixation, the simplicity and versatility of the splint make it useful in many circumstances where other means of fixation could be used. The screws are placed distant from the surgical site, thus preventing them from introducing infection or causing delayed healing. The mouth and surgical defect are left free of all apparatus so that there is no danger of impinging upon soft tissue flaps. The acrylic bar can be molded as necessary to avoid tubes, drains, or flaps and to provide access for secondary procedures. The strength of the splint permits the patient to function after surgery and thereby inhibits muscle contracture (fig. 13.15). Finally, the long-term stability of the splint permits it to remain firmly in place for as long as one to two years. This allows

**Figure 13.15**

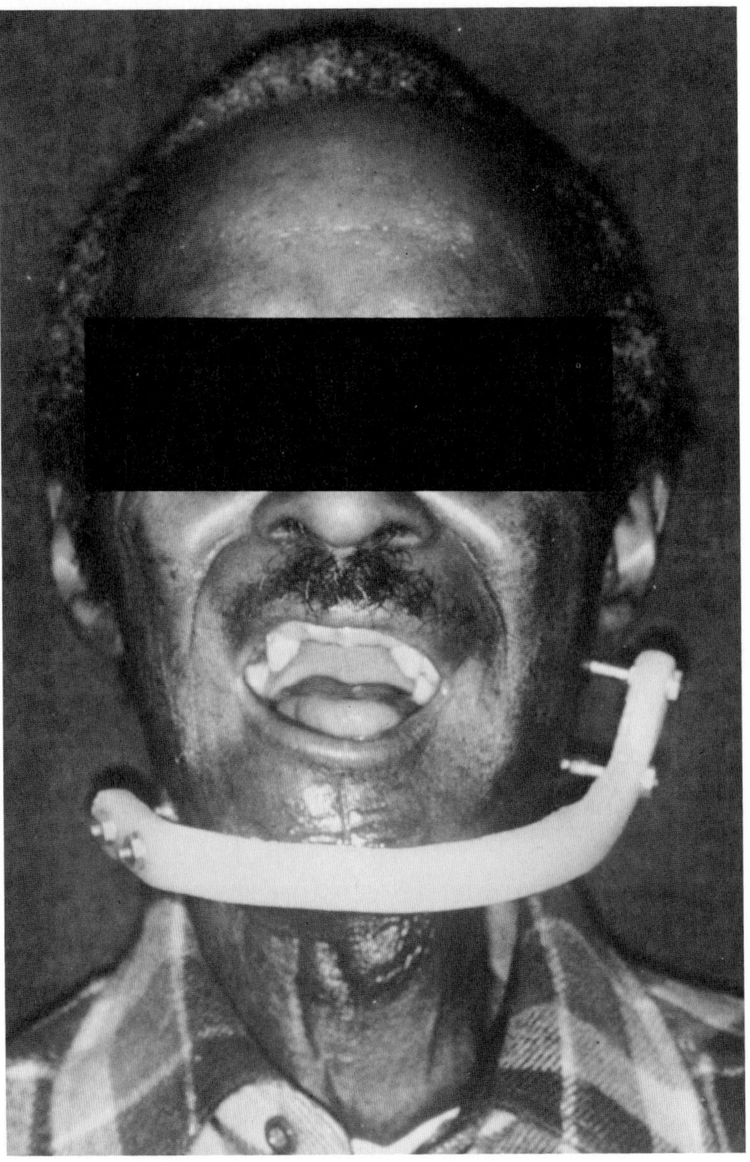

*Same patient shown in figure 13.13. There is no trismus or deviation on opening.*

secondary reconstruction to be delayed as necessary, while a great degree of lower facial form and function are maintained—a particular advantage for patients who retain a large complement of teeth. Once bone grafting has been accomplished, no additional fixation is generally needed.

## Primary Soft Tissue Closure versus Reconstruction

Surgical resection for oral carcinoma involves the removal of large areas of mucous membrane, and occasionally skin, in addition to bone and neck contents. Considerable morbidity can result from inadequate soft tissue reconstruction following such radical surgery. If mandibular reconstruction is to be performed, whether primarily or secondarily, it is possible only with adequate soft tissue coverage. Rarely will a tension-free primary closure be possible without distortion of normal anatomic relationships.

**Figure 13.16**

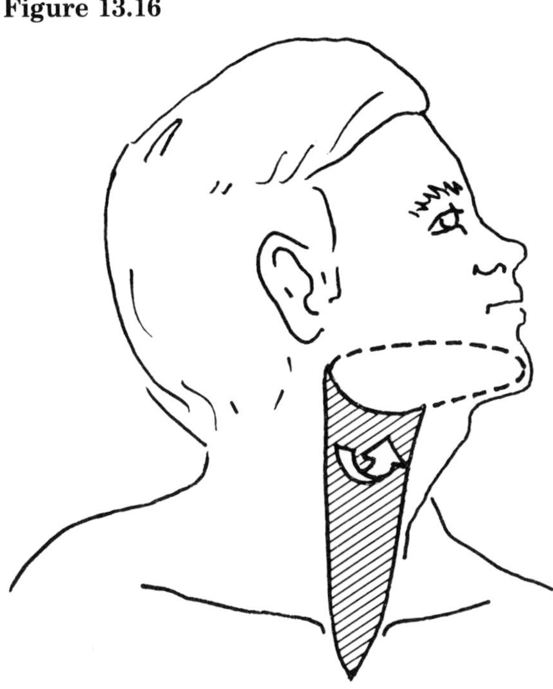

*Cervical flaps can be turned under to provide lining. Their usefulness is limited in irradiated necks or if there has been a radical neck dissection.*

## Local Mucosal Flaps

Mucosal flaps are random local flaps. While they provide the same type of tissue as that which has been resected, they are limited in size. Tongue and buccal mucosa are the most suitable donor sites.

Tongue flaps are the most versatile of these flaps because of their mobility and excellent blood supply (Chambers, Jaques, and Mahoney 1969). Small

**Figure 13.17**

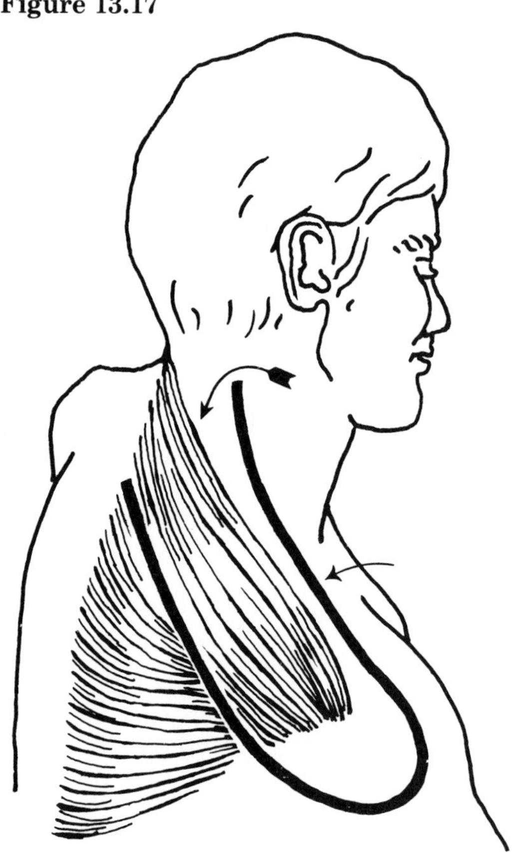

*Shoulder flaps are based on the mastoid-occipital area. They can be elevated to the level of the mid-clavicle* (short arrow) *without delay. The vascular supply can be increased by elevating the nuchal portion of the trapezius muscle* (long arrow) *with the flap. This produces a trapezius myocutaneous flap.*

defects may be covered by flaps elevated from the dorsal, ventral, or lateral surfaces and based either anteriorly or posteriorly. A disadvantage of the tongue flap is the possibility of its pulling loose during swallowing or other muscular activity.

## Local Skin Flaps

Many random regional flaps of neck and shoulder skin (figs. 13.16 and 13.17) may be used to line the oral cavity or to provide skin coverage (Bakamjian and Littlewood 1964; Edgerton and Des Prez 1957; Robson et al. 1976; Zovickian 1957). They can generally be constructed with a length to width ratio of 3 to 1; the use of fluorescein is a prudent measure to assess viability of the distal portions.

## Axial (Arterialized) Flaps

Axial pattern flaps offer many advantages to the reconstructive surgeon. They can be elevated without delay, unless it is desired to extend them beyond the vascular territory of their nutrient arteries. They may be designed with a large length-to-width ratio. Careful dissection of a narrow vascular pedicle can produce a wide arc of rotation. Segmental deepithelialization can

**Figure 13.18**

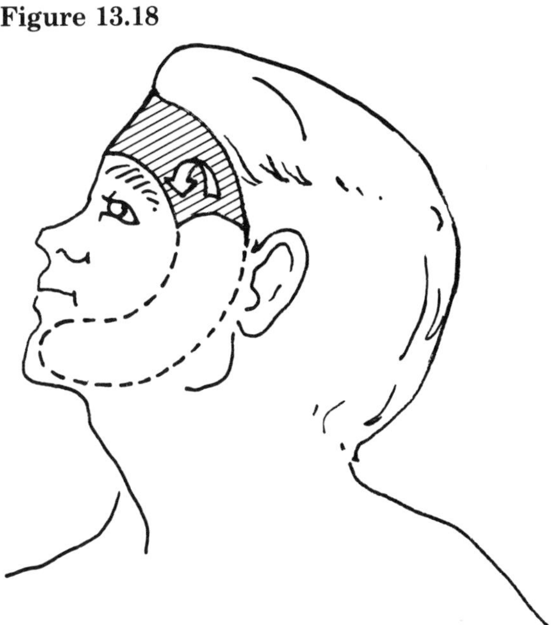

*The forehead flap can be used to line all areas of the oral cavity. It is based on the superficial temporal artery.*

permit the same flap to replace both skin and mucosa or can permit the proximal segment of the flap to be buried, thus avoiding an orocutaneous fistula and a second procedure for division of the flap.

The forehead flap (fig. 13.18) (McGregor 1963), deltopectoral flap (fig. 13.19) (Bakamjian 1965), cervicohumeral flap (fig. 13.20) (Mathes and Vasconez 1978), nasolabial flap (fig. 13.21) (Cohen and Edgerton 1971), and palatal island flap (Gullane and Arena 1977) are examples of axial flaps that are useful in head and neck reconstruction.

**Figure 13.19**

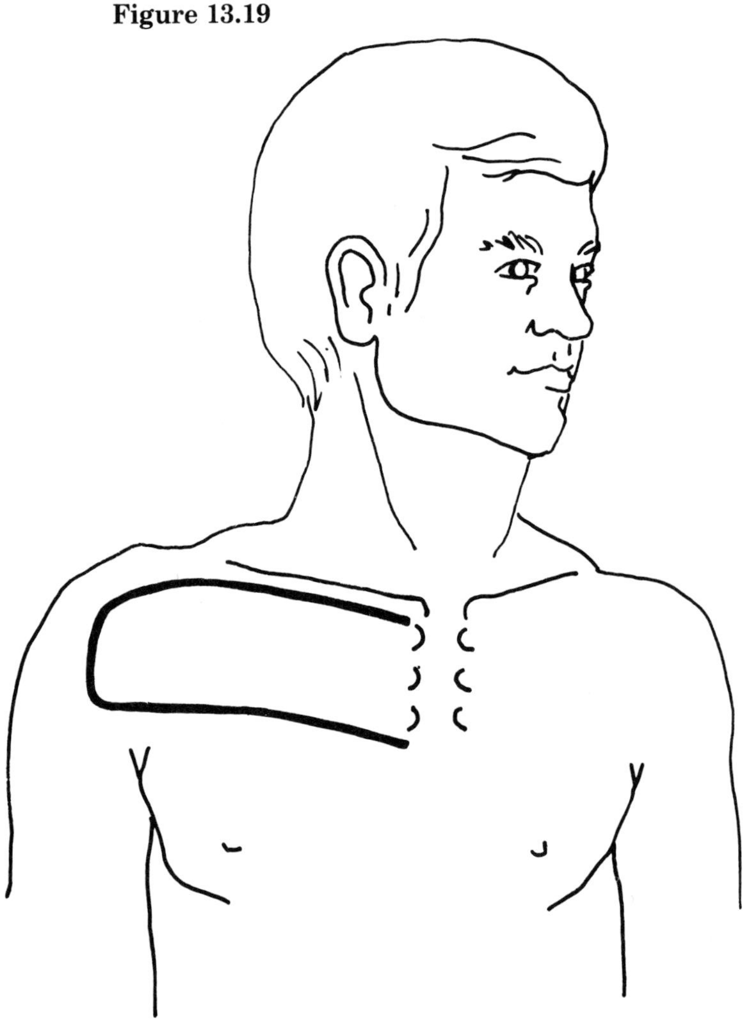

*The deltopectoral flap can be used to line all areas of the oral cavity. It is based on intercostal perforators of the internal mammary artery.*

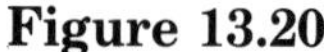

**Figure 13.20**

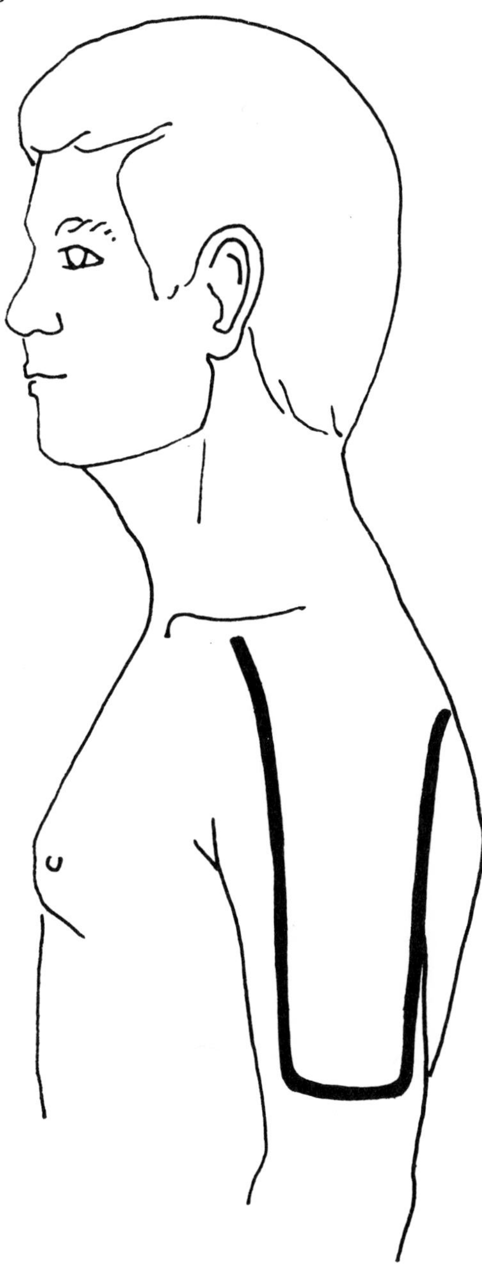

*The cervicohumeral flap can be used to line all areas of the oral cavity. It is based on the transverse cervical artery.*

**Figure 13.21**

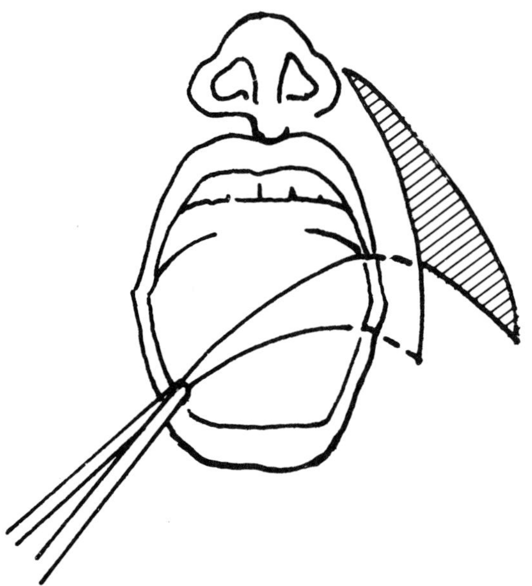

*The nasolabial flap, when based inferiorally, is supplied by the facial artery. It can be used to line small defects of the floor of the mouth.*

## Myocutaneous Flaps

In compound skin-muscle flaps (McCraw, Dibbell, and Carraway 1977), the muscle acts as a carrier for the cutaneous portion of the flap. Many muscles have a single dominant vascular supply that will permit them to survive when all other vessels are ligated. The skin overlying such muscles is perfused by perforating vessels and can therefore be elevated with the muscle. The flap may be detached completely, except for the dominant vascular pedicle, forming an island myocutaneous flap. The cutaneous portion of the flap may be extended beyond the vascular territory of the perforating vessels if it is delayed. Two cutaneous segments may be designed so that both skin and mucosa can be replaced by the same flap. The muscular portion of the flap provides bulk for filling large defects. Since the vascular pedicle is not secondarily divided, the flap is capable of bringing new vascularity into areas of radiation necrosis (Brown, Fryer, and McDowell 1951).

The pectoralis major (fig. 13.22) (Ariyan 1979), sternomastoid (fig. 13.23) (Owens 1955), trapezius (fig. 13.17) (McCraw, Dibbell, and Carraway 1977), and platysma (fig. 13.24) (Futrell et al. 1978) myocutaneous flaps are useful in head and neck reconstruction.

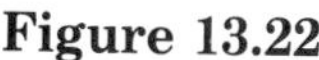

**Figure 13.22**

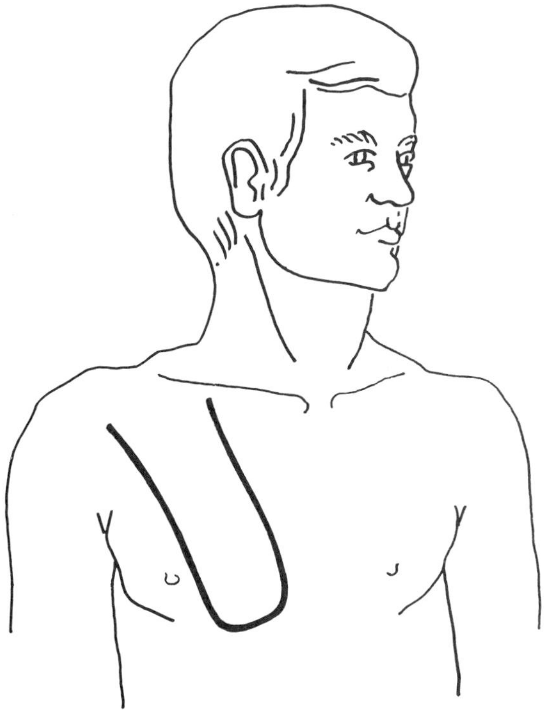

*The pectoralis major myocutaneous flap. Any part of the outlined area of skin can be carried by a thin segment of underlying muscle with its axial blood supply from the thoracoacromial artery. It can be used to line all areas of the oral cavity.*

## Free Flaps

Recent advances in microsurgery have permitted the transfer to distant sites of free composite flaps by microvascular anastomosis. There are many theoretical advantages to this type of flap transfer: it is accomplished in a single stage; donor sites can be chosen that minimize cosmetic deformity; and an orocutaneous fistula is avoided. Nevertheless, the role of the free flap in head and neck reconstruction has yet to be fully defined.

Despite occasional reports (Harashina, Fujino, and Aoyagi 1976; Panje, Bardach, and Krause 1976) of clinical successes, the few reported (Finseth, Kavarana, and Antia 1975) and many unreported failures of free flaps in the region of the oral cavity signal caution. Free flaps in the oral cavity are difficult to observe postoperatively for signs of vascular insufficiency; they are subject to salivary contamination, with inflammation and thrombosis of vessels (Ackland 1979). Further advances will be necessary if this technique is to supplant the methods for soft tissue reconstruction discussed previously.

**Figure 13.23**

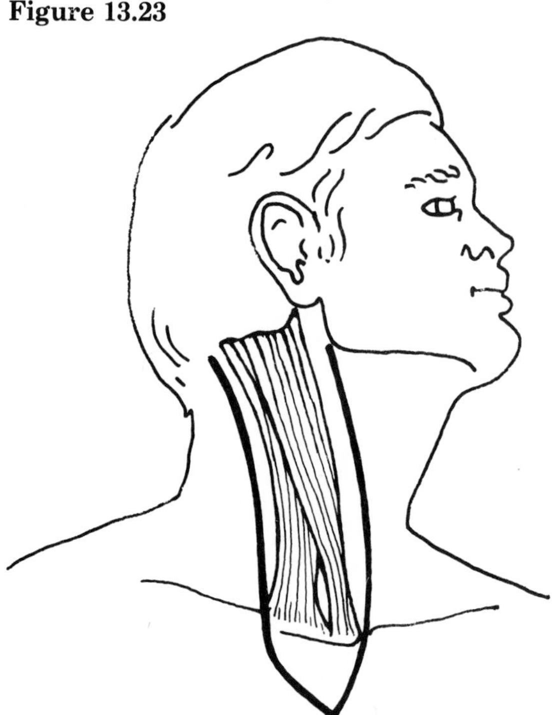

*The sternomastoid myocutaneous flap utilizes skin from the neck and upper chest. It can be used to line all areas of the oral cavity.*

# Preoperative versus Postoperative Radiotherapy

Combining the modality of radiotherapy with surgery in the treatment of head and neck cancer has vastly improved survival. Tumors may exhibit microscopic spread beyond resection margins. By controlling such micrometastases, radiotherapy increases control of the primary site (Perez, Marks, and Powers 1977). Moreover, radiotherapy is also effective in controlling subclinical metastases to the cervical lymph nodes (Berger et al. 1971). Recommendations for the dose of radiation, the timing relative to surgery, and the volume of tissue to be treated vary widely. Preoperative radiotherapy is more commonly used at present.

## Preoperative Radiotherapy

The rationale for planned preoperative radiotherapy is to control micrometastatic disease and to render any tumor cells that are released into the operative site or the circulation at the time of surgery incapable of implantation. Preoperative radiotherapy, however, results in an increase in both major and minor surgical complications (Flynn 1977; Joseph and Shumrick 1973).

**Figure 13.24**

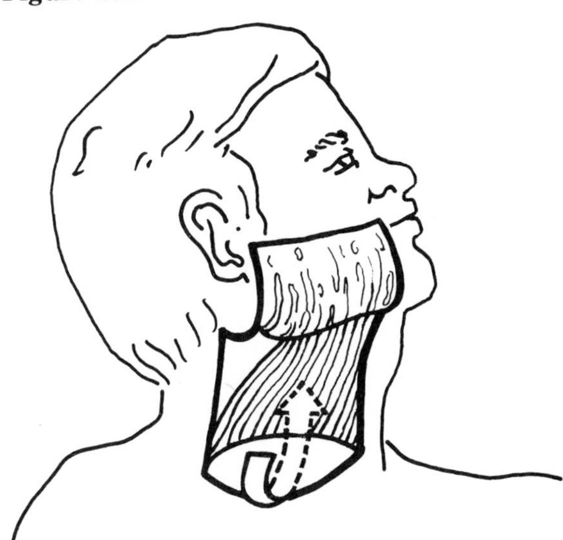

*The platysma myocutaneous flap is an island myocutaneous flap which utilizes skin from the lower neck. It can be used to line the cheek and lateral floor of mouth. It should be used with caution in irradiated necks.*

Following radiotherapy, the condition of the local soft tissues may be unfavorable for the support of a bone graft.

## Postoperative Radiotherapy

The rationale for planned postoperative radiotherapy is to control residual or micrometastatic disease following surgical extirpation of the tumor. Therapy is begun as soon as the surgical wound has healed. Fewer complications are encountered than with equal doses of preoperative radiation (Vanderbrouck et al. 1977). Higher doses than are normally given preoperatively may be well tolerated postoperatively (Donald 1978).

Preliminary data (Schwartz 1979) indicate that mandibular bone grafting may be successfully carried out in combination with postoperative radiotherapy (fig. 13.25).

# Cortical versus Cancellous Bone Grafts

Autogenous bone is the preferred material for most skeletal reconstruction. It is incorporated by the host tissues and is mechanically sound. Most importantly, bone grafting works.

In the process of bone grafting, the transplant assumes both an active

**Figure 13.25**

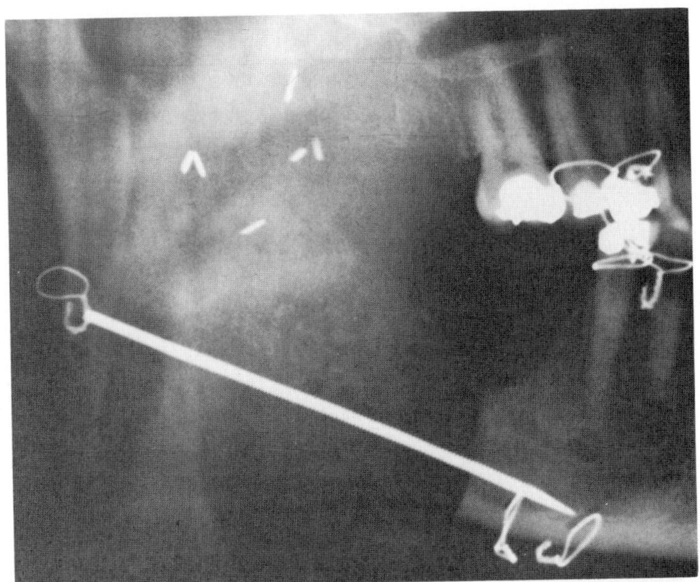

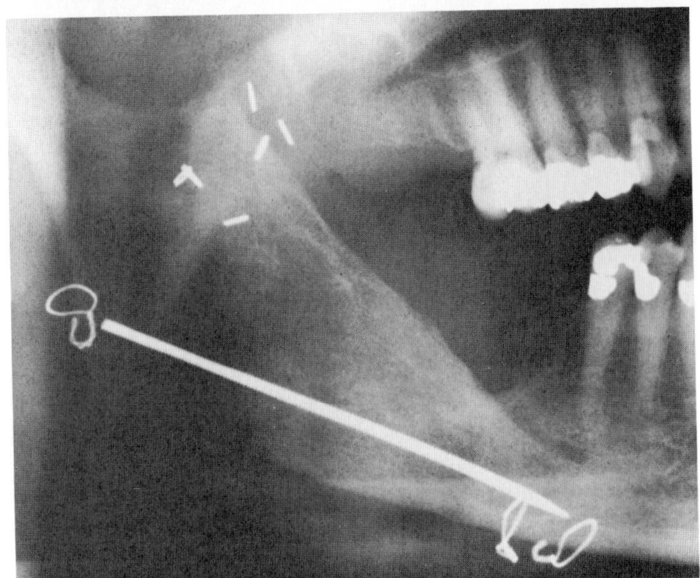

Top, *immediate postoperative radiograph of a mandible reconstructed by the technique illustrated in figure 13.31. Note that this patient received 5000 rad postoperative radiotherapy.* Bottom, *the same area after one year. There is excellent incorporation of the graft with effacement of the host-graft interface and a normal trabecular pattern.*

and a passive role. The active role involves the survival of cells with osteogenic potential in the transplant and the induction of cells with osteogenic potential in the host. Thus new bone originates from both transplanted and host tissues (Arora and Laskin 1964). The passive role is that of a template, which is resorbed and ultimately replaced by viable new bone (Boyne 1970).

Cortical bone grafts are revascularized slowly (Enneking et al. 1975). Only scattered surface cells survive transplantation. There are few interstices for the ingrowth of host tissues. Interior areas may remain non-viable for many years. Subject to irregular, often unfavorable remodelling, cortical bone grafts are not infrequently clinical failures (Gregory 1972).

Cancellous bone grafts are rapidly revascularized (Abbott et al. 1947). The large surface area presented by the open marrow spaces permits many cells to survive transplantation. Grafted bone marrow contributes many cells with osteogenic potential (Burwell 1964). The individual spicules of grafted bone are completely resorbed and replaced by viable new bone.

Allogenic bone may be treated by various means to reduce its antigenicity. Despite occasional reports (Pike and Boyne 1974) of the successful use of banked bone in reconstruction of the mandible, its clinical usefulness is still being debated. With the ready availability of sufficient autogenous bone for most mandibular reconstructions, further developments in immunosuppression and in the reduction of antigenicity will be necessary before the routine use of allogenic bone may be contemplated for anything but major limb reconstruction.

As has been mentioned above, cancellous bone grafts offer certain advantages over cortical bone grafts. Mowlem (1944) came to recognize this through the fortunate circumstance of having shattered a solid block of ilium that he had been sculpting to replace a hemimandible. Although he inserted the separate pieces with some reluctance, the result was so good that he soon found himself routinely fragmenting bone grafts to expose the cancellous surfaces. Clinical application of cancellous bone grafting to the mandible is, however, frought with technical problems—the graft can take no part in stabilizing the remaining mandibular fragments, and the particles of cancellous bone seek a dependent position in the surgical wound. Fibrous union frequently results (Anlyan and Manis 1968). Boyne (1970) improved the technique with his development of a Vitallium tray, which gives stability and imposes the complex mandibular contours upon the amorphous mass of cancellous bone particles. Simultaneously, the tray provides internal fixation for the remaining fragments of the mandible.

Solid cortico-cancellous bone grafts offer many of the advantages of both cortical and cancellous grafts. The donor bone is split in such a way that one surface of the graft is a solid cortical plate, while the opposite surface consists of cancellous bone from the medullary region. Such a graft can be stabilized by the routine techniques used for fracture fixation (fig. 13.26). The exposed cancellous surface favors rapid revascularization and incorporation of the graft (fig. 13.27).

**Figure 13.26**

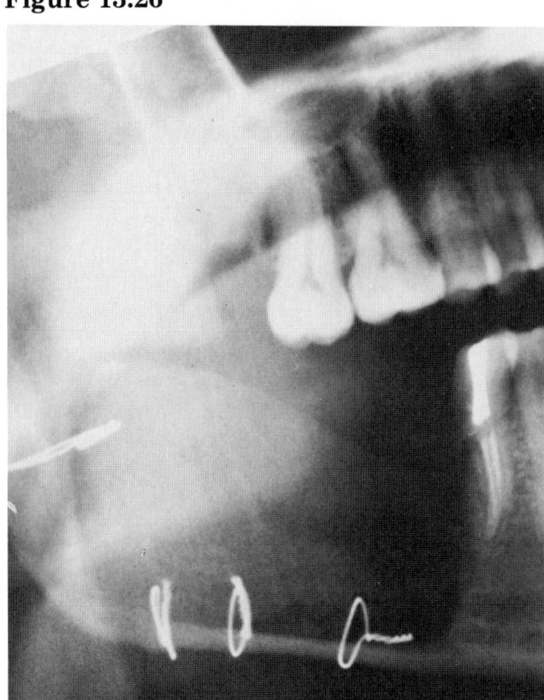

*A cortico-cancellous iliac bone graft is wired into the defect resulting from a radical marginal mandibular resection. Any deficiencies along the host-graft interface are packed with cancellous bone chips.*

It should be added that solid, full-thickness, vascularized bone grafts have been transferred to the mandible, either as part of a composite flap (Conley 1972) or by free transfer using microvascular anastomosis (Serafin, Villarreal-Rios, Georgiade 1977). These can be lengthy procedures requiring multiple stages. There is considerable donor site morbidity, as compared with routine bone grafts. Either rib or clavicle may be used, but neither can replace highly contoured areas of the mandible successfully. Thus these grafts are suited only for straight segmental reconstructions. Since routine methods are highly effective for such reconstructions, use of these techniques hardly seems justified at the present time.

## Donor Sites

The ilium is the best source for cancellous bone. Either the lateral or the medial cortical plate may be exposed above the anterior superior spine. A craniotome is then used to perforate the cortical bone in multiple overlapping sites so that cancellous bone can be scooped from the medullary cavity with a curette. This technique (Schwartz and Leake 1979) is accomplished very

**Figure 13.27**

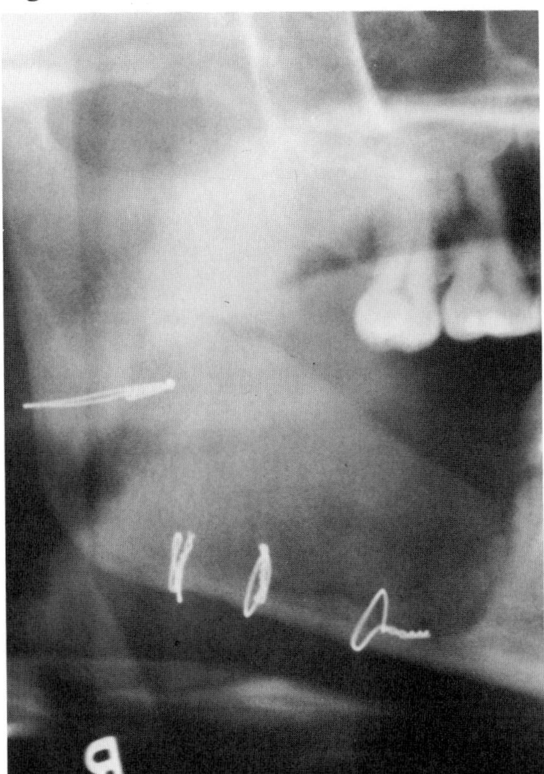

*Same case as figure 13.26. After one year, there is effacement of the host-graft interfaces. A normal trabecular pattern is visible in the area of the graft.*

rapidly as compared with methods that require the creation of a large window in the cortical plate. There is no resultant deformity if the iliac crest is left intact. A strong repair of the fascia lata assures an early return to normal ambulation.

The ilium is also the preferred source for large cortico-cancellous blocks. The required shape is best outlined in the cortical plate with one of the micro bone saws. A thin, curved osteotome is used to cleave the cortical plate and the underlying cancellous bone from the deep cortical plate. Penetration of both cortical plates should be avoided, as the underlying soft tissues may be injured. After the cortico-cancellous block of bone is removed, additional cancellous bone should be curetted from the medullary cavity. This is used to pack any small gaps between the transplant and the host bone (see figs. 13.26 and 13.27).

Split ribs are useful for highly contoured cortico-cancellous bone grafts, such as in the region of the mandibular symphysis. The right eighth, ninth, or tenth ribs may be approached through an inframammary incision. The incision is extended to the posterior axillary line if necessary. It is prudent to

**Figure 13.28**

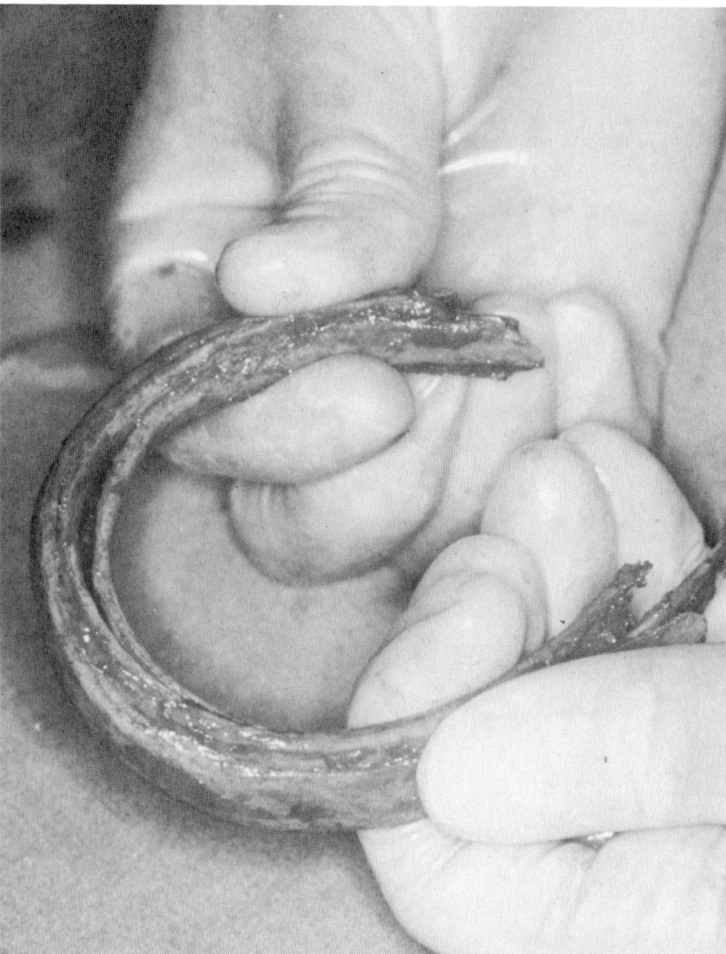

*Four cortico-cancellous laminae of split ribs have sufficient bulk and contour to reconstruct the symphysis and both horizontal rami.*

remove alternate ribs if more than one is required for the reconstruction. Care is taken to prevent penetration of the pleura as the rib is being removed. If this occurs, however, an airtight closure can generally be performed, and a chest tube is rarely needed. Resuturing of the periosteum often permits the rib to regenerate. To prepare the rib, the superior and inferior cortical bone is burred away. It is then easily split into two cortico-cancellous segments, using a thin osteotome. These grafts can be given considerable contour with bone-bending forceps, but they have little bulk. It is wise to use at least four thicknesses to prevent a stress fracture in the graft (fig. 13.28).

## Intermaxillary versus Monomaxillary Fixation Following Bone Grafting

Rigid intermaxillary fixation is not a requirement for union of mandibular bone grafts. The only absolute indication for intermaxillary fixation is for precise restoration of the occlusion when natural teeth remain in both maxillary and mandibular arches. If the bone graft is properly stabilized, patients who are edentulous, who have teeth in only one arch, or whose remaining teeth do not have a functional occlusion can generally be treated without intermaxillary fixation. Moreover, the splints that are used to immobilize edentulous jaws may serve to introduce oral contamination, either via circum-mandibular wires or by causing pressure necrosis of underlying mucous membranes.

## Metallic versus Nonmetallic Trays in Mandibular Reconstruction

The routine use of cancellous bone for mandibular reconstruction has become possible with the introduction of biocompatible trays which provide stability

**Figure 13.29**

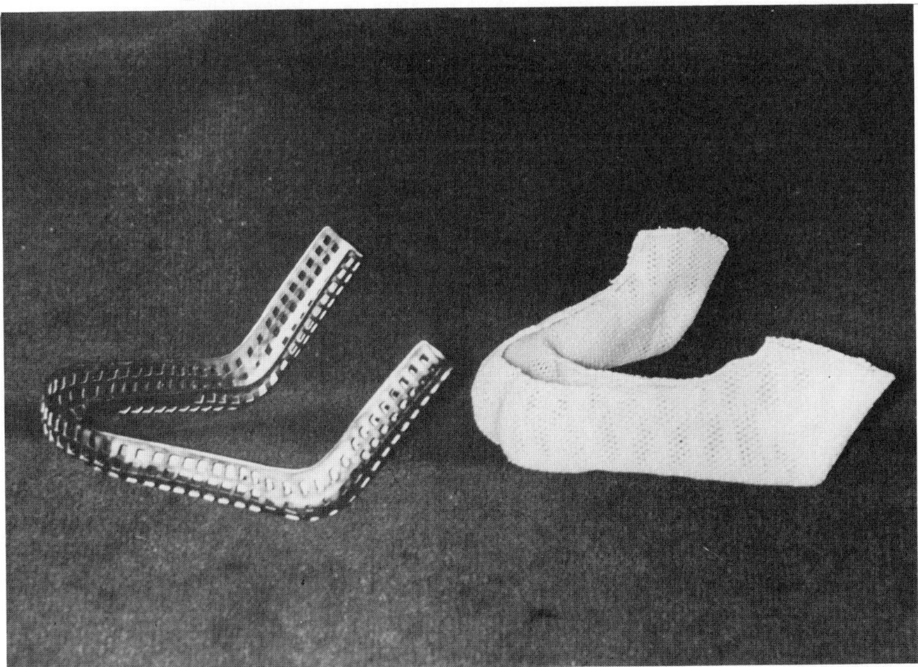

*Mandibular trays. A metallic prosthesis is pictured on the left and a Dacron/urethane prosthesis on the right.*

and impose anatomic form upon the amorphous mass of bone chips. Trays of titanium, Vitallium, tantalum, stainless steel, and a polyurethane-coated Dacron cloth mesh have been used for this purpose (fig. 13.29).

The technique combines the major advantages of grafting with autogenous cancellous bone with the minor disadvantages of implanting a prosthesis.

**Figure 13.30**

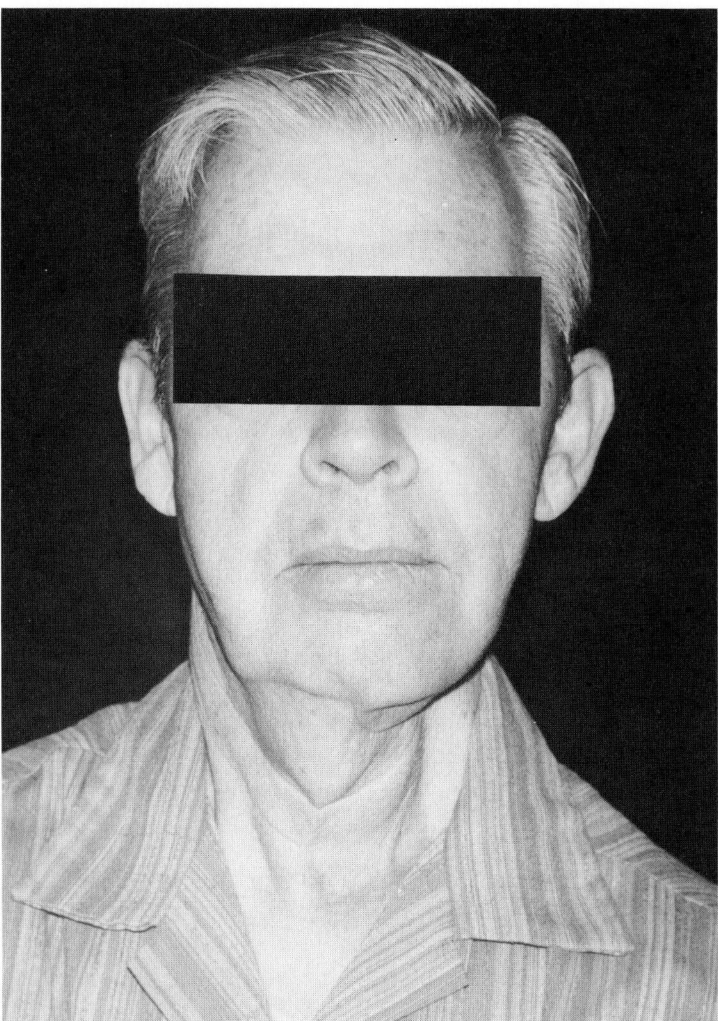

Left, *same patient as figure 13.6. He had undergone 7000 rad preoperative radiotherapy. After reconstruction with a cancellous bone graft in a Dacron/urethane tray, facial symmetry and the dental occlusion have been restored.*

The graft is rapidly replaced by viable new bone which assumes the shape of the tray. This produces a mandibular reconstruction that has optimal morphologic and mechanical characteristics (fig. 13.30). It is the preferred technique in most clinical situations.

All of the materials used to produce prosthetic mandibular trays have long histories of safe use in human implantation. The Dacron/urethane tray (Reyer-Schulte Corp., Goleta, California) developed by Leake (1974) (fig.

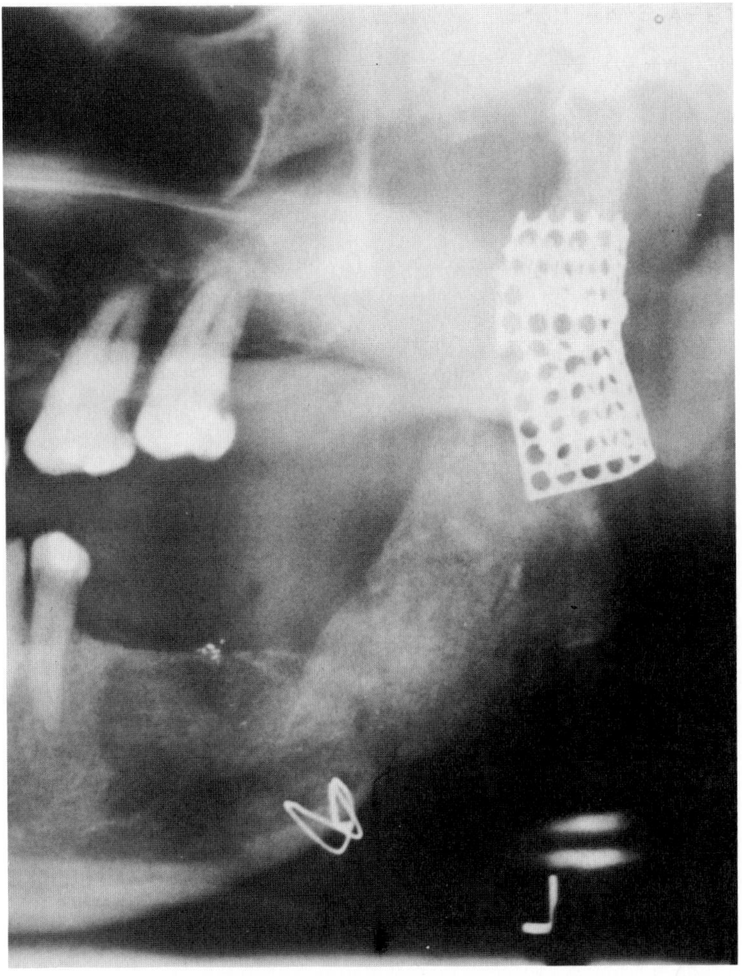

Right, *radiograph taken one year after reconstruction shows good incorporation of the graft. The condyle, which was in poor position and densely fibrosed (see fig. 13.7), was removed and replaced as a free graft. A small piece of Vitallium mesh was used to attach the condyle to the posterior border of the Dacron/urethane tray.*

**Figure 13.31**

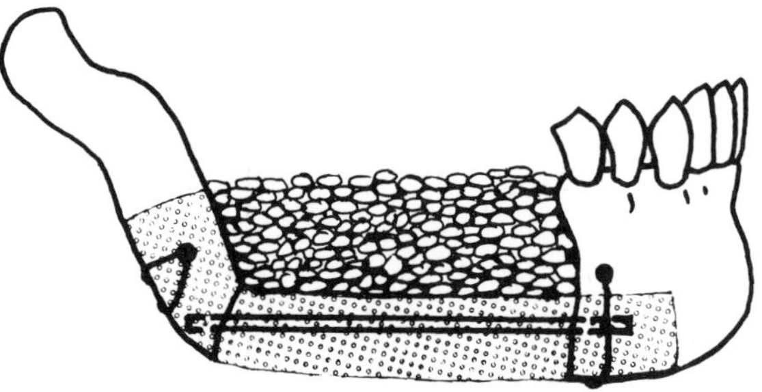

*Mandibular reconstruction using a Dacron/urethane tray. A Kirchner wire bridges the defect and provides extra stability, permitting the Dacron/urethane mesh to be trimmed back. The tray is fixed to host bone with ordinary surgical steel wire. Wires may be placed either around or through the mesh. The tray is tightly packed with cancellous bone chips; care is taken to pack around and below the Kirchner wire. After the tray is full, bone chips are packed above it to the desired height of the alveolar ridge.*

13.31) has proved to have many advantages over the metal trays. It can be custom-fabricated for individual cases and is easily adaptable in the operating room to the needs of a particular reconstruction. The Dacron/urethane tray requires no special armamentarium for insertion—it can be trimmed with scissors and affixed to the host bone with ordinary surgical steel wire. It is radiolucent, permitting unimpaired monitoring of grafts with radiographs or radionuclide scans (see figs. 13.25 and 13.30). There are no sharp edges to produce dehiscence of overlying soft tissues. The material does not significantly alter the dose when postoperative radiotherapy is used. The material has a modulus of elasticity less than that of cortical bone. It therefore does not absorb the functional stresses that are applied to the new bone that forms within the tray. It has a low thermal conductivity.

Metallic mandibular trays are difficult to modify significantly in the operating room. Trimming, adaptation to host bone, and fixation require a special instrument kit, wire, and bone screws, all of the same metal, to prevent the battery effect that results from contact between dissimilar metals. The radiopaque metal structure impairs routine radiographic and radionuclide imaging of the graft (fig. 13.32). The trays are thin to keep them lightweight, and the free edges are sharp. When irradiated, a metallic mandibular tray generates secondary electrons (Schwartz et al. 1979). This increases the local dose of radiation by about one-third, which may exceed the tolerance of overlying tissues and lead to exposure of the tray (Schwartz et al. 1979). Once

**Figure 13.32**

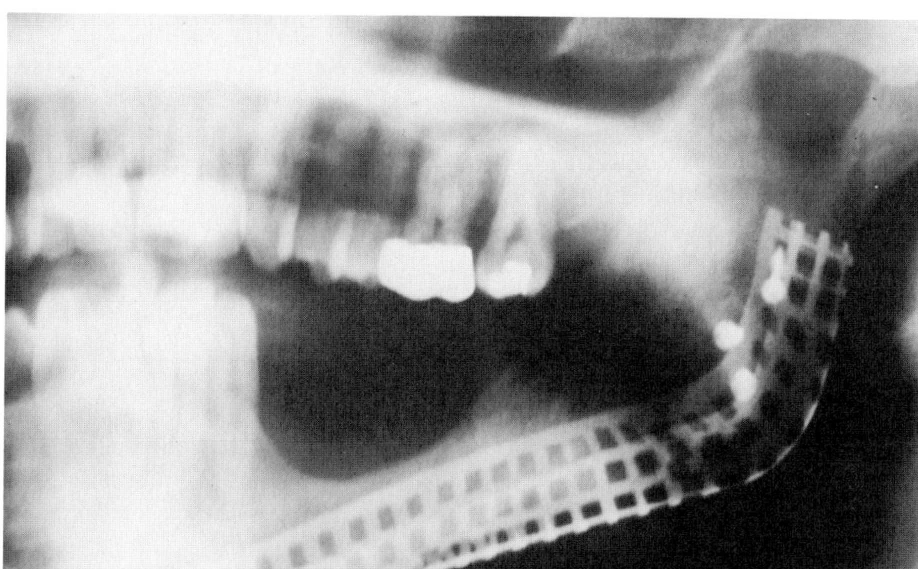

*Mandibular reconstruction using a metallic tray. After one year the bone above the level of the tray looks good, but it is impossible to assess the status of the bone contained within the tray.*

new bone has formed within a metallic tray, it has occasionally been noted to undergo gradual resorption. Since the modulus of elasticity of the metals exceeds that of cortical bone, the tray absorbs the functional stresses that are applied to the graft. This upsets the dynamic balance between bone formation and bone resorption, in favor of the latter (Tonino et al. 1976). External temperature changes may affect the tray and may cause discomfort to the patient.

The author has performed 21 mandibular reconstructions using the Dacron/urethane mandibular tray, with follow-up from one to four years. One patient's reconstruction failed because of a streptococcal infection in the fourth postoperative week; the patient was subsequently regrafted. There was no early dehiscence. Two patients underwent late removal of the tray: one at one year, after a super-erupted maxillary tooth literally bit through the insensate overlying mucosa; and one at two years, after a fixation wire became exposed beneath a denture flange. Both patients had fully consolidated grafts and experienced no further problems. Patients who had undergone preoperative radiotherapy presented no difficulties and evidenced excellent new bone formation (fig. 13.30). Patients who had had neck dissections did well, despite tightness of the skin over the surface of the tray. Patients who had had osteoradionecrosis did well. Two patients underwent postoperative radiotherapy, to a total dose of 5000 rad beginning six weeks after grafting, with excellent results (fig. 13.25).

In Boyne and Zarem's (1976) series of 53 cases in which titanium mandibular trays were used, 15% experienced wound dehiscence, 12% required removal of the tray, and 9% were considered failures. Seventeen percent of these patients required regrafting, usually because of poor contour or an inadequate alveolar ridge.

## Primary versus Secondary Reconstruction

A routine procedure when dealing with benign disease, primary mandibular reconstruction presents many difficulties in malignant disease, where large areas of mucous membrane have been resected along with the mandible. Millard's (1964) initial enthusiasm for primary reconstruction has waned as the failure rate in his series reached 30% (1970).

In general, primary reconstruction should be reserved for those cases where the intraoral defect can be closed with local tissues. Pedicle flaps with controlled orocutaneous fistulas do not reliably seal off the graft from the oral cavity.

Because of the potential for oral contamination, cortico-cancellous grafts are preferred in primary mandibular reconstruction. They require less foreign material for fixation, and they can survive a mild postoperative infection and go on to union. Cancellous bone grafts may be used in selected favorable cases.

In most instances it is prudent to plan a secondary reconstruction of the mandible. This allows time for the oral cavity to become closed off and for dead space to resolve. Should there be an infection, wound separation, or partial necrosis of a pedicle flap, the problem can be dealt with prior to bone grafting. Permanent histologic sections of resection margins can be reviewed prior to definitive reconstruction.

If pedicle flaps have been used to provide oral lining, bone grafting is conveniently performed at the time the pedicle is divided. This should be done six to eight weeks after the initial procedure to assure a well-vascularized bed for the graft and a tightly-sealed oral cavity.

## Conclusions

1. Current surgical techniques enable us to cure many cancers of the head and neck. Surgical cure, however, can result in severe functional, cosmetic, and psychological impairments. Patients with such impairments deserve consideration for rehabilitation.

2. Preservation of the mandibular arch is preferable to reconstruction; this is frequently accomplished without compromising an adequate tumor resection.
3. If resection must be carried out, mandibular reconstruction is simplified when the anatomic relationships of the remaining mandibular fragments are maintained.
4. With the mandibular remnants in anatomic position, reconstruction of the resected soft tissues is usually necessary. Axial pattern flaps and myocutaneous flaps are especially useful for introducing new vascularization and for providing bulk.
5. Survival rates for many cancers of the head and neck are improved by combining surgery with radiotherapy. Preoperative radiotherapy is associated with a high incidence of surgical complications. The incidence of surgical complications in postoperatively-irradiated patients is about the same as that seen in non-irradiated patients.
6. Cancellous bone grafts are preferable to cortical bone grafts in mandibular reconstruction. Cortico-cancellous grafts offer many of the advantages of both in certain cases.
7. Immobilization of the mandible is not necessarily a requirement for a successful bone graft. Intermaxillary fixation is only used to restore precisely the occlusion when teeth remain in both the mandible and the maxilla.
8. Cancellous bone grafts are given stability and anatomic form by biocompatible trays which are implanted with them. Dacron/urethane mandibular trays are preferable to metal mandibular trays.
9. Primary mandibular reconstruction should be attempted only in selected, favorable cases. Secondary mandibular reconstruction, following healing of all soft tissues and final histologic evaluation of surgical margins, is the procedure of choice.
10. A major tumor resection that includes the mandible and associated soft tissues in continuity with a radical neck dissection should be followed by immediate anatomic fixation of the mandibular fragments and soft tissue reconstruction. Secondary mandibular bone grafting follows, usually at the time that pedicle flaps are divided. The reconstruction is completed after 6 to 12 months with a vestibuloplasty that permits the wearing of a denture. With use of the appropriate surgical techniques and attention to technical detail, neither preoperative nor postoperative radiotherapy should affect the outcome of the reconstruction.

# References

Abbott, L. C. et al. The evaluation of cortical and cancellous bone as grafting material. *J. Bone Joint Surg.* 29:381–414, 1947.

Ackland, R. C. The free iliac flap. *Plast. Reconstr. Surg.* 64:30–36, 1979. Discussion by Harii, K. 64:257–258, 1979.

Anderson, R. An ambulatory method of treating fractures of the shaft of the femur. *Surg. Gynecol. Obstet.* 62:865–873, 1936.

Anlyan, A. J., and Manis, J. R. Re-evaluation of bone chip grafts for mandibular defects. *Am. J. Surg.* 116:606–609, 1968.

Ariyan, S. The pectoralis major myocutaneous flap. *Plast. Reconstr. Surg.* 63:73–81, 1979.

Arora, B. K., and Laskin, D. M. Sex chromatin as a cellular label of osteogenesis by bone grafts. *J. Bone Joint Surg.* 46A:1269–1276, 1964.

Bakamjian, V. Y. A two stage method for pharyngo-esophageal reconstruction with a primary pectoral skin flap. *Plast. Reconstr. Surg.* 36:173–184, 1965.

Bakamjian, V. Y., and Littlewood, M. Cervical skin flaps for intraoral and pharyngeal repair following cancer surgery. *Br. J. Plast. Surg.* 17:191–210, 1964.

Ballantyne, A. J.; McCarten, A. B.; and Ibanez, M. L. The extension of cancer of the head and neck through peripheral nerves. *Am. J. Surg.* 106:651–667, 1963.

Benoist, M. Experience with 220 cases of mandibular reconstruction. *J. Maxillofac. Surg.* 6:40–49, 1978.

Berger, D. S. et al. Elective irradiation of the neck lymphatics for squamous cell carcinomas of the nasopharynx and oropharynx. *Am. J. Roentgenol.* 111:66–72, 1971.

Bowerman, J. E. A review of reconstruction of the mandible. *Proc. Roy. Soc. Med.* 67:610–614, 1974.

Boyne, P. J. Autogenous cancellous bone and marrow transplants. *Clin. Orthop.* 73:199–209, 1970.

Boyne, P. J., and Zarem, H. Osseous reconstruction of the resected mandible. *Am. J. Surg.* 132:49–53, 1976.

Brown, J. B.; Fryer, M. P.; and McDowell, F. Permanent pedicle blood-carrying flaps for repairing defects in avascular areas. *Ann. Surg.* 134:486–494, 1951.

Burwell, R. G. Studies in the transplantation of bone. VII. *J. Bone Joint Surg.* 46B:110–140, 1964.

Chambers, R. G.; Jaques, D. A.; and Mahoney, W. D. Tongue flaps for intraoral reconstruction. *Am. J. Surg.* 118:783–786, 1969.

Cohen, I. K., and Edgerton, M. T. Transbuccal flaps for reconstruction of the floor of the mouth. *Plast. Reconstr. Surg.* 48:8–10, 1971.

Conley, J. *Cancer of the head and neck.* New York: Appleton-Century-Crofts, 1967.

Conley, J. Use of composite flaps containing bone for major repairs in the head and neck. *Plast. Reconstr. Surg.* 49:522–526, 1972.

Constable, J. D., and Bernstein, N. R.: Public and professional reactions to the facially disfigured which interfere with rehabilitation. *Scand. J. Plast. Reconstr. Surg.* 13:181–183, 1979.

Donald, P. J. Complications of combined therapy in head and neck carcinomas. *Arch. Otolaryngol.* 104:329–332, 1978.

Edgerton, M. T., and Des Prez, J. D. Reconstruction of the oral cavity in the treatment of cancer. *Plast. Reconstr. Surg.* 19:89–113, 1957.

Enneking, W. F. et al. Physical and biological aspects of repair in dog cortical bone transplants. *J. Bone Joint Surg.* 57A:232–252, 1975.

Finseth, F.; Kavarana, N.; and Antia, N. Complications of free flap transfers to the mouth region. *Plast. Reconstr. Surg.* 56:652–653, 1975.

Fleming, I. D., and Morris, J. H. Use of acrylic external splint after mandibular resection. *Am. J. Surg.* 118:708–711, 1969.

Flynn, M. B. Morbidity and mortality of mandibular resection for malignant disease. *Am. J. Surg.* 134:510–516, 1977.

Futrell, J. W. et al. Platysma myocutaneous flap for intraoral reconstruction. *Am. J. Surg.* 136:504–507, 1978.

Gilbert, H., and Kagan, A. R. Recurrence patterns in squamous cell carcinoma of the oral cavity, pharynx, and larynx. *J. Surg. Oncol.* 6:357–378, 1974.

Gregory, C. F. The current status of bone and joint transplants. *Clin. Orthop.* 87:165–177, 1972.

Gullane, P. J., and Arena, S. Palatal island flap for reconstruction of oral defects. *Arch. Otolaryngol.* 103:598–599, 1977.

Harashina, T.; Fujino, T.; and Aoyagi, F. Reconstruction of the oral cavity with a free flap. *Plast. Reconstr. Surg.* 58:412–414, 1976.

Joseph, D. L., and Shumrick, D. A. Risks of head and neck surgery in previously irradiated patients. *Arch. Otolaryngol.* 97:381–384, 1973.

Leake, D. L. Mandibular reconstruction with a new type of alloplastic tray. *J. Oral Surg.* 32:23–26, 1974.

Marchetta, F. C.; Sako, K.; and Murphy, J. B. The periosteum of the mandible and intraoral carcinoma. *Am. J. Surg.* 122:711–713, 1971.

Mathes, S. J., and Vasconez, L. O. The cervicohumeral flap. *Plast. Reconstr. Surg.* 61:7–12, 1978.

McCraw, J. B.; Dibbell, D. G.; and Carraway, J. H. Clinical definition of independent myocutaneous territories. *Plast. Reconstr. Surg.* 60:341–352, 1977.

McGregor, I. A. The temporal flap in intraoral cancer: its use in repairing the post-excisional defect. *Br. J. Plast. Surg.* 16:318–335, 1963.

McGregor, I. A. Problems of reconstructive surgery of the oral cavity. *J. Laryngol. Otol.* 91:445–465, 1977.

Millard, D. R. A new approach to immediate mandibular repair. *Ann. Surg.* 160:306–313, 1964.

Millard, D. R. et al. Interim report on immediate mandibular repair. *Am. J. Surg.* 118:726–731, 1969.

Millard, D. R. et al. Composite lower jaw reconstruction. *Plast. Reconstr. Surg.* 46:22–29, 1970.

Morris, J. H. Biphase connector, external skeletal splint for reduction and fixation of mandibular fractures. *Oral Surg.* 2:1382–1398, 1949.

Mowlem, R. Cancellous bone chip grafts. *Lancet* 247:746–748, 1944.

Owens, N. A compound neck pedicle designed for the repair of massive facial defects. *Plast. Reconstr. Surg.* 15:369–389, 1955.

Panje, W. R.; Bardach, J.; and Krause, C. J. Reconstruction of the oral cavity with a free flap. *Plast. Reconstr. Surg.* 58:415–418, 1976.

Parkhill, C. A new apparatus for the fixation of bones after resection and in fractures with a tendency to displacement. *Trans. Am. Surg. Assn.* 15:251–256, 1897.

Perez, C. A.; Marks, J.; and Powers, W. E. Preoperative irradiation in head and neck cancer. *Semin. Oncol.* 4:387–397, 1977.

Pike, R. L., and Boyne, P. J. Use of surface-decalcified allogenic bone and autogenous marrow in extensive mandibular defects. *J. Oral Surg.* 32:177–182, 1974.

Robson, M. C. et al. The undelayed Mütter flap in head and neck reconstruction. *Am. J. Surg.* 132:472–475, 1976.

Schwartz, H. C. Effects of radiation on cancellous bone grafts. Paper read at the International Association for Maxillofacial Surgeons, September 1979, Los Angeles, California.

Schwartz, H. C. et al. Interface radiation dosimetry in mandibular reconstruction. *Arch. Otolaryngol.* 105:293–295, 1979.

Schwartz, H. C., and Leake, D. L. Use of a craniotome for obtaining cancellous bone and marrow from the ilium. *Ann. Plast. Surg.* 3:576–577, 1979.

Serafin, D.; Villarreal-Rios, A.; and Georgiade, N. G. A rib-containing free flap to reconstruct mandibular defects. *Br. J. Plast. Surg.* 30:263–266, 1977.

Terz, J. J. et al. Primary reconstruction of the mandible with a wire mesh prosthesis. *J. Maxillofac. Surg.* 6:105–108, 1978.

Tonino, A. J. et al. Protection from stress in bone and its effects. *J. Bone Joint Surg.* 58B:107–113, 1976.

Towers, J. F., and Wilson, J. S. P. Simple reconstruction of the mandible following resection. *Proc. Roy. Soc. Med.* 67:607–609, 1974.

Vanderbrouck, C. et al. Results of a randomized clinical trial of preoperative irradiation versus postoperative in treatment of tumors of the hypopharynx. *Cancer* 39:1445–1449, 1977.

Zovickian, A. Pharyngeal fistulas: repair and prevention using mastoid-occiput based shoulder flaps. *Plast. Reconstr. Surg.* 19:355–372, 1957.

# Chapter 14

# *Dental Extractions in the Irradiated Patient*

John Beumer III

Radiation therapy has been used with increasing frequency in recent times in the management of neoplasms of the head and neck region. For some tumors radiation therapy is the treatment of choice while it is employed for others in combination with surgery or sometimes with chemotherapy. Postradiation oral sequelae are significant, well known, and can result in needless morbidity. Notable advances have been made in recent years that have resulted in decreased incidence of radiation caries and osteoradionecrosis. Many questions, however, remain unanswered, and much research remains to be done. The literature regarding evaluation of dentition and extraction of teeth remains indeterminate and confusing. It is the intent of this chapter to summarize and collate the available data and clinical experience of those active in this field so as to present an organized, rational approach to the issue of dental extractions in the pre- and postradiation patient.

## Preradiation Dental Extractions: Review of the Literature

Most patients developing osteoradionecrosis are those with teeth present prior to the beginning of radiation therapy. Hence, many questions arise relative to dental evaluations prior to initiation of radiation treatment. How does one manage the dentulous patient prior to therapy? Which teeth, if any, should be extracted, and how should they be extracted? How long should one wait until beginning radiation therapy after dental extractions? These are difficult questions, and historical reviews of the literature indicate much controversy. Some clinicians have recommended full mouth extraction prior to therapy whereas others prefer to extract only those teeth within the primary beam. Still others discourage preradiation extraction of teeth insofar as dental pathology permits. We feel that a number of factors should be considered before deciding on dental extraction in any particular patient. Our experience indicates that the clinician should not rely on specific rules for guidance when arriving at such decisions. Obviously, before making a determination consultation with the radiation therapist is mandatory.

Prophylactic extraction of teeth within the radiation field has been considered by some clinicians as a means of reducing the incidence of bone necrosis (Del Regato 1939; Daland, 1941; Silverman and Chierci 1965). Others propose that preradiation extractions increase the risk of bone infections (Wildermuth and Cantril 1953; Quick 1959; Carl, Schaaf, and Sako 1973; Daley and Drane 1972), but specific data available indicating the risks of osteoradionecrosis and its relation to timing of extractions, dose levels, and radiation fields employed are scanty and often are misleading. Consequently, many important issues remain controversial: (1) the wisdom of elective preradiation extractions within the field and the risk of bone necrosis in these patients, (2) the time interval between dental extraction and radiation therapy necessary to organize the wound sufficiently to prevent a bone necrosis from developing, and (3) the factors involved in delivery of the radiation therapy which may predispose to bone necrosis in patients requiring dental extractions prior to radiation therapy.

A review of the literature will answer a few of these questions. Wildermuth and Cantril (1953) reported 6 patients developing bone necroses out of 14 requiring dental extractions prior to therapy. The time interval between extraction and commencement of therapy was 9.5 days in the osteoradionecrosis group and 15.3 days in the non–bone necrosis group. Orthovoltage was used and dose levels ranged from 4100 to 6300 rad in those requiring dental extractions. Six patients requiring postradiation dental extractions did not develop osteoradionecrosis. Based on this data, they suggested that extractions prior to radiation were not prudent. Daley and Drane (1972) reported that 22 of their 74 bone necrosis cases occurred at the site of preradiation dental extractions. Average healing time before radiation was 11.1 days. Thirteen of these patients had 10 or more days of healing and five patients had 2 weeks or more. They suggested that only completely unsalvageable teeth should be removed prior to radiation. They felt that if extractions were difficult or rapid tumor growth required immediate commencement of radiation, teeth should not be considered for elective removal. They recommended that if extractions were necessary, the healing period should be two to three weeks. Starcke and Shannon (1977) reported no bone necrosis in 62 patients requiring preradiation extractions. The average time interval between extractions and radiation was 25.3 days (range: 5 to 72 days). Only 15 out of 62 enjoyed healing periods of less than 15 days. Dose levels were somewhat low, as 36 of the 62 patients received less than 6000 rad. No patient received more than 7000 rad. The authors concluded that dental extractions, by themselves, are not associated with an increased incidence of bone necrosis. They suggested that the time interval between dental extraction and radiation therapy is not critical. Bedwinek and colleagues (1976) felt that elective dental extraction prior to therapy increases the risk of bone necrosis. During a period of elective dental extraction when 203 patients were treated with radiation therapy, 24 patients developed bone necrosis from preradiation extractions. During a subsequent period of so-called dental conservation (178 patients were evaluated), four developed bone necroses secondary to preradiation extraction. Unfortunately, the delineation between the period of elective dental extraction and the period of dental conservation was not well defined. Likewise, in neither group were data provided indicating the number of patients requiring preradiation extractions without developing bone necrosis.

There are a few animal studies aimed at clarification of these issues, but they are difficult to extrapolate to clinical practice. Stein, Brady, and Raventos (1957), using rats, extracted maxillary molars and implanted radon seeds lateral to the tooth sockets at the time of extraction and at various time intervals ranging from 4 to 20 days thereafter. Severe tissue changes were noted when the radiation sources were implanted immediately or within four days following extraction. On the basis of their observations Stein and associates suggested that 7 to 14 days were necessary for healing before radiation therapy could be started. Shearer (1967) felt, based on a study using dogs, that radiation could be contemplated as early as three days following extraction. In selected groups of dogs he extracted teeth on days 3, 7, 10, 14, and 21 prior to commencement of radiation. After extraction an aggressive alveolectomy was performed and primary closure obtained. The dogs received their fractionated radiation therapy over a six-week period using the cobalt 60 apparatus. Total dose delivered was 6000 rad measured in air. He reported that the timing of extractions had little influence on organization and healing of the surgical sites.

In our review (Beumer, Curtis, and Harrison 1979) the risk of bone necrosis directly referable to dental extractions prior to radiation therapy was

**Table 14.1**
Osteoradionecrosis at Extraction Sites

| | |
|---|---|
| Number of Patients | 94 |
| Osteoradionecroses at extraction sites (spontaneous) | 12 |
| Osteoradionecroses at extraction sites secondary to denture irritations | 2 |
| Delayed healing | 3 |
| Mandibular teeth extracted in field | 313/(86 patients) |
| Maxillary teeth extracted in field | 147/(31 patients) |
| Teeth extracted out of field | 183/(31 patients) |

12.7% (12 of 94 patients). In two additional patients bone necroses at preradiation extraction sites were precipitated by mucosal irritation associated with complete dentures. Eighty-six of the 94 patients had mandibular teeth within the primary beam extracted (table 14.1). All necroses were detected in the mandible and, in 11 of the 14, external radiation therapy was delivered via bilateral opposed mandibular fields which encompassed the entire body of the mandible (tables 14.2 and 14.3). Eleven out of 28 patients treated with opposed mandibular fields requiring preradiation dental extractions developed an osteoradionecrosis, whereas only 3 of 38 patients developed a bone necrosis where the fields terminated anteriorly at the first bicuspid region (table 14.2). In addition, for those patients whose therapy was delivered via bilateral opposed mandibular fields, the average dosage was significantly higher in the necrosis group (7400 rad vs 6284 rad) (table 14.4). There was a small difference in healing time (time interval between extractions and radiation therapy) between these two groups. When considering the entire

**Table 14.2**
Radiation Fields Including the Mandible

| Radiation Field | Number of Patients | Number of Osteo-radionecroses | Percentage |
|---|---|---|---|
| Opposed mandibular | 28 | 11 | 39 |
| Opposed mandibular to 4 \| 4* | 38 | 3 | 8 |
| Opposed mandibular to 6 \| 6 | 9 | 0 | 0 |
| Unilateral mandibular 6 \| 6 | 4 | 0 | 0 |
| Unilateral mandibular 4 \| 4 | 5 | 0 | 0 |
| Unilateral mandibular 1 \| 1 | 2 | 0 | 0 |
| Totals | 86 | 14 | 16 |

*Throughout the tables in this chapter, the following system for denoting dental anatomy is used:

| | Left | Right |
|---|---|---|
| **Maxilla** | 87654321 | 12345678 |
| **Mandible** | 87654321 | 12345678 |

with the numbers representing teeth as they number laterally from the midline.

The following abbreviation system may be used: 6 is the sixth tooth to the right of the midline on the maxilla. 3 is the third tooth to the left of the midline on the mandible. Alternatively, the anatomy may be listed as mandible 66 (without the bars to denote maxilla versus mandible or right versus left) and indicates the sixth tooth to the right and the left on the mandible.

**Table 14.3** Osteoradionecrosis Occurring at Preradiation Sites in Squamous Cell Carcinoma

| Tumor Site | Dose (Rad) | Modality | Radiation Fields (External Therapy) | Teeth Extracted in Field | Site of Bone Necrosis | Onset after Therapy (Months) | Healing Time for Extraction (Days) | Course |
|---|---|---|---|---|---|---|---|---|
| Lateral tongue | 5000<br>3000 | Linear accelerator<br>Peroral cone | Opposed mandibular | upper: │8; lower: 78│ | 8┐ | 0* | 12 | Patient died after 12 months; osteoradionecrosis was present but had improved with conservative measures |
| Floor of mouth | 5700<br>2700 | Linear accelerator<br>Implant | Opposed mandibular | upper: 76│; lower: 7│ | 6┐ | 4 | 1 | Still present after 40 months but reduced in size with conservative measures |
| Floor of mouth | 5579 | $^{60}Co$<br>Implant | Opposed mandibular | upper: 765│; lower: 57│ | 6┐ | | | Still present after 36 months and enlarging after hyperbaric therapy |
| Alveolar ridge | 5700 | Linear accelerator | Opposed mandibular | upper: │34; lower: │123 | ┌23 | 0 | 8 | Patient died with metastatic disease; osteoradionecrosis present, but stable |
| Floor of mouth | 5000 | $^{60}Co$ | Opposed mandibular | upper: 76521│1; lower: 246│ | 1┐ | 1 | 0 | Still present; enlarged and progressed to pathologic fracture following radical neck dissection |
| Floor of mouth | 5940 | $^{60}Co$ | Opposed mandibular | upper: 765434│1234; lower: 567│ | 6┐ | 5 | 9 | Healed in 12 months with conservative measures |
| Alveolar | 6600 | Linear accelerator | Opposed mandibular | upper: 75434│12; lower: 467│ | 7┐ | 1 | 10 | Still present at last follow-up; present for 52 months; no enlargement with conservative measures |
| Retromolar pad | 6530 | $^{60}Co$ | Opposed facial | 7┐ | 7┐ | 13 | 6 | Patient died of a cerebrovascular accident 21 months after onset of necrosis; no enlargement with conservative measures |
| Floor of mouth | 7080 | Linear accelerator | Opposed mandibular | 76543┐ | 6┐ | 4 | 6 | Patient died of metastatic disease 8 months after osteoradionecrosis onset; progressive enlargement with conservative measures |
| Floor of mouth | 6686 | $^{60}Co$ | Opposed mandibular | upper: 7│; lower: 3│ | 6┐ | 4 | 6 | Osteoradionecrosis still present and had progressed to pathologic fracture |
| Soft palate | 6000 | $^{60}Co$ | Right and left facial to upper: 4│4; lower: 4│4 | upper: 8│4; lower: 567│ | 7┐ | 0 | 9 | Still present; no change with conservative measures |
| Floor of mouth | 5640<br>3206 | Linear accelerator<br>Implant | Opposed mandibular | upper: │67; lower: │7 | ┌7 | 2 | 7 | Still present; no change with conservative measures |
| Soft palate (bilateral) | 7000 | Linear accelerator | Right and left facial to upper: 4│4; lower: 4│4 | ┌6 | ┌6 | 7 | 14 | Healed in 6 months with conservative measures |
| Floor of mouth | 6525 | Linear accelerator | Opposed mandibular | upper: 76543│; lower: 7│ | 7┐ | 11 | 15 | Healed in 13 months with conservative measures |

*Exposure developed during radiation therapy.

**Table 14.4**
Opposed Mandible Fields

| | Number of Patients | Dose Range | Average | Healing Time (Days) |
|---|---|---|---|---|
| Osteoradionecrosis | 11 | 5700–8500 | 7400 | 7.5 |
| Nonosteoradionecrosis | 17 | 5000–7700 | 6284 | 9.0 |

group of 94 patients, however, there was no significant difference in healing time for extraction sites between the necrosis and non-necrosis groups, particularly when the averages were computed at the 90% confidence level (table 14.5). All but one bone necrosis developed in patients with healing periods of 14 days or less. Healing time was less than two weeks in 80% of the non-necrosis patient populations (table 14.6).

The following criteria were used in identifying teeth within the field for extraction. When significant portions of the body of the mandible were within the radiation field, teeth were carefully scrutinized. All teeth within the field demonstrating periapical pathology were extracted. Those mandibular molars with roentgenographic evidence of furcation involvement were almost always extracted. Caries did not indicate the need for extraction unless there was roentgenographic evidence of pulpal exposure and/or significant pain. Maxillary teeth were seldom removed even when within the radiation field, except where dental pathology was severe or the teeth involved were symptomatic. When teeth were extracted, mucoperiosteal flaps were reflected, and radical alveolectomies were performed to permit primary closure without tension. Patients were covered with antibiotics during the immediate postextraction period.

In our review radiation fields and dose were important factors contributing to the incidence of osteoradionecrosis following preradiation dental extractions within the field. When eliminating the group of patients treated with opposed mandibular fields, the incidence was small (4%) and the morbidity slight (two healed and one remained stable with local conservative measures). On the other hand, the incidence in the group where the entire

**Table 14.5**
Healing Time: Extraction to Radiation Therapy

| | | Time in Days | | |
|---|---|---|---|---|
| Patient Group | Number of Patients | Range | Average | 90% Confidence Limits |
| Osteoradionecrosis | 14 | 6–15 | 7.8 | 8.5 |
| Nonosteoradionecrosis | 80 | 26–55 | 9.3 | 9.1 |

**Table 14.6**
Healing Time for Extraction Sites

| **Healing Time** | **Patients** | **Bone Necrosis** |
|---|---|---|
| Extractions during therapy | 6 | 2 |
| 0 to 7 days before therapy | 25 | 3 |
| 8 to 14 days before therapy | 26 | 6 |
| More than 14 days before therapy | 13 | 1 |

body of the mandible was heavily irradiated was rather high (39%) and changes relative to extraction criteria appear to be in order. When doses in excess of 6500 rad with this field set-up are to be employed, 14 to 21 days healing time will insure better organization of the extraction wound and will probably reduce the risk of bone necrosis. If healing periods of this length cannot be provided it may be best to defer dental extractions in the mandible altogether. The 25-day average healing time reported by Starcke and Shannon (1977), although apparently eliminating the risk of necrosis secondary to preradiation extractions, would appear to compromise the chance of cure in some patients. Few radiation therapists are willing to wait this long before beginning therapy. It should be emphasized that the extraction sites should be examined carefully for epithelialization before commencing radiation. Difficulty with the extractions, and variable patient responses, may result in a lengthening or shortening of the healing period.

In our view the concept of prophylactic preradiation dental extraction appears to be sound, particularly if extractions are reserved for those teeth exhibiting advanced pathology. Wholesale extraction of teeth within the radiation field probably is not indicated. Extraction of impacted mandibular third molars, prior to radiation, is not advocated in most patients. Such extractions often necessitate removal of much bone, thus creating large defects requiring prolonged periods for healing. Patients with partially erupted mandibular third molars represent a particularly difficult and perplexing clinical problem because of the risk of pericoronitis. Fortunately, the majority of these patients are below age 40 and most have Hodgkin's disease and other types of lymphomas. The dose and small volume of mandible included within the radiation field results in less compromise of the vasculature of the mandible and salivary glands. Our clinical experience indicates that the incidence of osteoradionecrosis in patients receiving 4500 to 5000 rad has been negligible. Operculectomy is useful in selected cases.

## Criteria for Preradiation Dental Extractions

Based on the preceding discussion we feel that the following issues must be addressed before deciding upon extraction of teeth prior to radiation therapy.

**Figure 14.1**

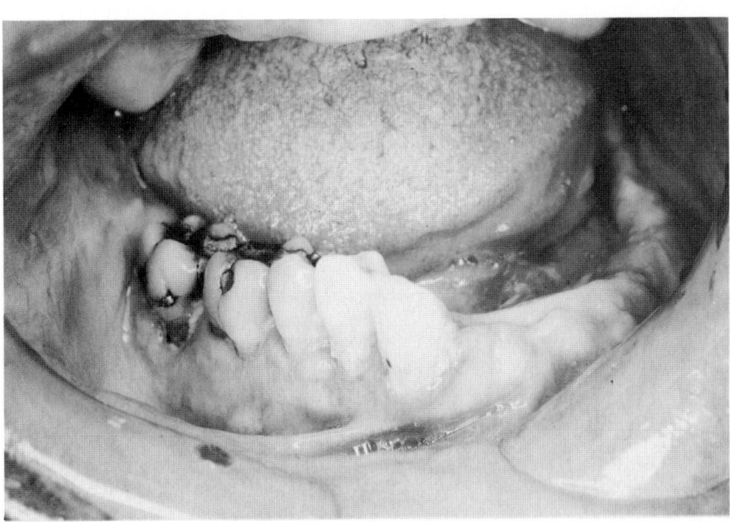

*Patient with advanced periodontal disease clinically demonstrating furcation involvement of mandibular molars.*

## Condition of the Residual Dentition

The clinician's primary goal should be to place the patient's dentition in optimal condition so that high-risk dental procedures will not have to be performed in the immediate postradiation period. All teeth with a questionable prognosis should be extracted before radiation. Teeth with advanced carious lesions (with pulpal exposure), periapical infection, and significant periodontal bone loss are most suspect. The patient's periodontal status is most important in this assessment. Dentitions with significant periodontal deficiencies are difficult to maintain and are susceptible to caries and infection. An aggressive extraction philosophy is recommended in the management of dentitions with severe periodontal involvement. We believe furcation involvement of mandibular molar teeth in the radiation field is grounds for preradiation extraction in most patients. This finding is best confirmed by a dentist by the use of periodontal probes and appropriate dental roentgenographs (figs. 14.1 and 14.2). The presence of moderate caries is less important, since in most instances it is restorable and can be controlled with appropriate oral hygiene measures and topical fluoride applications. Obviously, mandibular teeth within the radiation field should receive the closest scrutiny.

**Figure 14.2**

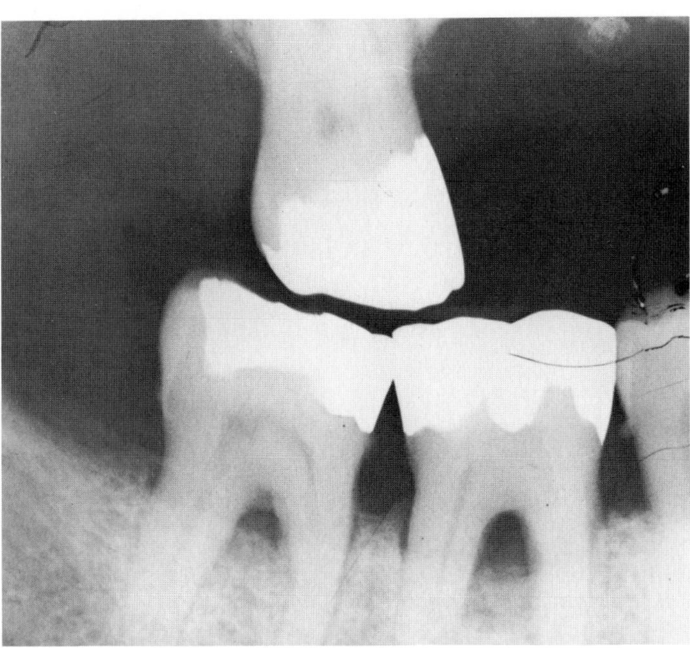

*A dental roentgenograph often reveals a furcation involvement* (arrow) *which is not clinically observable.*

## Dental Awareness of the Patient

This factor is a most important consideration when evaluating a patient for dental extractions prior to therapy. After radiation treatment with reduced salivary output, hygiene becomes increasingly difficult. Trismus, impaired motor functions, and surgical morbidities may also compromise oral hygiene procedures. Patients must possess the motivation and the physical ability to maintain their dentition properly. Without the patient's help and cooperation, the risk of complications is increased immeasurably. The less motivated the patient, the more aggressive one should be in extraction of teeth prior to therapy. The awareness and motivation of the clinician are of no less importance. Oral hygiene (fig. 14.3) at the time of initial examination of the patient is often a reliable indicator of future performance. If oral hygiene and dental health are to be maintained, patients must understand the implications of their radiation therapy and be disposed to carry out the prescribed procedures. These instructions must be reiterated constantly, for patients often forget or fail to grasp the issues with a single presentation.

**Figure 14.3**

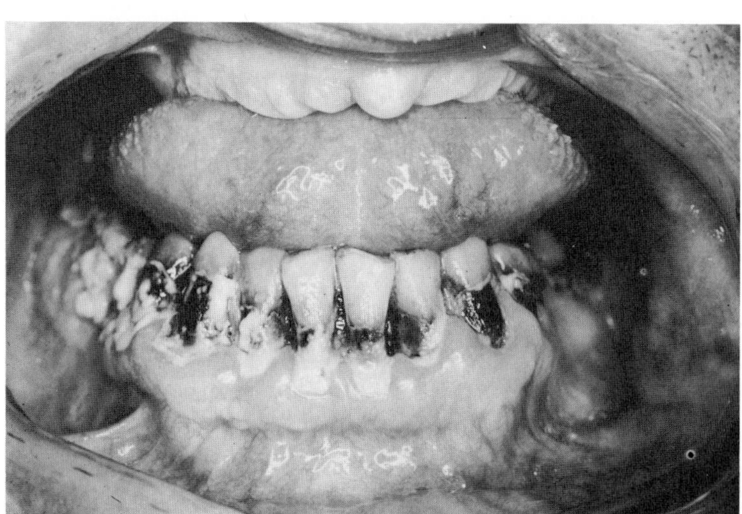

*Patient with unsatisfactory oral hygiene. Risk of caries and bone necrosis is greater.*

## Immediacy of Treatment

Often the status and behavior of the tumor will preclude preradiation dental extractions, for delays secondary to healing of the extraction sites could significantly compromise control of disease. The dentist, radiation therapist, and patient must therefore accept the attendant risk of complications and attempt to maintain oral health at an optimum level. Control of the tumor obviously is the most important consideration.

## Mode of Therapy

Radiation is delivered to the tumor either by an external source or by implanting radioactive materials within it. In external therapy the radiation beam often must traverse important structures before reaching the tumor, and consequently such tissues as salivary gland, periodontium, and bone may be damaged. When radiation sources are implanted within the area occupied by tumor, however, the radiation is more confined. Rarely is salivary gland function significantly compromised by implantation techniques. Consequently, radiation caries is not a significant problem in patients treated with interstitial radiation therapy. In these patients, extraction of teeth after radiation therapy does not involve high risk unless the teeth are adjacent to the implant. Osteoradionecrosis is rare except when the implant is located in close proximity to the bone. Pretreatment extractions are considered when teeth with significant pathology are located close to the implant site.

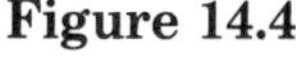

**Figure 14.4**

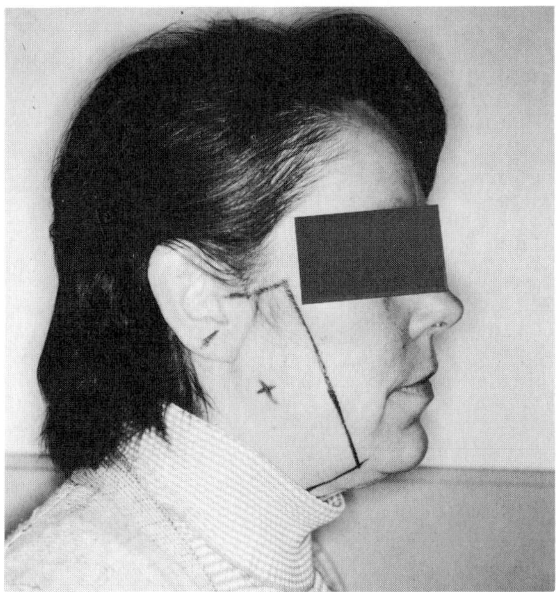

*Radiation field encompasses the parotid and submaxillary salivary glands.*

When external radiation therapy is employed, close scrutiny of the dentition is mandatory because salivary glands and bone will be exposed to high doses of radiation. Depending upon fields and dose, this obviously increases the risk of complications (caries, bone and soft tissue necroses). Hence a more aggressive program is used in removing teeth prior to therapy. The majority of patients are treated with external beam therapy. When both external and interstitial therapy are used, decisions regarding extraction of teeth are dictated by the amount and character of the external therapy and the site of the implant.

## Radiation Fields

The risk of caries or necrosis is dependent upon the radiation fields. For instance, in lesions situated in the nasopharynx and posterior soft palate, where the field is directed superiorly and posteriorly and includes both parotid glands (fig. 14.4), the risk of postradiation caries is high because of the profound xerostomia that results. Clinical experience, however, reveals the incidence of bone necrosis to be low in this group. We therefore advocate a conservative philosophy when considering extraction of teeth in such patients. Our experience reveals that in this group of patients postradiation extractions in both mandible and maxilla may be effected with minimal risk.

In lesions situated in the lateral tongue and floor of the mouth, the radiation fields will be quite different (fig. 14.5). In these lesions the entire body of the mandible is within the field of radiation, but the superior portions of both parotid glands are usually spared. Thus, salivary flow, although reduced, is not as profoundly impaired when compared to more posterior superior radiation fields. Radiation caries has not proved to be as prevalent in this group of patients, although the incidence of osteoradionecrosis, in our view, is higher. The clinician must attempt to place the patient's dentition in optimal condition so that extractions need not be performed in the immediate postradiotherapy period.

Where the radiation beam includes the major salivary glands and a significant portion of the body of the mandible—as in base of tongue, tonsillar pillar, and retromolar trigone carcinomas—radiation-induced xerostomia is severe and the blood supply to the mandibular body is also compromised. Clinical experience indicates that the incidence of caries and osteoradio-

**Figure 14.5**

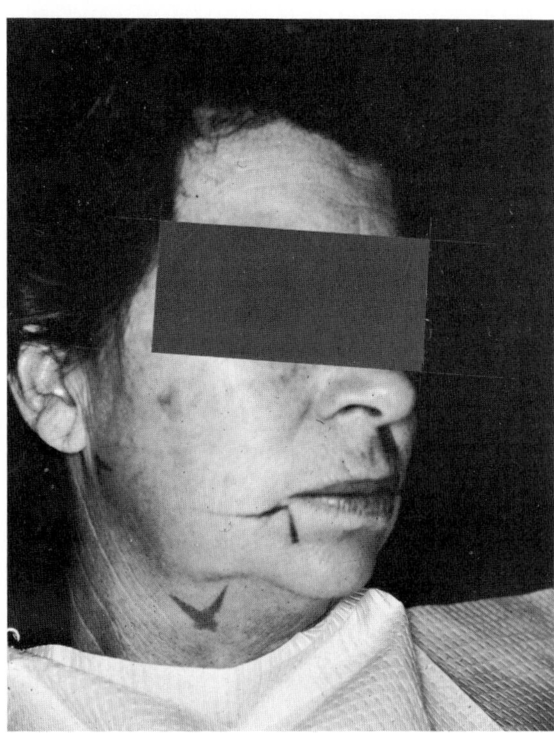

*Opposed mandibular fields. Much parotid tissue is spared.*

necrosis is high in this group (Grant and Fletcher 1966). We believe that a more aggressive approach to extraction of teeth is justified in these patients, especially in cases involving mandibular molars within the radiation field and showing advanced periodontal disease.

## Mandible versus Maxilla

Almost all osteoradionecroses occur in the mandible (Beumer, Silverman, and Benak 1972; Daley and Drane 1972; Bedwinek 1976). Osteoradionecrosis of the maxilla is rare, and a conservative approach regarding extraction of teeth in the maxilla therefore seems justified. In addition, we feel that extraction of maxillary teeth within the radiation field can be performed after radiation therapy with little risk of a bony infection. A far different situation exists in the mandible, where exposure of bone and infection after therapy can lead to loss of large segments, resulting in significant morbidity. Consequently, a more aggressive management approach is advocated when evaluating mandibular teeth for extraction prior to therapy. Particular attention should obviously be directed to the mandibular molars when they are within the radiation beam.

## Prognosis for Tumor Control

Tumor prognosis can be of predominant importance in patients where palliation and relief of symptoms are the primary goal of the radiation therapist. Teeth ordinarily extracted in a patient with a more favorable prognosis are not extracted in terminal patients. If the clinician feels that the remaining teeth will cause patients unnecessary pain and discomfort during their remaining days, they probably should be extracted. If, however, extractions could compromise the functional or emotional well-being of the patient, they probably should be deferred.

## Dose

The higher the dose the higher the incidence of postradiation sequelae. In patients treated to the highest level of tolerance a more aggressive program of extracting teeth prior to therapy is indicated. Conversely, in patients treated more conservatively, a less aggressive approach is indicated. For example, for patients with lesions to be treated by means of a combined approach (radiation followed by a surgical resection), the radiation therapist may be more conservative. The dose level often will be lower than that normally used for cure. The lower dose allows the surgeon to operate with decreased risk of complication. Therefore, a more conservative approach in extracting teeth from these patients is justified prior to therapy.

The type of tumor will also dictate the radiation levels employed in treatment. Patients treated for Hodgkin's disease receive dosages which reach 4500 to 5000 rad, whereas patients with squamous cell carcinoma of the oral cavity receive 6500 to 8000 rad. Although osteoradionecroses have been reported at the lower radiation levels, occurrence at these dose rates is extremely rare. In addition, lymphomas and Hodgkin's disease occur in a younger population of patients whose capacity for repair is greater. Clinical experience indicates that posttherapy extractions involve less risk in this particular patient population.

## Surgical Procedures

When dental extractions are performed in the preradiation period, clinical experience and the literature indicate that the following factors should be observed for best results: (1) Radical alveolectomy should be performed and primary closure obtained. Meticulous care should be exercised in tending the tissue flaps. Good surgical technique will pay great dividends in reducing the incidence of complications. (2) Teeth should be removed in segments within the field of radiation. It is far easier to perform an appropriate alveolectomy and attain adequate soft tissue closure by extracting teeth in segments. When individual teeth are extracted, closure is difficult to obtain without excessive tension on tissue flaps. (3) Some authors advocate administering antibiotics during the healing period. It is difficult to assess the benefit prophylactic antibiotics provide in these situations. They probably are effective when extractions result in excessive trauma. (4) In most patients, 7 to 10 days are adequate for healing before therapy is begun. This period may be extended or shortened depending upon progress made by the patient, ease or difficulty of the surgery, proposed dose, and radiation fields. When the whole body of the mandible is to be included in the radiation field, healing time should probably be extended in excess of two weeks.

It should be emphasized that preradiation extractions should be accomplished with minimal trauma to flaps, and closure should be effected without excessive tension. The lingual flap in the mandible is most susceptible to mishandling during the surgical procedure, and perforation or thinning often leads to a bony exposure after radiation therapy. It should be reemphasized that within the field the periosteum will be the predominant source of vascularity after therapy and all efforts should be made to avoid mishandling it during the surgical procedure.

## Postradiation Extractions

The risk of bone necrosis secondary to dental extractions in the postradiation period has been debated by many clinicians. Many issues remain unresolved, including incidence of necrosis, timing of extraction relative to the end of radiation therapy, and the surgical approach most desirable when performing extractions.

The risk of bone necrosis following extraction of teeth within the radiation field has been reported to be as high as 100% (Daley and Drane 1972) and as low as 0% (Wildermuth and Cantril 1953; Solomon et al. 1968; Carl, Schaaf, and Sako 1973). Interpretation of the data provided in these studies is difficult, however, because of imprecise definitions of osteoradionecrosis and poor documentation of radiation doses and radiation fields.

A recent review at the University of California, Los Angeles (Beumer, Curtis, and Harrison 1979) has revealed new information but has not settled all of the issues. In this study bone necrosis was defined as exposed bone within the radiation field of at least two months' duration not accompanied by local neoplastic disease. In this study the incidence of bone necrosis following dental extractions within the radiation field after therapy was 12% (table 14.7). One additional patient developed bone necrosis precipitated by mucosal irritation from complete dentures at a posttherapy extraction site. Three have healed, three are still present but are improving, and two proceeded to pathologic fracture and formation of oral cutaneous fistulae eventually requiring resection. In an additional three patients, healing was delayed following extraction but mucosal coverage was complete within two months following surgery (table 14.8). There was no perceptible difference relative to dose, radiation fields, modalities of therapy, and the risk of bone necrosis between the group developing bone necrosis and the group that did not.

Evidence derived from animal studies implies that some revascularization does take place within the radiated tissues after therapy (Hoffmeister, Macomber, and Wong 1969), and indeed many clinicians have reported that fewer bone necroses occur after, rather than before, two years have elapsed since the completion of radiation therapy (Daley and Drane 1972; Beumer, Silverman, and Benak 1972; Hoffmeister, Macomber, and Wong 1969). Consequently an attempt was made to defer extraction of teeth as long as possi-

**Table 14.7**
Postradiation Extractions Time Interval:
Radiation Therapy to Extraction
(50 Patients, 57 Extraction Procedures)

| Time Lapse between Therapy and Extraction | Number of Surgical Extraction Procedures | Number of Osteoradionecroses Directly Referrable to Extractions (No./%) |
|---|---|---|
| 0 to 12 months | 12 | 0 |
| 13 to 24 months | 11 | 4/36 |
| 25 to 36 months | 14 | 0 |
| More than 36 months | 20 | 3/15 |
| Totals | 57 | 7/12 |

**Table 14.8**
Osteoradionecrosis at Posttherapy Extraction Sites

| Tumor Site and Diagnosis | Dose | Modality | Radiation Fields | Teeth Extracted in Field | Time of Extraction (Months after Therapy) | Site of Necrosis | Follow-up |
|---|---|---|---|---|---|---|---|
| Squamous carcinoma Floor of mouth | 6975 | $^{60}Co$ | Opposed mandibular | $\overline{432 \mid 23}$ | 24 | $\overline{43 \mid 34}$ | Enlarged with conservative measures eventually requiring resection |
| Tonsil | 6700 | Linear accelerator | 2 right to 1 left facial to $\underline{4 \mid 4}$ | $\overline{765 \mid 567}$ | 60 | $\overline{6 \mid 56}$ | Still present but improving with conservative measures 12 months after onset. |
| Mucoepi-dermoid Parotid | 5579 | $^{60}Co$ | Right facial to $\frac{4 \mid}{4 \mid}$ | $\overline{765 \mid}$ | 96 | $\overline{76 \mid}$ | Enlarged with conservative measures leading to pathologic fracture and oral cutaneous fistula eventually requiring resection |
| Squamous carcinoma Soft palate | 6600 | $^{60}Co$ | Right and left facial to $\frac{4 \mid 4}{4 \mid 4}$ | $\overline{7 \mid}$ | 40 | $\overline{7 \mid}$ | Healed with conservative measures and hyperbaric therapy 24 months after onset |
| Squamous carcinoma Base of tongue | 7000 | Linear accelerator | Right and left facial to $\frac{4 \mid 4}{4 \mid 4}$ | $\overline{765 \mid 567}$ | 24 | $\overline{76 \mid}$ | Still present; no change with conservative measures 9 months after onset |
| Squamous carcinoma Maxillary sinus | 6700 | Linear accelerator | Right and left facial to $\underline{1 \mid 1}$ | $\underline{12 \mid}$ | 20 | $\underline{2 \mid}$ | Healed with conservative measures 13 months after onset |
| Squamous carcinoma Floor of mouth | 7333 | Linear accelerator | Opposed mandibular | $\overline{\mid 4567}$ | 18 | $\overline{\mid 4}$ | Still present; no change with conservative measures after onset |
| Squamous carcinoma* Floor of mouth | 6580 | $^{60}Co$ | Opposed mandibular | $\frac{875 \mid 67}{421 \mid 123}$ | 20<br>36<br>65 | $\overline{\mid 2}$ | Secondary to denture irritation; healed with conservative measures following removal of dentures |

*Precipitated by denture irritation.

ble in the hope of reducing the risk of necrosis. In our study, however, the time lapse between the end of radiation therapy and dental extraction seemed to have little effect on the risk of osteoradionecrosis (table 14.7). The fact that three necroses occurred more than three years following completion of radiation therapy indicates that tissue effects are relatively irreversible when significant portions of the mandible are included within the radiation fields. When the situation otherwise permits, we suggest root canal therapy be attempted before considering dental extraction.

Some clinicians feel that when extractions are necessary they should be performed with minimal trauma (Carl, Schaaf, and Sako 1973; Hayward et al. 1969). Others propose that mucoperiosteal flaps should be reflected, radical alveolectomies performed, and primary closure be obtained for best results (Beumer, Silverman, and Benak 1972). All agree that prophylactic antibiotic coverage is useful. In our study of 43 patients upon whom radical alveolectomies were performed and primary closure attained, three developed necrosis. In eight patients teeth were extracted atraumatically with only minimal removal of bone and without obtaining primary closure. Four of these patients developed osteoradionecrosis.

In summary, in the mandible we attempt to employ conservative dental measures, such as root canal therapy, before considering dental extraction of teeth within the radiation field. When mandibular teeth require extraction in the postradiotherapy patient, we perform them in association with radical alveolectomy, primary closure and provide antibiotic coverage. The risk of necrosis while employing this philosophy has run about 10%. In radiation fields in which the whole body of the mandible is included, we do not feel that deferring extractions for undetermined periods will significantly improve local vascularity. In other field set-ups in which only a portion of the mandibular body is included within the field, vascularity locally may improve and justify deferring surgery until at least one year has elapsed after therapy. Recent evidence indicates that hyperbaric oxygen therapy will reduce the incidence and severity of postradiation extraction complication (Hart and Maimous 1976).

The risk of complications secondary to extraction of teeth after radiation therapy in the maxilla is exceedingly small. Because of the greater vasculature in the maxilla, healing is usually rapid and risk of necrosis slight. We feel that radical alveolectomies are neither necessary nor technically practical, particularly in posterior maxillary teeth. If a necrosis does occur in the maxilla its resolution is almost always effected with conservative measures resulting in little morbidity for the patient.

## Osteoradionecrosis

The incidence of osteoradionecrosis, although apparently declining since the advent of supervoltage radiation therapy, has not done so dramatically. The relatively lower radiation absorption resulting from this equipment apparently is being partially offset by the increased dose levels employed with current techniques. Preradiation evaluations and dental prophylactic measures probably are responsible for whatever reduction can be documented. Recent studies assign the risk to be somewhat less than 10% of all those treated. This overall figure is quite misleading, for in some lesions the risk of necrosis can be quite high. Risk is dependent upon size and location of the lesions, volume of mandible within the radiation field, dose level, and health of the dentition, among other factors.

When the primary tumor is adjacent to or overlies bone, the risk of necrosis is significantly increased. Often, particularly in large lesions, rapid destruction of tumor results in a direct bone exposure. Even if the mucosa does regrow it often is thin and atrophic and thus much more susceptible to perforation. The size of the primary has long been thought to be an important indicator of the risk of necrosis. In the Bedwinek and associates (1976) study, T3 lesions had double the rate of spontaneous necrosis of T2 lesions, and five times the incidence of T1 lesions.

The volume of the mandible within the radiation field is undoubtedly a prime factor relating to predisposition to bone necrosis. In our study, 30 out of 50 patients were treated with bilateral opposed mandibular fields, thus including the entire body of the mandible within the primary beam (Beumer, Curtis, and Harrison 1979). The postradiation avascularity of the mandible is doubtlessly more profound and irreversible when such fields are employed. In 11 out of 14 patients developing osteoradionecrosis from preradiation extractions, opposed mandibular fields were employed (table 14.2).

Retromolar trigone and base of tongue-tonsillar pillar lesions likewise seem to imply increased risk because of the nature and extent of the radiation fields. The bilateral fields employed include most of the major salivary glands and extend anteriorly to include much of the body of the mandible. This regimen results in substantial reduction in salivary output as well as significant compromise of the vascularity of the body of the mandible. Indeed, in one report the incidence of bone necrosis was 37% following irradiation of tumors in those areas where similar radiation fields were employed (Grant and Fletcher 1966).

Obviously, as the dose increases, tissue changes become more profound and irreversible, leading to increased incidence of bone complications. Total dose, however, by itself is not always an accurate indicator of tissue response. The number of fractions, dosage per fraction, and time period over which the therapy is delivered are all important variables to be considered when evaluating biologic effects. Hence the NSD (nominal single dose) index may be a valuable predictor of tissue response (Ellis 1968). This index is an attempt to account for the variables of delivery so as to indicate more accurately what is the true biologic response. Theoretically, normal tissue tolerance in the head and neck has been postulated to be in the range of 1800 ret (rad therapeutic equivalent). The NSD index does have some limitations, the most important being that it does not incorporate a necessary and vital tolerance parameter into the equation-volume included within the radiation field. The NSD index may prove to be a valuable instrument in delineating risks of complications, but more detailed studies need to be completed before all-encompassing suppositions can be made. In our study, the numbers of osteoradionecroses occurring at levels less than 1800 and the high percentage of patients retaining mucosal integrity with NSDs above 1800 indicate that individual tolerance to radiation is an important cofactor (Beumer, Curtis, and Harrison 1979).

The development of new, more adaptable radioactive sources and recent advances in implantation techniques and dosimetry have enabled the therapist to implant a greater variety of oral cavity neoplasms. Implantation techniques normally are of advantage because exposure to bone, salivary glands, and mucosa is minimized. In floor of mouth lesions, however, the implant inadvertently may be placed quite close to the mandible. In our series those bone necroses secondary to interstitial therapy for anterior and lateral floor of mouth lesions proved to be the most intractable to the conservative forms of treatment. Four out of the five progressed to pathologic fracture and progressive loss of significant segments of the mandible. They were not responsive to irrigations, antibiotics (local and systemic), or hyperbaric oxygen therapy.

Most osteoradionecroses appear to develop from either preradiation or postradiation extractions. In our study those developing spontaneously were most often associated with mandibular molars demonstrating severe periodontal bone loss. As previously suggested, furcation involvement of mandibular molars is grounds for preradiation extraction. Such clinical presentation usually indicates a history of dental neglect, and if such dentitions are left intact the most stringent oral hygiene is required to prevent complications.

Extractions of teeth either prior to or after radiation increase the risk of necrosis. Definitive data defining the risk are scanty and difficult to interpret. We suggest that a conservative philosophy be adhered to when considering teeth for extraction prior to therapy. After radiation is completed all conservative measures available should be considered before proceeding with dental extractions.

In our study (Beumer, Curtis, and Harrison 1979) most osteoradionecrosis developed within the two years after radiation therapy (29 of 50), but the substantial number of cases appearing after the second year indicate that tissue changes resulting from radiation are long-lasting. Other studies support this finding (Daley and Drane 1972).

## Treatment

A conservative approach is advocated in the management of osteoradionecrosis. Most bone exposures can be controlled with local irrigation, topical application of antibiotic packings, and selective use of systemic antibiotics.

In our UCLA study only 4 of 50 patients have required mandibular resection to control infection. Stringent oral hygiene measures must be demanded of the patient, and close follow-up by the clinician is necessary. Depending upon the extent and severity of the exposure these patients are monitored from twice a week to once per month. Those projections contributing to irritation of adjacent structures should be smoothed, but aggressive surgical sequestration is not indicated. Only those bone sequestrae which are loose should be removed. If healing is progressing adequately mucosa or granulation tissue will be found underneath the loose sequestrations. Zinc oxide and neosporin packings have been advocated by some clinicians.

Patience on the part of the clinician during the follow-up of these patients is of primary importance. Bone exposures in irradiated tissues require extended periods for healing. Healing is accomplished by natural sequestration, and, because of the relative avascular nature of the affected bone, osteoclastic activity and resorption of nonvital bone may take many months or even years. Antibiotics are usually necessary only to control acute flare-up of local infection. It is not advised that patients with bone exposures be placed on systemic antibiotics for months. Doing so results in little benefit because of the compromised vasculature of the local area and may lead to the promotion of resistant organisms.

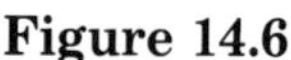

**Figure 14.6**

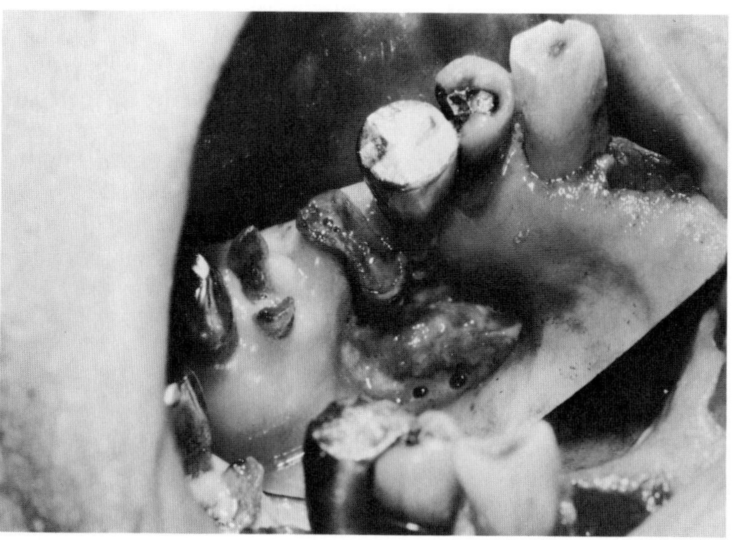

*Bone exposure following external radiation therapy for an anterior floor of mouth carcinoma.*

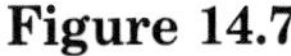

**Figure 14.7**

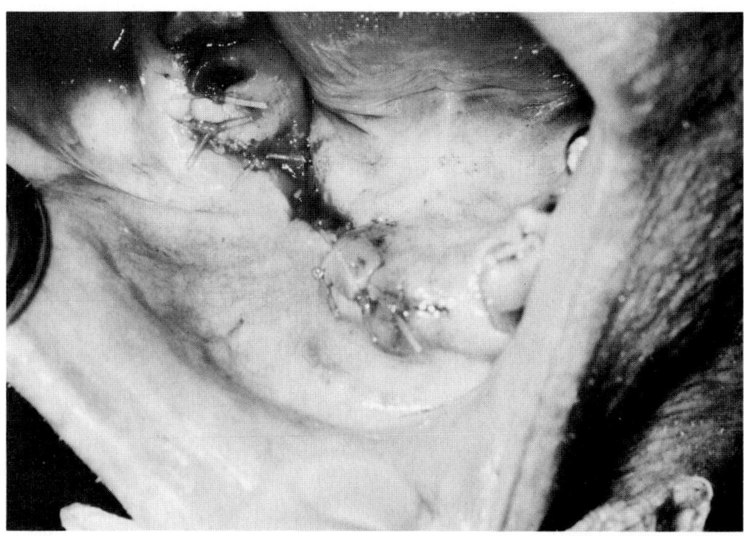

*After 20 treatments of hyperbaric oxygen, teeth were extracted and the wound debrided.*

A most exciting development in the treatment of osteoradionecrosis is the advent of hyperbaric oxygen therapy. Investigative studies have indicated increased osteoblastic and osteoclastic activity in hyperbaric environments. Hart and Maimous (1976) reported on 46 patients with osteoradionecrosis of the mandible treated with this technique. Patients with bone necrosis were exposed to two atmospheres of oxygen in a hyperbaric chamber for two hours per session. One course of therapy extended for 120 hours. Nine-aminoacridine was used to irrigate the local area daily, and the patients were placed on systemic tetracyline once oral suppuration had been controlled. Neomycin packings were used on purulent oral wounds. Surgical procedures (extraction, removal of sequestra, debridement) were performed between the twentieth and fortieth treatments. Alpha-tocopherol (100 mg daily) was administered during the treatment course.

All patients were candidates for mandibulectomy according to Rankow and Weisman's formula. After the first series of hyperbaric treatments, 37 of 46 patients were free of symptoms including elimination of all bony exposure intraorally. Nine patients had teeth extracted with radical alveolectomy, and all sites healed without complication. Five of these patients had immediate dentures inserted with a temporary denture reliner. These prosthetic restorations were employed without complication. In four patients mandibular bone grafts were placed to restore a discontinuity defect. All four were successful. It should be noted that this series of osteoradionecroses was comprised of those patients with the most serious and extensive exposures. Nineteen patients, for instance, had pathologic fracture of the mandible and 15 had oral cutaneous fistulae prior to hyperbaric therapy.

It is difficult to assess what role the local procedures (daily irrigations, antibiotic packings) played in the success enjoyed by these clinicians. Obviously local procedures are important, but this study makes it impossible to assess accurately these variables since no controls were used. It should be noted that in the absence of regular aggressive local wound debridement hyperbaric oxygen has been less successful. Surgical debridement and extraction of teeth are best effected after at least 20 hours of therapy (figs. 14.6, 14.7, and 14.8).

**Figure 14.8**

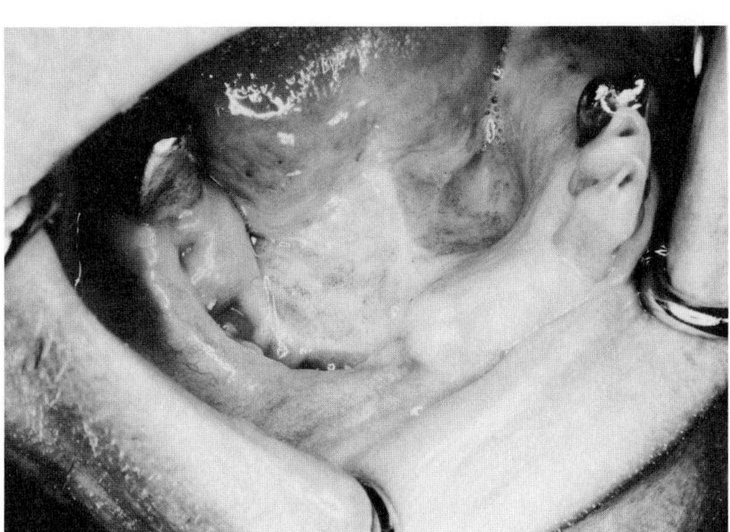

*Patient three months following hyperbaric treatment. The bone exposure is resolved.*

# References

Bedwinek, J. M. et al. Osteonecrosis in patients with definitive radiotherapy for squamous cell carcinomas of the oral cavity and naso- and oropharynx. *Radiology* 119:665–667, 1976.

Beumer, J., III.; Curtis, T. E.; and Harrison, R. E. Radiation therapy of the oral cavity: sequellae and management, part 2. *Head Neck Surg.* 1:392–408, 1979.

Beumer, J., III; Silverman, S.; and Benak, S. B. Hard and soft tissue necroses following radiation therapy for oral cancer. *J. Prosthet. Dent.* 27:640–644, 1972.

Carl, W.; Schaaf, N. G.; and Sako, K. Oral surgery and the patient who has had radiation therapy for head and neck cancer. *Oral Surg.* 36:651–659, 1973.

Daland, E. M. Surgical treatment of postirradiation necrosis. *Am. J. Roentgenol.* 46:287–301, 1941.

Daley, T. E., and Drane, J. B. *Management of dental problems in irradiated patients.* Houston: University of Texas Press, 1972.

Del Regato, J. A. Dental lesions observed after roentgen therapy in cancer of the buccal cavity, pharynx, and larynx. *Am. J. Roentgenol.* 42:404–410, 1939.

Ellis, R. Relationship of biologic effect to dose-time fractionation factors in radiotherapy. In *Current topics in radiation research,* vol. 4. Amsterdam: North Holland Publishing Co., 1968.

Grant, B. P., and Fletcher, G. H. Analysis of complications following megavoltage therapy for squamous carcinoma of the tonsillar area. *Am. J. Roentgenol.* 96:28–36, 1966.

Hart, G. B., and Maimous, E. G. The treatment of radiation necrosis with hyperbaric oxygen. *Cancer* 37:2580–2585, 1976.

Hayward, J. R. et al. The management of teeth related to treatment of oral cancer. *Cancer* 19:98–106, 1969.

Hoffmeister, F. S.; Macomber, W. B.; and Wong, M. K. Radiation in dentistry—surgical comments. *J. Am. Dent. Assoc.* 78:511–516, 1969.

Quick, D. The treatment of intraoral malignant disease. In *Clinical therapeutic radiology,* ed. U. V. Portman. New York: Thomas Nelson, 1959.

Shearer, H. T. Effect of cobalt-60 radiation on extraction healing in the mandible of dogs. *J. Oral Surg.* 25:115–121, 1967.

Silverman, S., and Chierci, G. Radiation therapy of oral carcinoma. I. Effects on oral tissues and management of the periodontium. *J. Periodontol.* 36:478–484, 1965.

Solomon, H., et al. Extraction of teeth after cancerocidal doses of radiation therapy to the head and neck. *Am. J. Surg.* 115:349–351, 1968.

Starcke, E. N., and Shannon, I. L. How critical is the interval between extractions and irradiation in patients with head and neck malignancy? *Oral Surg.* 43:333–337, 1977.

Stein, M.; Brady, L. W.; and Raventos, A. The effects of radiation on extraction wound healing in the rat. *Cancer* 10:1167–1180, 1957.

Wildermuth, O., and Cantril, S. T. Radiation necrosis of the mandible. *Radiology* 61:771–785, 1953.

# Chapter 15

# *Cervical Lymph Node Metastases: The Place of Radiotherapy*

Peter J. Fitzpatrick and
Barry S. Tepperman

There are 20 to 30 lymph nodes on either side of the neck, extending from the base of the skull to the clavicle (fig. 15.1). The lymph nodes in superficial and deep groups are mainly situated in chains below the ramus of the mandible in close approximation to the carotid sheath and above the clavicle. These lymph nodes drain the superficial tissues and deep structures of the head and neck. In this study, we numbered the groups of nodes because of their different clinical behavior, prognosis, and treatment. Group 1 includes the submental and submaxillary nodes; groups 2, 3, and 4 the upper, middle and lower cervical nodes; and group 5 the nodes in the posterior triangle. When tumors metastasize through the lymphatics, not all of the nodes trap cancer cells and develop into regional metastases.

## The Treatment of Metastatic Cervical Lymph Nodes

The definition of an optimal therapeutic approach, preferably with minimal necessary treatment, requires an impartial and objective analysis of the advantages and disadvantages of the different treatment methods available. These are mainly surgical or radiotherapeutic or a combination of both, and their various merits have been vigorously debated for half a century and they have been the subject of many reports.

---

This chapter represents the combined efforts of many people. We are grateful to the various members of the radiotherapy staff of the Princess Margaret Hospital for allowing us to review their patients. Many surgeons referred these patients, and without their cooperation and help this chapter could not have been assembled. In particular we wish to thank Mrs. Shaheen Khan for the computerization of results and statistical help. Over 400 pages of computer printouts and tables were generated in order to tabulate the information recorded here. Without the secretarial assistance of Miss Evelyn Eisenreich, this chapter would not have been completed. To all these, we offer our grateful thanks.

**Figure 15.1**

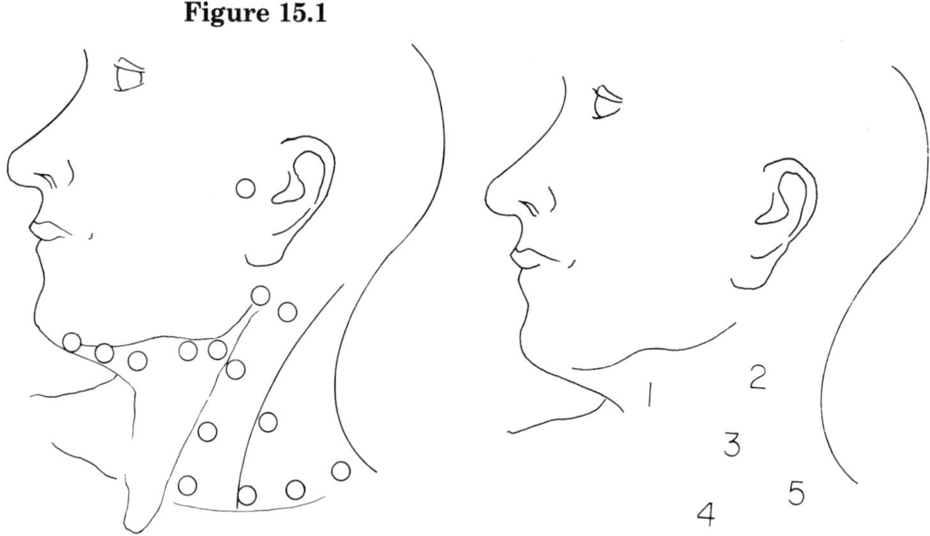


*The main chains of lymph nodes in the neck. Group* 1 *includes the submental and submaxillary nodes; groups* 2, 3, *and* 4 *the upper, middle, and lower deep cervical nodes; group* 5 *includes nodes in the posterior triangle of the neck.*

The standard radical neck dissection was first described by Crile in 1906. This operation removes the lymph-bearing structures of the neck from the mandible to the clavicle and from the midline to the trapezius. There have been many modifications of the standard operation to improve cosmesis and function while controlling metastatic disease. The operation is usually confined to one side of the neck, although bilateral dissections are performed in selected cases. The operation is considered therapeutic when palpable disease is detected, elective when nodes involved histologically are removed before they become palpable, and deferred when impalpable nodes subsequently become palpable. The indications for these operations vary with the site, extent, and control of the primary tumor and the patient's age and general condition. The success of these operations varies from center to center and report to report. Failure is most commonly associated with coincidental failure of treatment at the primary site. In general an elective neck dissection for occult metastases will control the neck for about half of all patients whereas therapeutic or deferred neck dissections only control one-third of all cases (Mustard and Rosen 1963; Som 1973). The failures die from uncontrolled regional metastatic disease in some distress and discomfort and disfigured by extensive and often mutilating surgery. To improve these results, both pre- and postoperative radiation have been tried with limited success.

It is a common practice to irradiate lymph node fields draining cancer sites in the head and neck. The treatment is therapeutic when the aim is to destroy malignant cells in clinically involved nodes and prophylactic when the object is to sterilize presumed microscopic tumor deposits. Radiotherapy has a poor reputation in many quarters for its curative effect on metastatic cervical nodes. Indeed, it seldom controls nodes that are fixed or greater than 3 cm in diameter. There is good evidence, however, that therapeutic radiation will control about one-third of clinically malignant nodes and that prophylactic radiation can prevent the development of overt metastases in about half of all patients (Hanks, Bagshaw, and Kaplan 1969; Berger et al. 1971; Wizenberg et al. 1972; Million 1974; Schneider, Fletcher, and Barkley 1975; Fu, Lichter, and Galante 1976).

The damaging effect of radiation on lymph nodes depends upon the amount of radiation received. With doses up to 3000 rad there is a reduction in the number of lymphocytes and some shrinkage of the follicles. As the dose increases the follicles are destroyed, and by 4000 rad no recognizable lymphoid tissue is seen. The small lymphocytes intimately concerned with the immune response disappear, and this reduction in the lymphocyte population may theoretically reduce the quantitative response to the tumor. The final appearance following high-dose radiation is an unrecognizable fibrosed and hyalinized lymph node (Burge 1975; Henk 1975).

There is a steady relationship between the extent of the primary tumor and the presence of significant lymph nodes either at the time of diagnosis or subsequently. There is also a constant relationship between lymph node size and the likelihood of control by radiation, which is dependent on the size and fixity of the nodes rather than the number involved. Metastatic squamous cell carcinoma in the lymph nodes is not more radioresistant than the primary tumor from which it is derived. It is therefore sound clinical practice to irradiate the primary tumor and regional nodes en bloc (Hanks, Bagshaw, and Kaplan 1969; Wizenberg et al. 1972; Schneider, Fletcher, and Barkley 1975; Fu, Lichter, and Galante 1976). The radiation field extends from the mandible to the clavicle and from the midline anteriorly to the line of the transverse cervical processes posteriorly. The tissues of the neck should be adequately irradiated to a depth of 3 cm, but treatment is individualized according to need. Laryngeal and spinal cord shields should be used to limit the radiation to these structures when a tumor dose in excess of 4500 rad is prescribed. The primary tumor must be adequately encompassed, and if it crosses the midline then the cervical lymph nodes on both sides of the neck should be irradiated. In general, higher doses of radiation are required to destroy gross tumor whereas smaller doses will eliminate the better-oxygenated occult micrometastases.

To determine the place of megavoltage radiation and optimum time-dose relationships in the treatment of metastatic cancer in the neck two groups of patients were reviewed in detail. These were a series of patients with cervical metastases from an unknown primary tumor (Fitzpatrick and Kotalik 1974) and another with squamous cell carcinoma arising in the floor of the mouth.

**Figure 15.2**

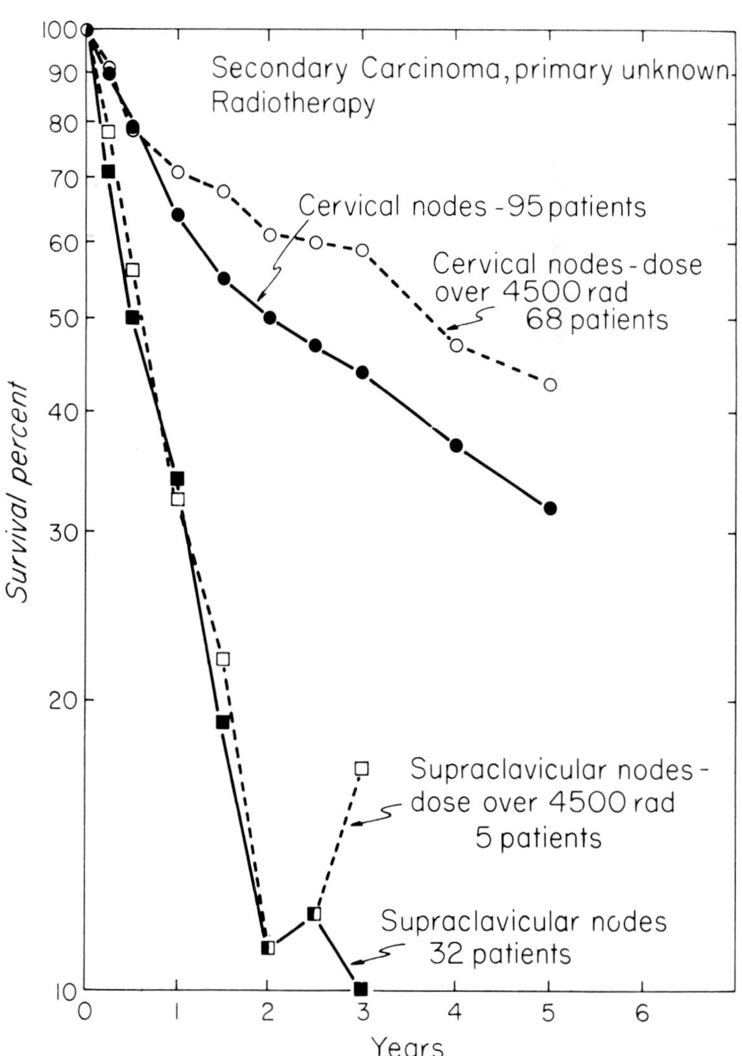


*The crude survival for 233 patients with secondary carcinoma in the neck but no known primary tumor is divided into cervical and supraclavicular groups. Patients with cervical disease alone and treated to 4500 rad or more had a better prognosis, with a five-year survival of 43%.*

## Cervical Metastasis from an Unknown Primary Tumor

It is now established that over 70% of patients with metastatic cancer in the neck in whom there is no detectable primary tumor have in fact a cancer somewhere within the head and neck. Common occult sites include the nasopharynx, tonsil, base of tongue, and pyriform fossa. These are the probable primary sites in 90% of patients when the metastases are in the upper or midcervical region. Because of these facts it is logical to treat a block of tissue that includes the cervical node metastases in continuity with the probable primary tumor sites.

Among 233 patients whose first symptom of disease included a lump in the neck 95 patients had disease limited to the upper or middle neck and a histologic diagnosis of undifferentiated or squamous cell carcinoma. The patients were treated by radiotherapy, and the five-year crude survival was a disappointing 32% (fig. 15.2), although a subgroup of 68 patients treated in this manner to 4500 rad or more had a better prognosis, with a five-year survival of 43%. During this period the five-year survival for carcinomas of the nasopharynx and oral cavity was 30% and 40% overall.

## Squamous Cell Carcinoma of the Floor of the Mouth

Squamous cell carcinoma of the mouth metastasizes through the lymphatics, piercing the mylohyoid muscle to the first-echelon nodes in the submental or submaxillary regions. Tumor cells then spread in a fairly orderly manner to the upper and midcervical nodes situated on the superficial surface of the internal jugular vein. Untreated or uncontrolled the tumor cells enter the jugular vein via lymphaticovenous communications and seed metastases in the lungs and elsewhere. Few patients die as a result of distant metastases. The most common cause of death is failure to control the primary tumor and regional metastases.

Between 1958 and 1975, 377 patients with squamous cell carcinoma were seen. Radiation was the primary treatment in 330 (87.5%) patients. The median age was 60 years, and males predominated over females 4 to 1. Classified by the UICC (1978) system, 235 (62%) patients had T1 or T2 lesions, and in 242 (64%) patients the cervical nodes were not palpable. The clinical stage of the lymph nodes and the level of cervical involvement are shown in table 15.1. The majority of patients had mobile homolateral metastases in the submental or submaxillary regions.

In order to study the force of regional metastases on prognosis, a multivariate analysis was carried out with the aid of a computer. One-third of the patients are found to have cervical node metastases, another third develop

**Table 15.1**
The Clinical Stage (UICC 1978) and Level of Metastatic Cervical Nodes among 377 Patients with Squamous Cell Carcinoma of the Floor of the Mouth

| Nodes | Patients | Level 1 | 2 | 3 | 4 | 2 Sites |
|---|---|---|---|---|---|---|
| N0 | 242 (64%) | | | | | |
| N1 | 75 | 59 | 14 | 7 | 1 | 1 |
| N2 | 23 | 12 | 7 | 3 | 2 | 7 |
| N3 | 37 | 25 | 8 | 5 | 0 | 7 |
| Totals | 377 | 96 | 29 | 15 | 3 | 15 |

NOTE: Ninety-seven patients have nodes at one level only. Two-thirds of patients do not have detectable metastases at diagnosis.

them later, and in the remaining third metastases are never detected. The development of regional metastases implies a guarded prognosis (fig. 15.3). When the regional nodes remain uncontrolled the five-year survival is 17.5%, compared to 33% when the metastases are destroyed. Failure to control regional metastases is soon apparent, with 97% detected within two years and over half within three months following primary treatment.

**Figure 15.3**

377 Patients { 135 (36%) N1, N2, N3
91 (24%) N + later
226 (60%) N + anytime

| Nodes | | | 5-Year Survival |
|---|---|---|---|
| | Controlled | 69 | 33% |
| | Uncontrolled | 157 | 17.5% |

| Months | Patients (157) | Cumulative Failure (%) |
|---|---|---|
| < 3 (residual) | 92 | 59 |
| 3–6 | 27 | 76 |
| 6–24 | 33 | 97 |
| > 24 | 5 | 100 |

*Squamous cell carcinoma of the floor of the mouth. Metastases in regional nodes are present in one-third of patients at diagnosis and subsequently develop in another third. Survival is doubled when they are controlled.*

**Table 15.2**
Squamous Cell Carcinoma of the Floor of the Mouth (377 Patients): Control Regional Nodes—First Treatment

| Nodes | Surgery | Radiation | Combined | Total | Percentage |
|---|---|---|---|---|---|
| N0 | 12/16 | 163/219 | 8/12 | 183/247 | 74 |
| N1 | 3/8 | 22/58 | 2/4 | 27/70 | 39 |
| N2 | 0/2 | 1/19 | 0/2 | 1/23 | 4 |
| N3 | 0/2 | 5/34 | 0/1 | 5/37 | 14 |
| Totals | 15/28 (54%) | 191/330 (58%) | 10/19 (53%) | 216/377 | 57 |

NOTE: Different treatment modalities produce comparable results in all clinical stages.

Radiotherapy was used in treating the regional nodes in the majority of patients, although some were managed by surgery or a combination of surgery and radiation (table 15.2). The control rates of metastatic disease in the lateral neck ranged from 74% for those in whom the first examination failed to reveal enlarged nodes to 14% in whom the nodes were fixed. Overall, the different treatment modalities produced similar results and an overall control rate of 57%.

There were 114 patients who had metastatic cervical nodes at the time of diagnosis and who were treated by external radiation. The techniques varied, and the radiation doses ranged from 2000 rad in two weeks to 6000 rad in six weeks. When the data were analyzed in 500-rad steps, no obvious difference in control was found among the different groups. Therefore the results are summarized into patients receiving more or less than 5000 rad

**Table 15.3**
Squamous Cell Carcinoma of the Floor of the Mouth (114 Patients): Radiotherapy of Metastatic Nodes

| | | Control | |
|---|---|---|---|
| Nodes | Patients | < 5000 Rad | ⩾ 5000 Rad |
| N1 | 62 | 7/15 | 20/47 |
| N2 | 20 | 0/7 | 2/13 |
| N3 | 32 | 1/17 | 2/15 |
| Totals | | 8/39 (20%) | 24/75 (32%) |

NOTES: $P = 0.08$.
Radiation doses over 5000 rad probably achieve better control of metastatic cervical nodes.

**Figure 15.4**

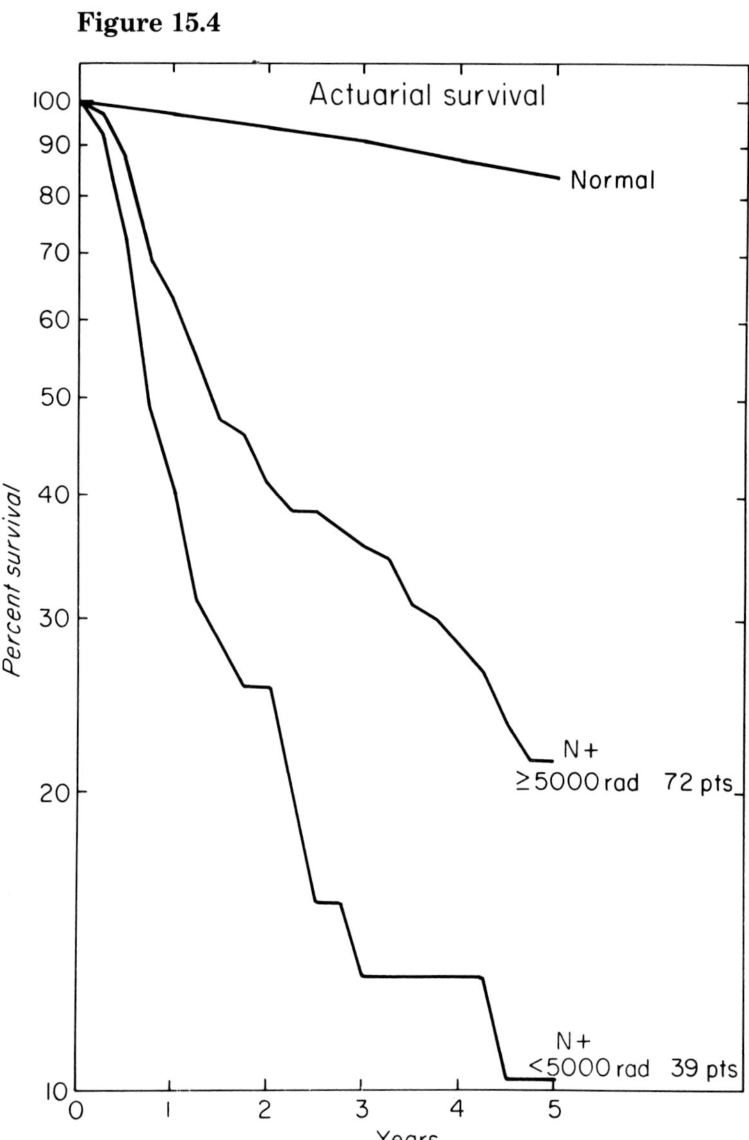


*Among patients with metastatic cervical nodes from squamous cell carcinoma of the floor of the mouth, radiation doses over 5000 rad achieved better control and survival.*

(table 15.3). The differences are not statistically significant, but we have a strong impression that radiation doses in excess of 5000 rad achieve better tumor control. These results correlate with the higher five-year survival (24%) of patients with metastatic nodes treated to 5000 rad or more, com-

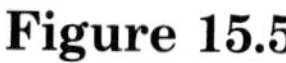

**Figure 15.5**

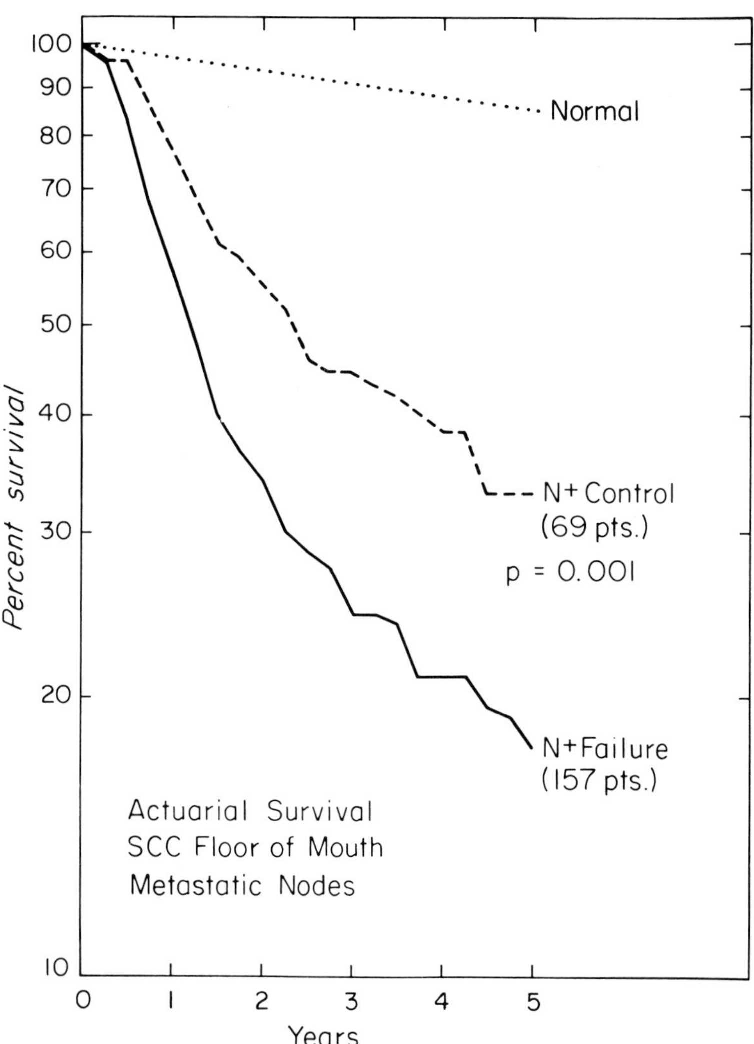


*Patients who have their metastatic nodes controlled have a better survival at all times than do those who fail.*

pared to survival of only 10% among those who received a lower dose (fig. 15.4).

The treatment of metastatic lymph nodes uncontrolled by the first planned treatment is disappointing (fig. 15.5). Surgery provides the best results, with 61% control in selected cases. When used after failure of initial treatment, radiation is usually palliative. Only 12.5% of the patients man-

**Table 15.4**
Squamous Cell Carcinoma of the Floor of the Mouth (115 Patients): Salvage of Metastatic Nodes

| | Surgery | Radiation | Combined |
|---|---|---|---|
| Residual ≤ 3 months | 16/31 (51%) | 0/20 (0%) | 4/19 (21%) |
| Recurrent | 14/18 (77%) | 4/12 (33%) | 8/15 (53%) |
| Totals | 30/49 (61%) | 4/32 (12.5%) | 12/34 (35%) |

NOTE: When the first planned treatment fails to control regional nodes, surgery, sometimes combined with radiation, provides the best chance of salvage.

aged in this way were controlled. The treatment of uncontrolled cervical metastases was superior by all modalities in those patients who developed metastases after their initial treatment when compared to patients with residual disease at three months (table 15.4). The results of any method of treatment, however, were inferior when the primary tumor was uncontrolled.

Because of the reduced prognosis once cervical metastases are established some patients undergo prophylactic treatment by neck dissection or radiation to prevent their appearance. Fifty-seven patients received prophylactic cervical radiation; these included 42 patients with clinically negative N0 necks and 15 with metastases limited to the upper neck N1 (fig. 15.6). Fewer metastases developed in the first group, and radiation doses over 5000 rad were more successful in preventing their development. Among 187 patients in whom the initial examination failed to reveal cervical metastases, however, and in whom an expectant attitude with observation was adopted, only 44 (24%) subsequently developed metastatic nodes. While suggesting that prophylactic radiation is beneficial in destroying micrometastases in a clinically negative (N0) neck, the difference is not statistically significant.

These groups are not strictly comparable because in the N1 group the primary tumor already had confirmed metastatic potential. In two-thirds of the patients without cervical metastases, disease in the lateral neck never develops, and there was a significant advantage in those patients receiving more than 5000 rad. Among those patients (N1) with disease limited to the upper neck there was no apparent advantage in prophylactic radiation. Among the 187 patients without cervical metastases (N0) who were closely observed without prophylactic treatment, cervical metastases failed to appear in 76%. This finding is not significantly different from that for patients who received prophylactic radiation at all dose levels.

## Discussion

The objective of this study was to research two groups of patients with head and neck cancers to determine the place of megavoltage radiation in the treatment of cervical lymph node metastases. It is not our purpose to review the literature but to make definitive conclusions from our own clinical material. In retrospective studies, clinical reviews are handicapped equivalent to the shortcomings of the clinical records, and these limitations must be kept in mind when the results are considered. The first clinical record is the most important and should include a carefully completed staging sheet with the consensus of two experienced observers. The difficulties we encountered in this retrospective analysis confirm the importance of carefully controlled prospective clinical trials. The controversy that exists as to the best primary method for treating metastatic lymph nodes will continue. There is good evidence, however, that radiation is a curative agent and that moderate doses will selectively destroy neoplastic cells while in most instances sparing damage to the normal structures. Although we could not establish statistical significance we have a strong impression that 5000 rad in 20 treatments delivered in one month constitute optimal radiotherapy. The data both for control of secondary carcinoma from an unknown primary and for treatment of clinically involved nodes from carcinoma of the floor of the mouth suggest the need for a radiation dose exceeding 4500 rad.

Survival is determined by the inherent biology of the tumor, which can be modified by treatment. Radiation is equally effective in controlling the primary cancer and regional metastases, so there is little reason to divide the initial treatment between radiotherapy and surgery. Treatment should always be individualized according to the variables of host, tumor, and best

**Figure 15.6**

| | | Control | $<$ 5000 Rad | $\geq$ 5000 Rad |
|---|---|---|---|---|
| 57 Patients Radiation | N0 | 27/42 (64%) | 17/37 (46%) | 17/20 (85%) $P = 0.004$ |
| | N1 | 6/15 (40%) (lower neck) | 3/10 (30%) | 4/5 (80%) $P = 0.04$ |

143/187 (76%) N0 Patients Observed Alone Never Develop Metastatic Nodes

N0 Patients Expectant vs Prophylactic Tx, $P = 0.1$

*Prophylactic neck radiation. Some patients with squamous cell carcinoma of the floor of the mouth never develop cervical node metastases. Prophylactic radiation of the neck with doses over 5000 rad provides the best chance of destroying occult metastases.*

available treatment. It is important to select and give patients with a favorable prognosis radical therapy. When cervical metastases are present, the lymph nodes should be included with the primary tumor in the radiation field and receive the same dose. If the metastases are fixed, or larger than 3 cm in diameter, boost radiation or surgical dissection is necessary to achieve control. With the exception of patients with early T1 primary tumors, prophylactic neck radiation is recommended to destroy micrometastases and reduce the incidence of cervical metastases and the guarded prognosis once they develop. The regional control of a cancer is reflected in improved survival, but it is reasonable to limit radiation to the primary tumor and first-echelon nodes and to adopt an expectant attitude in regard to the lower cervical nodes. When this is treatment policy, patients must be examined by competent observers at monthly intervals for at least two years. The detection of metastases requires immediate intervention.

Overall, the results of treating metastatic cervical lymph nodes are disappointing. The results are worse when the first planned treatment fails, either at the primary site or at the regional lymph nodes. Currently, clinical trials are in progress to assess the efficacy of radiosensitizers in combination with radiation when compared to radiation alone. Other studies include the use of combination chemotherapy, prior to and concomitant with radiation. It is hoped that these new approaches will improve the results in head and neck cancer, which have remained essentially unchanged during the past 30 years.

## References


Ash, C. L. Oral cancer: a twenty-five year study. *Am. J. Roentgenol.* 87:417–50, 1962.

Berger, D. S. et al. Elective irradiation of the neck lymphatics for squamous cell carcinomas of the nasopharynx and oropharynx. *Am. J. Roentgenol.* 111:66–72, 1971.

Burge, J. S. Histological changes in cervical lymph nodes following clinical irradiation. *Proc. R. Soc. Med.* 68:77–79, 1975.

Fitzpatrick, P. J., and Kotalik, J. F. Cervical metastases from an unknown primary tumor. *Radiology* 110:659–663, 1974.

Fu, K. K.; Lichter, A.; and Galante, M. Carcinoma of the floor of mouth: an analysis of treatment results and the sites and causes of failures. *Int. J. Radiat. Oncol. Biol. Phys.* 1:829–837, 1976.

Hanks, G. E.; Bagshaw, M. A.; and Kaplan, M. S. The management of cervical lymph node metastasis by megavoltage radiotherapy. *Am. J. Roentgenol.* 105:74–82, 1969.

Henk, J. M. Radiosensitivity of lymph node metastases. *Proc. R. Soc. Med.* 68:85–86, 1975.

Million, R. R. Elective neck irradiation for TXNO squamous carcinoma of the oral tongue and floor of the mouth. *Cancer* 34:149–155, 1974.

Mustard, R. A., and Rosen, I. B. Cervical lymph node involvement in oral cancer. *Am. J. Roentgenol.* 90:978–989, 1963.

Schneider, J. J.; Fletcher, G. H.; and Barkley, H. T., Jr. Control by irradiation alone of non-fixed clinically positive lymph nodes from squamous cell carcinoma of the oral cavity, oropharynx, supraglottic larynx, and hypopharynx. *Am. J. Roentgenol.* 123:42–48, 1975.

Som, M. L. Elective neck dissection for carcinoma of the tongue and floor of mouth. *Trans. Am. Acad. Ophthalmol. Otolaryngol.* 77:82–85, 1973.

Wizenberg, M. J. et al. Radiation therapy in the management of lymph node metastases from head and neck cancers. *Am. J. Roentgenol.* 114:76–82, 1972.

# Chapter 16

# *Modified Neck Dissection with and without Radiation*

# Richard H. Jesse

Crile, in 1906, developed the operation known as radical neck dissection, and until recently the procedure has gone relatively unchallenged as the optimum method for control of cancer metastatic to the cervical nodes. The procedure was popularized by Martin and associates at Memorial Sloan-Kettering Hospital in New York and by a paper (1951) describing in detail their refinements of the original Crile method of radical neck dissection. The procedure, as described, removed all of the tissue between the mandible above, the clavicle below, the anterior midline, and the anterior border of the trapezius lying between the platysma muscle and the deep layer of the deep cervical fascia. Removed, therefore, were the sternomastoid muscle, the spinal accessory nerve, and the jugular vein—in addition to the lymph nodes.

Martin subscribed to a number of dicta, among which was the rule that if one side of the neck was entered for any reason a radical neck dissection would be performed. Before criticizing this procedure, one must keep in mind the type of patient material Memorial Sloan-Kettering Hospital was receiving. The state of the art regarding cure of head and neck cancer was in its infancy. Many patients delayed in obtaining medical advice and many physicians (not knowing of the recent advances) prescribed courses of treatment which were less than optimal. Therefore, in Martin's day, many of the cases of head and neck cancer were inoperable and the majority of the operable ones showed advanced neck staging. This meant that small lymphatics often contained cancer cells and that the disease had often spread out into surrounding connective tissue. Because of this, Martin realized that to enter a neck without cleaning it out invited bizarre recurrences.

Rigid dicta, however, must change with the times, and in the late 1950s and early 1960s Bocca and Pignato (1967), Ballantyne (personal communication), and others began to realize that one could follow anatomic principles in removing the nodes of the neck and spare the spinal accessory nerve and the sternomastoid muscle in most instances. They recognized the fact that neither of these structures contained lymph nodes and that they became involved with cancer only when the nodal metastases were large enough to break the capsule of the node and enter into the surrounding connective tissue. Patients were coming to the surgeons with neck metastases staged in the less advanced categories. The concept of removing nodal groups rather than the entire contents of a neck became an exciting clinical research exercise.

Two other somewhat related studies contributing to the information were started in the early 1960s. Jesse and MacComb (1962) did a retrograde study on tongue cancer using a TNM staging system in an attempt to form a common language by which treatment regimens could be compared. While a number of different classifications were promulgated over the ensuing 15 years, the American Joint Commission for Cancer Staging and End-Results Reporting finally produced a manual culminating with a refinement in 1978, which is accepted by most groups engaged in the study and care of the head and neck patient. The second factor was the realization that most undisturbed squamous cancers of the head and neck area metastasize in a reasonably predictable fashion. It was noted by Skolnick and associates (1976), for example, that squamous cancer of the supraglottic and glottic larynx rarely spread to nodes in the posterior triangle. The culmination of the distributions of neck metastasis was accomplished by Lindberg (1972), who mapped out all clinically positive cervical nodes and found that cancers originating in certain anatomic sites rarely spread to certain cervical nodes, whereas certain nodal groups are prone to receive metastases from other specific anatomic sites.

The radiation therapy concepts were also changing, perhaps at a somewhat slower rate than surgical concepts. Metastatic cervical nodes in the neck were generally not treated with radiation therapy if the neck was operable. The inoperable patient was generally referred to the radiation therapist for palliative treatment. Meaningful palliation was probably not achieved unless the dose of radiation delivered for this purpose approached that necessary for cure. The second change in concept was one of including the entire neck, or at least the ipsilateral side of the neck, in very laterally-placed primary lesions within the treatment field. Berger and colleagues (1971) showed a 12% recurrence within the neck if only a portion of the neck was covered, as opposed to 3.7% if the entire neck was within the field. The third concept was that the reduction of the size of the metastatic tumor in the neck would make the surgeon's job easier when removing it. A companion concept implied that many of the cancer cells, both in the lymph nodes and in the lymphatic ducts, would be destroyed by this practice, leaving less residual material for the surgeons to spread during the procedure.

Another concept, having to do not exclusively with cervical node metastasis but with radiation therapy in general, was the idea that moderate doses of radiation secured an almost 100% cancer kill at the periphery of the lesion whereas a very high dose was necessary for securing the relatively anoxic portion of the cancer in the center of the node. Surgeons, on the other hand, had exactly the reverse problem: they could usually remove the central portion of the node, but the peripheral extensions often escaped them or attached themselves to areas which they would choose not to remove.

The question of whether the radiation therapy should be delivered pre- or postoperatively has been argued between surgeons and radiotherapists and has still not been answered. Preoperative radiation therapy was attractive because it effected a good cancer cell kill prior to any surgical procedure and theoretically, therefore, there were fewer cells to squeeze into the general circulation to set up metastases. On the other hand, the surgeons rebelled to some extent in trying to secure healing in patients who had had the necessary 5000 rad or more delivered over large cervical fields. Extra days of hospitalization, blow-out of the carotid artery, and large skin sloughs at incisions all attested to the undesirability of this procedure from the surgeon's standpoint. Postoperative radiation therapy was designed to secure a cancer kill both at the periphery of the surgical excision and including those cells that might remain in the middle of the surgical field. The idea of postoperative radiation was somewhat abhorrent to radiation therapists, partly because they were not used to it and partly because it appeared to violate the principles of radiologic therapy they had been taught. From the patient's standpoint, performing the surgery first was tolerated better in most cases. Time spent in hospitals was shorter, and there were fewer lasting complications. The only real problem was that surgeons were often slow in getting their patients' wounds to heal, often doing multiple staged procedures for repair and thereby delaying the initial visit to the radiotherapists far beyond the optimal time for postoperative radiation therapy. In instances such as these, the cancer had a chance to begin regrowth, and this made the procedure fall into disfavor among both groups of physicians.

A surgeon and other members of the treatment team must ask themselves the question, "If it can be performed, why do we think that a functional neck dissection is superior to the radical procedure?" Certainly the radical procedure is easier, both from the standpoint of the dissection and the time required to perform it. Often the answer comes from those members of the treatment team who consistently rationalize that patients do not care whether they have lost the spinal accessory nerve or the sternomastoid muscle. One can only believe that these physicians do not consistently see patients in follow-up over many years. It has been our experience that in the first two or three years, patients will not generally complain about the drop shoulder incidental to the loss of the spinal accessory nerve, or the flat neck produced by removing the sternomastoid muscle. During this time they are more worried about whether the cancer will recur than about function or appearance. When they can be assured that the cancer has a relatively small chance of recurring, they begin to complain about the inability to lift an arm and also about their cosmetic appearance. Not too many years ago, most patients afflicted with head and neck cancer requiring radical neck dissection did not expect to return to a gainful occupation or to be seen extensively in public. With modern treatment and rehabilitation techniques, the patient often expects to go back to work. Individuals who make their living as laborers, painters, steelworkers, and in other occupations requiring lifting or prolonged work over the horizontal level of the shoulder often find themselves in severe pain at the end of the working day. Women constantly complain that their dresses cannot be made to fit well, that they look lopsided in a bathing suit, and that one side of their neck is thin in comparison to the other side. If surgeons can be assured that the functional procedure with or without radiation therapy is at least equal to the radical procedure in eliminating cancer within the neck, they should, for their patients' well-being, perform the slightly more difficult procedure.

Results of large series using radical neck dissection as the sole planned procedure for metastasis in the neck are available. Beahrs and Barber (1962) and Strong (1969) reported 26.5% and 36.5% recurrence, respectively, after radical neck dissection performed at their institutions. Strong further broke this down according to the histologic findings of the lymph nodes within the surgical specimens and determined a 71% recurrence when the nodes were multiple and at different levels.

If surgeons only succeed 66% to 75% of the time using their most radical procedure, they should ask themselves whether they can do better with another type of treatment. We must hasten to add that a functional neck dissection will obviously do no better than the radical procedure if used as the only treatment modality. Strong reported a series of patients who were to undergo radical neck dissection, half of whom received 2000 rad of radiation preoperatively on five successive days prior to radical neck dissection. Even this moderate dose of preoperative radiation reduced recurrence in the dissected neck of patients with multiple metastatic nodes at different levels from 71% to 37.5%. Based upon these data, it is relatively safe to assume that combinations of radiation therapy and surgery are superior to either modality used exclusively.

In our opinion, there is little if any difference in recurrence within the neck whether radiation is given pre- or postoperatively. If this is true, we do not need to delineate between the two in future considerations within this chapter. The concept that the limits of each modality can be reduced to achieve the same results is important. If 5000 rad in five weeks to 5500 rad in five and one-half weeks does take care of peripheral microscopic extensions of cancer within the neck, then this dose need not be exceeded. This decreases the possibility of complications of high-dose radiotherapy. By the same token, the surgeon need not remove wide areas of normal tissue beyond those in which microscopic disease is present or those nodal groups which, because of the placement of the primary, are at low risk for metastases.

This, then, forms the basis of our premise, that is, that in most cases a functional neck dissection preceded or followed by 5500 rad in five and one-half weeks of radiation offers the optimum treatment both from the standpoint of recurrence and that of patient comfort.

There are certain dicta the surgeon must observe to obtain the desired result.

1. Surgeons who occasionally operate upon patients with cancer should probably do the classic radical neck dissection rather than a functional procedure, because they may not have the surgical expertise or the intimate knowledge of patterns of metastatic spread which is all important in doing a lesser procedure.
2. The surgeons should remove all gross disease. The concept of even 90% tumor reduction is unacceptable, and will almost certainly result in treatment failure regardless of the dose of radiation employed.
3. In patients with cervical metastases whose primary is to be treated by radiation therapy, one or both sides of the neck, depending on the laterality of the primary cancer, should also receive a dose of at least 5000 rad in five weeks.
4. The side of the neck originally containing the clinically positive metastatic node must then be dissected whether or not there is clinically positive disease palpable at the end of radiation therapy. It is well recognized that this practice will result in negative histologic reports of the neck contents in perhaps 60% of patients. Since surgeons cannot tell which patient group will have the 60% sterilized necks and which will have the 40% unsterilized necks, they must be prepared to follow this dictum. The only exception to this rule might be a node less than 2 cm, single, lying in the first echelon of nodes expected for the primary cancer in question, receiving 6000 rad in six weeks or more, and disappearing within four weeks after treatment.
5. If cancer has broken out of the capsule of the lymph node and invaded either the sternomastoid muscle or the eleventh nerve, one or both of these structures must obviously be resected, turning the procedure into a radical neck dissection. The patient should therefore be forewarned that while a functional neck dissection will be attempted, the dictates of the tumor will be the deciding factor.

The choice of functional neck dissection is wide and is dictated by the clinical evaluation of the neck, the findings at surgery, and the surgeon's intimate knowledge as to which nodal groups are at high risk for harboring cancer. The type of functional neck dissection varies depending upon which node groups are to be removed. The most radical procedure can remove all nodal groups between the mandible above, the clavicle below the anterior midline, and the anterior border of the trapezius. Generally this would be the procedure of choice in a patient whose primary was in the oral cavity, oropharynx, or the hypopharynx and whose neck is staged $N2_b$ or greater. In some instances, such as that of a patient whose primary cancer is in the supraglottic larynx and whose neck is stage N1 or $N2_a$, the posterior triangle can be virtually ignored since it is almost never at risk. For patients with N1 neck staging whose primary is in the lateral oral cavity, resection of all the nodes above the omohyoid muscle is usually all that needs to be planned. For patients whose lesion approaches the midline, that is, palate, dorsum of the oral tongue, anterior floor of the mouth, and epiglottis, bilateral functional procedures are preferred rather than large unilateral operations. A compendium of all preferred surgical procedures is not within the scope of this chapter. It requires study of metastatic patterns, the experience of the surgeon, and constant review of data, particularly in those instances in which treatment has failed.

Extensive data regarding the results of functional neck dissection have only been available since about 1970. At that time only about 17% of the neck dissections done at our institution were functional in nature, but by 1976 88% of the patients were receiving the lesser procedures. From 1970 through 1975, neck dissections were performed at our institution on 440 patients with squamous cell carcinoma of the oral cavity, oropharynx, supraglottic larynx, and hypopharynx (Jesse, Ballantyne, and Larson 1978). One hundred thirty patients who did not have recurrence in the neck were excluded from the analysis because they died of other causes prior to the 24 months. Comprising the excluded group were 50 patients in whom the primary was never controlled, 27 patients who died from a complication of treatment, 33 patients who had an intercurrent disease or a second primary cancer, and 20 patients who were lost to follow-up or whose cause of death was unknown. Three hundred ten patients comprised the group for analysis. Twenty-four months was chosen as the cut-off point since our experience shows that 88% of recurrent neck cancer becomes manifest by that time. The series was not randomized and included some elective neck dissections in patients with necks staged N0. The choice of treatment was generally determined according to the surgeon's decision.

Three types of neck dissections are defined, two of which are functional procedures, and one the classic Crile procedure. In the following table, those classified as eleventh nerve spared had removal of all nodal groups within the neck, while those classified as regional procedures had only certain nodal groups removed. Recurrence in the neck, according to the procedure performed, is seen in table 16.1. Each of the four primary sites was studied individually. Twenty-six (19%) of the 140 patients with oral cavity cancer developed recurrence within the dissected neck. No statistical difference among the three surgical procedures was found, and this was true whether the patients were treated electively or therapeutically. The records of the 26 patients in whom a failure in the neck was recorded were examined in detail. In 10 of the 26 patients, a possible explanation for recurrence was found, while in 16 none was evident. The reasons included late recurrence of the primary cancer (one patient), failure to receive postoperative radiation therapy (six patients), and a poor choice of a regionally dissected neck (three patients).

Eight (15%) of the 53 patients with oropharynx cancer developed recur-

**Table 16.1**
Failure to Control Cancer in the Neck

| Dissection | Number of Patients | Percentage of Recurrence |
|---|---|---|
| Radical (classic) | 115 | 16 |
| Regional | 117 | 11 |
| Functional (eleventh nerve spared) | 24 | 3 |

rence within the dissected neck. Again, there was no statistical significance among the procedures, and this was true even if only the patients treated therapeutically were considered. Four of the eight patients in whom failure was recorded had an adequate reason for recurrence, whereas no possible explanation was identifiable in four patients. Two patients would today have received postoperative radiation; one had a late recurrence of the primary cancer, and the choice of procedure for one patient was not wise.

Two (3%) of the 27 patients with primary cancer in the supraglottic larynx experienced recurrence within the dissected neck. There were no failures in the electively treated group. No human judgment errors were found in this group, and all recurrences could be attributed to advanced neck disease.

Three (6%) of the 50 patients with hypopharynx cancer developed recurrence within the dissected neck. Again, no failures were recorded in patients treated electively. Two of the three patients with recurrence had necks staged $N2_b$ and did not receive postoperative radiation therapy.

As more data accumulate, the principle of adding radiation therapy to the surgical procedure has changed. Today the patient whose neck is staged $N2_a$, $N2_b$, or $N3_b$ (in which one side is $N2_a$ or greater) receives pre- or postoperative radiation therapy, the order depending on the choice of treatment for the primary lesion. In the earlier years in which these data were accumulated, this was not a universal practice; therefore, some patients who today would receive radiation therapy did not receive it under the old practice. The concept regarding the neck staged $N3_a$ (fixed node) has also changed. During the years these data were being generated some patients with $N3_a$ nodes underwent surgery as the initial procedure. When it became evident that cancer was being rather consistently left behind and that even high doses of radiation therapy administered postoperatively did not appear to be of significant benefit, the policy was changed. Today the patient with neck staged $N3_a$ is irradiated to approximately 5500 rad in five and one-half weeks. A reevaluation is done at that time, and if the surgeon believes the node can be removed without leaving cancer within the neck, the procedure is carried out. In the majority of cases, however, the surgeon has not felt comfortable in being able to predict total removal of the node, and the radiation therapy is administered to doses of 7000 rad or higher in seven weeks.

We rest our case, therefore, regarding the desirability of functional neck dissection where it can be performed, with the belief that there is no statistical difference between the functional and classical procedure when chosen by the experienced surgeon. The fact that over 90% of the patients we treat undergo a functional procedure is proof that we believe in our data. A study has been initiated by the Radiation Therapy Oncology Group in which either classical radical neck dissection or functional dissection will be performed in a randomized trial. In our opinion, this may or may not answer the question. First, it is a retrogressive step to submit half of a patient population to removal of the eleventh nerve and sternomastoid muscle if they do not require it. Second, the randomization is left up to a computer and takes away the judgment of the surgeon, which we think is extremely important. If this study, however, shows a significant difference between the surgical procedures, we would be willing to modify our stance.

## References


American Joint Commission for Cancer Staging and End-Results Reporting. *Manual for staging of cancer,* eds. O. Beahrs, D. Carr, and P. Rubin. Chicago: The Commission, 1978.

Beahrs, O. H., and Barber, K. W. The value of radical neck dissection in the management of carcinomas of the lip, mouth, and larynx. *Arch. Surg.* 85:65–72, 1962.

Berger, D. S. et al. Elective irradiation of neck lymphatics for squamous cell carcinoma of the nasopharynx and oropharynx. *Am. J. Roentgenol.* 111:66–72, 1971.

Boca, E., and Pignato, O. A conservation technique in radical neck dissection. *Ann. Otol. Rhinol. Laryngol.* 76:975–987, 1967.

Crile, G. W. Excision of cancer of the head and neck. *JAMA* 47:1780–1786, 1906.

Jesse, R. H., Ballantyne, A. J.; and Larson, D. L. Radical or modified neck dissection: a therapeutic dilemma. *Am. J. Surg.* 136:516–519, 1978.

Jesse, R. H., and MacComb, W. S. Squamous carcinoma of the tongue: the importance of staging. *Am. J. Surg.* 103:352–357, 1962.

Lindberg, R. D. Distribution of cervical lymph node metastases from squamous cell carcinoma of the upper respiratory and digestive tracts. *Cancer* 29:1446–1449, 1972.

Martin, H. et al. Neck dissection. *Cancer* 4:441–499, 1951.

Skolnick, E. M. et al. Posterior triangle in radical neck surgery. *Arch. Otolaryngol.* 102:1–4, 1976.

Strong, E. W. Preoperative radiation and radical neck dissection. *Surg. Clin. North Am.* 49:271–276, 1969.

# Chapter 17

# *The Classical Radical Neck Dissection*

Elliot W. Strong

The clinical significance of metastases to cervical lymph nodes from primary cancers of the head and neck cannot be overemphasized. In 1941, Martin described the likelihood of cervical nodal metastases from various head and neck sites, documented the major influence of such metastases upon ultimate prognosis, and pointed out that such metastases were most ominous when detected on initial examination. Many other studies have subsequently confirmed these facts and have further amplified the significance of the presence, as well as the extent, of such nodal metastases (Strong 1969; Farr and Arthur 1972; Spiro et al. 1974; Lee and Krause 1975; Kalnins et al. 1977). In addition, Merino, Lindberg, and Fletcher (1977) confirmed that the incidence of distant metastases from squamous cancers of the head and neck varied with the stage of the disease, but was more closely related to the extent of lymph node metastasis (N) than to the stage of the primary tumor (T). In every patient with head and neck cancer, the status of the regional lymph nodes must be considered in the choice of the ultimate treatment plan.

## Historical Review

In the medical writings of the early 1800s there was little reference made to the treatment of head and neck cancer once it had spread to what was usually referred to as cervical "glands." Chelius in 1847 stated that "the neighboring lymphatics and glands become hard and painful," but once the tumor had involved the submaxillary gland, complete removal of the disease was impossible. In the same year, Warren described an operation for removal of metastatic lymph nodes from the upper neck. In 1880 Kocher described the removal of a cancer of the tongue through the submaxillary triangle, clearing out the upper neck. Later he described a wider resection of cervical lymph nodes and introduced the Y incision which carries his name. In 1900, Butlin advised the removal of cervical lymphatics through the Kocher incision and even mentioned the routine elective excision of these tissues in the treatment of tongue cancer (Martin et al. 1951). It remained for George Crile, Sr., to design and perform a systematic operative procedure for the removal of cervical lymphatics and lymph nodes based upon anatomic principles. In 1906 he described his experience with a series of 132 operations and made some rather remarkable observations and contributions. He advocated endotracheal anesthesia and advised wide en bloc sharp dissection with complete removal of sternocleidomastoid muscle, internal jugular vein, spinal accessory nerve, soft tissues of the various triangles of the neck, and, when involved, the submaxillary salivary gland. He recognized the frequent need for tracheostomy and performed composite resections and even bilateral neck dissections, in stages, with an overall mortality of only 8%. He also advocated temporary occlusion of the common or external carotid artery for hemostasis but recognized the risks thereof. He described the relative rarity of distant as opposed to cervical lymph node metastases and recognized the vagaries of local lymphatic dissemination in the neck. Based upon this experience, he stated that incomplete excisions of advanced metastatic disease did more harm than good, and that in his hands "the radical block dissection [showed] itself to be four times more effective than the less radical."

Martin and associates (1951) reemphasized the importance of regional lymph nodes in head and neck cancer and outlined the indications for, and the anatomy and technique of, radical neck dissection. Subsequent reports have amplified the surgical technique (Beahrs, Gossel, and Hollinshead 1955; Bakamjian, Miller, and Poole 1977). On the basis of more recent studies of the distribution of cervical metastatic head and neck cancer (McGavran, Bauer, and Ogura 1961; Lindberg 1972; Shah and Tollefsen 1974; Skolnick et al. 1976; Razack et al. 1978) some authors (Dayal and DaSilva 1971; Bocca 1975; Lingemann et al. 1977; Chu and Strawitz 1978; Jesse, Ballantyne, and Larson 1978) have advocated a less radical surgical procedure. The validity and effectiveness of such procedures have yet to be documented in prospective controlled randomized studies. This chapter will confine itself to a discussion of the classical operation. Jesse discusses the conservative or modified procedure elsewhere in this volume.

## Definition

The classical radical neck dissection is an operative procedure which attempts to remove as thoroughly as possible the lymph nodes and lymphatics from the anterior and lateral neck likely to be involved by metastatic cancer. The margins of resection are the lower border of the mandible superiorly to the clavicle inferiorly, and the midline anteriorly to the anterior border of the trapezius muscle posteriorly. The specimen also routinely includes the entire sternocleidomastoid muscle, the jugular vein, spinal accessory nerve, and the submaxillary salivary gland with all the surrounding soft tissue en bloc. Any lesser procedure may be classified as partial, modified, functional, or conservative—but not (classical) radical—neck dissection.

The classical procedure may be extended by resection of additional structures and tissues as indicated by the extent of metastatic disease. These may include skin and platysma, adjacent lymph nodes (parotid, retroauricular and suboccipital, retropharyngeal, paratracheal and superior mediastinal, or contralateral submaxillary), portions of the adjacent muscles (digastric, strap, trapezius, levator scapulae, scalene, myelohyoid), bone (portions of mandible, mastoid, hyoid, clavicle), soft tissues (parotid, thyroid), nerves, and blood vessels. Such procedures should be designated extended radical neck dissections.

When neck dissection is performed in the absence of clinical involvement of lymph nodes (N0) it has been termed prophylactic or elective. The latter is more appropriate and much preferred, since the procedure does not prevent metastases or recurrence. Therapeutic neck dissection is performed for the removal of clinically (or pathologically) involved cervical lymph nodes (N+). Palliative neck dissection refers to that procedure whose indication is the relief of signs or symptoms with the usual implication that it is not expected to be curative. Such procedures are rarely justified and should be performed only after careful consideration of alternative forms of treatment and frank, honest, complete discussion with the patient and his or her family. Radical neck dissection may be safely performed bilaterally, either simultaneously or staged. While some (McGuirt, McCabe, and Krause 1979) suggest no increase in complications with simultaneous bilateral radical neck dissection, it has been our experience (Moore and Frazell 1964) and also that of others (McQuarrie et al. 1977) that the morbidity and mortality of bilateral neck dissection done simultaneously are greater than when the procedure is staged. The one compelling indication for simultaneous performance is the inability to resect the cancer by separate procedures without transecting tumor.

## Indications

The indications and contraindications for radical neck dissection are not absolute, but must be flexible depending upon the extent of the metastatic disease, the patient's general condition, history of any previous treatment, and the patient's wishes. These are summarized in table 17.1. The prime indication is the presence—either potential, suspected, or proved—of metastatic tumor involving cervical lymph nodes. The detection of such nodal metastases is primarily based on clinical grounds, depending on deviation from normal size and consistency of the lymph nodes at risk. Unfortunately, there are no diagnostic studies which with certainty will rule out the presence of metastatic cancer in clinically negative lymph nodes. Attempts to visualize cervi-

**Table 17.1**
Indications and Contraindications to Radical Neck Dissection

| Indications | Contraindications |
|---|---|
| Resectable cervical lymph nodes clinically or pathologically involved with metastatic tumor. | Uncontrolled (or uncontrollable) primary tumor. |
| High likelihood of occult involvement of cervical lymph nodes by metastatic tumor. | Unresectable cervical metastases. |
| Necessity of surgical entry into neck to resect primary tumor. | Invasion of unresectable structures. |
| Inability to assess adequately status of cervical lymph nodes. | En cuirasse involvement of skin and subcutaneous tissues. |
| Inability to maintain close patient follow-up postoperatively. | Phrenic or sympathetic nerve invasion. |
| Unlikely control of tumor by any other therapeutic modality. | Invasion of structures whose resection poses an unacceptable operative risk. |
| | Documented distant metastases. |
| | Medical conditions which preclude general anesthesia. |
| | Lack of patient understanding and/or refusal of therapy. |

cal lymphatics by lymphangiographic techniques (Fisch and Sigel 1964) have been described, but are too cumbersome and unreliable to be of any practical use. If positive, needle aspiration biopsy is reliable, but if negative it does not rule out the presence of metastatic cancer. It is virtually impossible clinically to detect minimal cancer deposits in normal-sized lymph nodes. Thus even the most experienced examiners will have significant errors in their clinical assessment of regional lymph nodes (Sako et al. 1964; Spiro et al. 1974). It would appear that such errors can be minimized with increasing experience of the examiner and careful and repeated examinations of the patient, but they cannot be totally eliminated.

The treatment of the clinically negative neck remains controversial. Many authors have studied and reported their experience, but conclusive statistically valid studies have yet to be reported (Spiro and Strong 1973; Lee and Krause 1975; Naham, Bone, and Davidson 1977). Shear, Hawkins, and Farr (1976) retrospectively studied a group of 898 patients with oral and oropharyngeal squamous carcinoma and subdivided them on clinical grounds into groups of low, intermediate, and high risk for cervical metastases. Using these clusters, the authors concluded that they could project the logistically transformed probability of cervical metastases with a high degree of accuracy. Similarly, many authors (McGavran, Bauer, and Ogura 1961; Spiro and Strong 1971; Lindberg 1972; Farr and Arthur 1972; Shah and Tollefsen 1974; Razack et al. 1978) using similar clinical data, but without statistical efforts, have estimated the likelihood of subsequent nodal metastases in the clinically negative neck. Unfortunately, clear evidence for improved survival following the elective dissection of the clinically negative but pathologically positive neck over those both clinically and pathologically positive for early metastases is lacking (Spiro and Strong 1973; Lee and Krause 1975). It seems reasonable to assume, however, that better local control can be achieved by resection of minimal rather than obvious metastatic tumor, which should be of some benefit to the patient. At what point the surgeon advises elective radical neck dissection will vary from individual to individual, but generally in those patients whose risk of metastatic tumor has exceeded 20%, we have advised elective ipsilateral radical neck dissection.

It seems appropriate to complete the radical neck dissection whenever resection of the primary tumor necessitates dissection into the lateral neck. This obviates the uncertainties surrounding the evaluation of postsurgical induration in the operated neck, and the operative procedure is technically easier. Clinical, but undocumented, experience suggests that frequently the metastatic disease appearing subsequently in the nondissected but previously operated neck is associated with the surgical scar, sometimes delaying its detection and rendering its adequate subsequent resection more difficult and less successful.

In those patients whose necks are difficult to evaluate either because of short stature, heavy muscular development, or primary lesion interfering with careful neck examination, it seems appropriate to advise elective radical neck dissection. Similarly, when the primary tumor, particularly one of parotid or thyroid origin, is massive and encroaches upon the soft tissues of the neck, elective radical neck dissection is justified not only because of the increased risk of occult nodal metastases, but to effect more adequate resection of the bulky primary tumor. In those patients at significant risk of nodal metastases who will not be available for careful follow-up observation, elective neck dissection as part of the initial surgical treatment is justified. Also, whenever the histology of the tumor is other than squamous or epidermoid carcinoma, and the patient is at risk of nodal metastases or direct extension into the neck, elective neck dissection is advisable, with the hope of achieving greater likelihood of cure. In these patients, adjunctive therapy will often be unavailable or ineffective.

The contraindications to neck dissection may be somewhat less controversial. It seems obvious that persistent uncontrolled cancer at the primary site and/or documented distant metastases will indicate that the disease is incurable and that the patient would not benefit from radical neck dissection. If, however, the neck metastases are ulcerated, foul-smelling, and symptomatic, there may be some palliation, admittedly often shortlived, to be derived from the removal of the bulky tumor in exchange for a cleanly healed wound. It should be pointed out that histologic confirmation of suspected distant metastases should be obtained wherever possible, before denying the patient the possibility of cure of neck metastases by radical neck dissection. The progression of certain head and neck tumors, most notably well-differentiated thyroid and certain salivary gland cancers, is sufficiently slow to justify radical local therapy in the presence of known pulmonary metastases. Such metastases may be apparently stable and asymptomatic for years, while the primary lesion represents the most morbid portion of the disease. Since a common cause of death from fatal thyroid cancer is the presence of uncontrolled central neck disease (Silliphant, Klinck, and Levitin 1964), it appears justified to advise radical treatment of the local and regional disease in selected such cases. Pulmonary metastases from epidermoid carcinoma are seldom solitary or stable, thus indicating a much more grave prognosis with less likelihood of lasting benefit from radical local and regional surgery. The real possibility of a second primary cancer of the lung in these high-risk patients should be investigated whenever a solitary pulmonary shadow is detected.

The surgical resectability of metastatic cancer in cervical lymph nodes is open to controversy and often depends upon the attitude and aggressiveness of the surgeon. Massive, rigidly-fixed tumor is clearly not resectable with any expectation of cure. Minimal skin involvement, especially after previous open biopsy, can be readily encompassed surgically but admittedly indicates more advanced local disease. Major skin involvement with *peau d'orange* indicates extensive retrograde lymphatic spread, usually far beyond what is clinically apparent, with little if any likelihood of cure. In view of their anatomic location, involvement of either phrenic nerve or sympathetic chain suggests deep infiltration of tumor through the deep cervical fascia with little likelihood of local control from surgical excision alone. Isolated hypoglossal, vagus, or marginal mandibular nerve involvement by critically located small metastatic tumor deposits may be resectable with reasonably adequate surgical margins, however. Such involvement by fixed metastatic tumor at the base of the skull would be surgically incurable, but in the middle neck by mobile metastatic disease would be worthy of surgical exploration. We have not hesitated to sacrifice part or all of the carotid arterial system if it was assumed that the metastatic cancer could not otherwise be controlled. The external carotid artery and its branches may be resected unilaterally or bilaterally with impunity, but interruption of the common or internal carotid carries a significant risk of death or major neurologic sequelae (Heller and Strong 1979). Attempts to predict preoperatively the safety of carotid resection have had some success (Gee et al. 1975), but this is not available intraoperatively. Attempting to peel tumor off the vessel by dissection in the subadventitial plane will leave residual tumor in many such patients (Huvos, Leaming, and Moore 1973). Ultimately, such patients have a high incidence of local recurrence as well as distant metastases (Kennedy, Krause, and Leavy 1977), emphasizing the poor prognosis of this clinical setting and the need for adjunctive therapy, probably both local and systemic. Thus the surgeon must balance the risk of carotid resection against the risk of failure to control the cancer.

There may be no medical contraindications to life-saving surgery, but certainly the operative risk is greatly increased by certain medical conditions, most notably recent acute myocardial infarction or acute hepatitis. Certainly with these two conditions the risk of general anesthesia is greatly increased, and alternate nonsurgical treatment should be sought. With the help of the patient's internist, most chronic medical conditions can be stabilized, and the patient can be optimally prepared for safe general anesthesia and surgery.

The wisdom of encouraging radical surgery in the mentally incompetent or unwilling and uncooperative patient is doubtful and under most circumstances should be avoided. Only when the patient's wholehearted cooperation and understanding have been obtained can the surgery, postoperative course, and subsequent rehabilitation proceed optimally and satisfactorily.

Large midline primary cancers or bilateral or contralateral lymph node metastases do not contraindicate radical neck dissection. In the former instance, if the primary tumor is truly midline—relatively rare—and both sides of the neck are free of clinical evidence of metastases, it is more appropriate to observe the neck rather than to perform bilateral classical neck dissections electively. Generally we have not hesitated to advise radical neck dissection on clinical grounds without histologic confirmation of metastatic disease involving ipsilateral cervical lymph nodes. The patient must understand and accept the possibility of a pathologically negative specimen, however. In view of the morbidity of second neck dissection, we have preferred to obtain histologic confirmation of metastatic disease before proceeding with the surgery. Generally this can be obtained by needle aspiration biopsy, but failing that, open biopsy may be performed just prior to the definitive procedure. The extent of primary tumor, particularly of larynx or thyroid origin, may necessitate bilateral radical neck dissection in the absence of clinically involved lymph nodes, solely to obtain adequate resection of the massive primary tumor.

# Surgery

## Anatomy

The lymphatic anatomy of the head and neck is diagrammatically illustrated in figure 17.1. A scheme for the description of cervical metastatic disease has been in use in this institution for many years and has the advantages of simplicity and brevity. This is depicted in figure 17.2. The submental and submaxillary (submandibular) triangles comprise level I. The internal jugular chain is arbitrarily divided into equal thirds, level II being the superior, level III the middle, and level IV the lower third. The posterior triangle is represented by level V. Using this scheme, the extent of cervical metastatic disease can be briefly and concisely described and related to prognosis as indicated below.

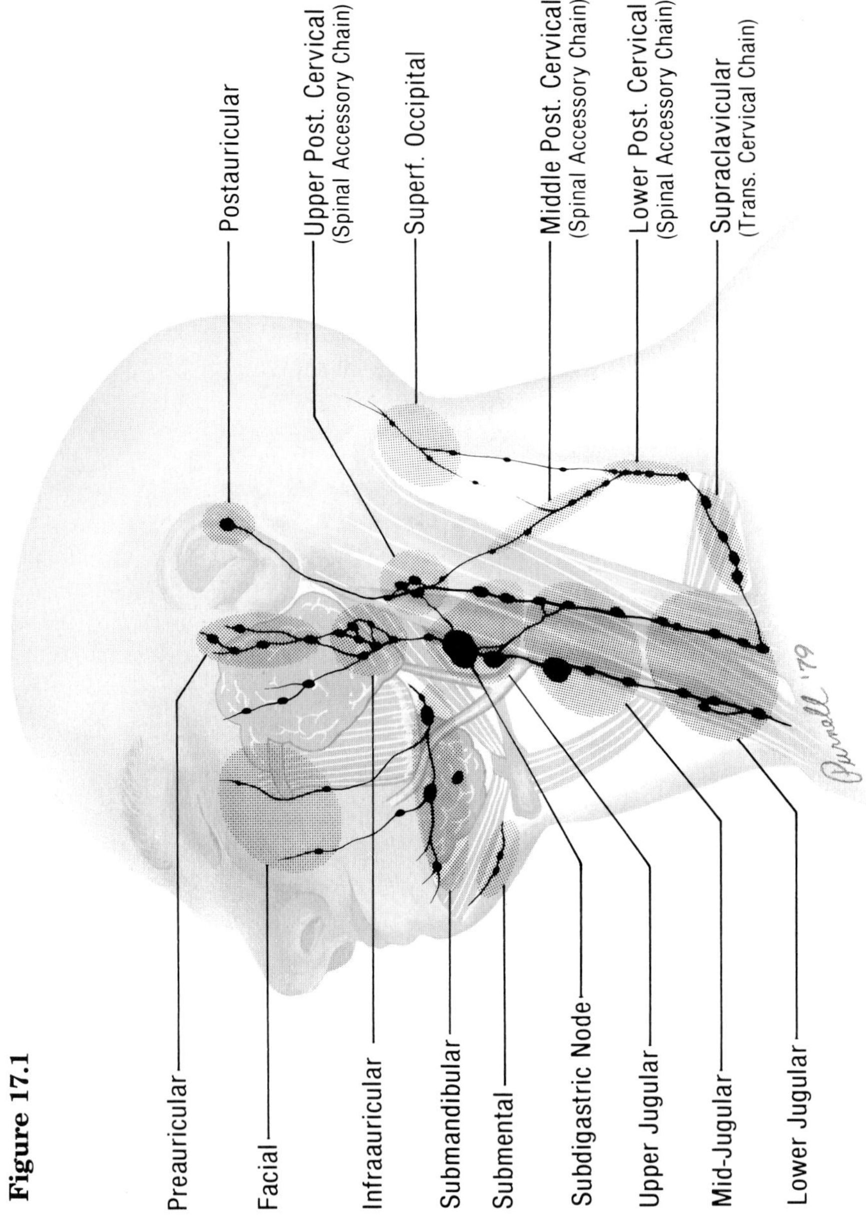
Postauricular
Upper Post. Cervical
(Spinal Accessory Chain)
Superf. Occipital
Middle Post. Cervical
(Spinal Accessory Chain)
Lower Post. Cervical
(Spinal Accessory Chain)
Supraclavicular
(Trans. Cervical Chain)
Preauricular
Facial
Infraauricular
Submandibular
Submental
Subdigastric Node
Upper Jugular
Mid-Jugular
Lower Jugular
Purnell '79

**Figure 17.1**

**Figure 17.2**

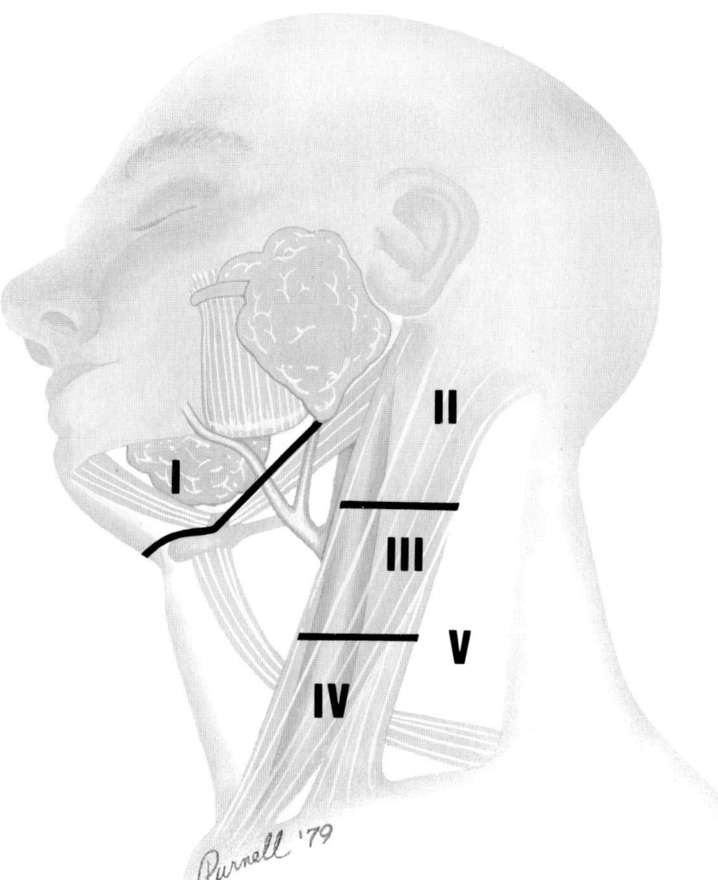


*Simplified diagrammatic system for description of lymph node metastasis.*

## Incisions

The choice of incisions for radical neck dissection will depend on the configuration of the patient's neck, the location and extent of the primary tumor (if present) and the nodal metastases, the history of any previous treatment, particularly radiotherapy or previous open biopsy, the need for possible reconstructive procedures, and the experiences and preferences of the surgeon. Figure 17.3 depicts some of the incisions that have been described. Generally,

**Figure 17.3**

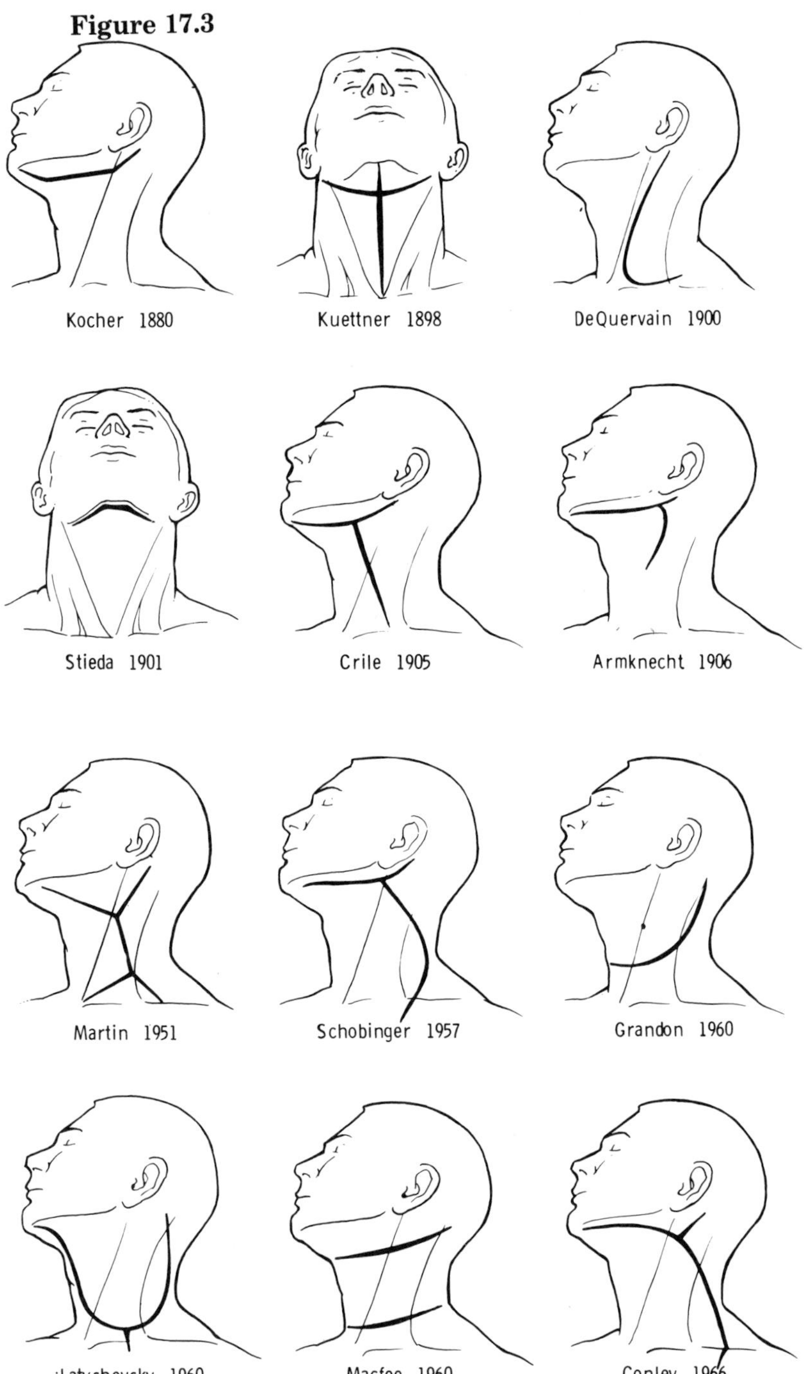


*Selected incisions described for radical neck dissection.*

incisions whose components cross rather than parallel the carotid artery are preferred. Transverse incisions tend to heal better and are more acceptable cosmetically, but may not provide optimum surgical exposure. Vertical incisions over the carotid artery, particularly in the previously irradiated patient, are to be condemned, since the risk of wound necrosis and carotid artery exposure with subsequent hemorrhage is increased. The blood supply to the cervical skin runs largely vertically, descending from branches of the facial and sternomastoid arteries above and ascending from branches of the transverse cervical and suprascapular artery from below (Freeland and Rogers 1975). Best use of this blood supply may be made with a single transverse incision, but this will not permit the insertion of distant flaps, either from below or above, for reconstruction of the oral cavity or pharynx. A modified T incision with the vertical limb well posterior and gently curved to lessen postoperative contracture is popular. The double horizontal parallel incisions of McFee (1960) violate all the principles of cutaneous blood supply, but survive because of the broad-based bipedicle construction, even in those patients previously heavily irradiated, with good cosmetic and functional results. It also permits the ready incorporation of inferiorly based flaps (deltopectoral, pectoralis myocutaneous) for reconstruction. Whatever the choice of incision, it must afford adequate exposure to permit the necessary surgery without difficulty, and it should produce a satisfactory cosmetic result with minimum risk of postoperative complications.

## Technique

Radical neck dissection is a precise anatomic exercise which, to be successful, must be performed with careful technique, controlled sharp dissection, careful handling of tissues, and meticulous hemostasis. Ideally, any surgeon who undertakes the biopsy or excision of a cervical mass should be psychologically and technically prepared to complete the radical neck dissection, if indicated, during the same procedure, since it probably offers the patient the best chance of control of the neoplastic disease. Preliminary biopsy before diagnosis and definitive treatment has been shown to produce higher incidence of complications, specifically wound necrosis, regional recurrence, and distant metastases, than with patients having definitive treatment of neck nodal disease without such biopsy (McGuirt and McCabe 1978). No neck surgery must ever be instituted without the patient's having first undergone complete and thorough head and neck and general examination, searching for any possible primary neoplasm. Needless to say, the patient's full understanding and informed consent, to the extent of his or her ability to comprehend, must be obtained prior to any such surgery.

In performing radical neck dissection, it has been our usual plan to preserve the platysma and digastric muscles unless the extent of metastatic tumor contraindicates it. Generally the dissection is begun inferiorly and posteriorly, and the specimen is swept upward and forward, including as its deep margin the deep layer of deep cervical fascia. Whenever possible, the immediately adjacent motor nerves to the levator scapulae and scalene muscles should be identified and preserved. All the dissection is done sharply, with minimal blunt dissection. The electrocautery is helpful in elevating the skin flap, incising through muscle, and coagulating minute bleeding points. Considerable experience is required for its proper use; care must be taken not to inflict thermal injury to normal structures or produce excess necrosis of those coagulated areas. Detailed knowledge of normal anatomy and its variations is mandatory for an expeditious, complete, and safe dissection. Every attempt should be made to obtain adequate surgical margins, and liberal use of frozen section examination of any suspicious tissue is encouraged. Intraoperative, interstitial implantation of locally unresectable tumor may be indicated. Areas of residual unresectable tumor should be adequately labeled with radiopaque clips to aid the radiotherapist in directing postoperative therapy. Removal of adjacent lymph node groups outside the usual radical neck dissection margins will be indicated by the location and extent of the primary tumor, with its expected pathways of lymphatic dissemination. Carotid artery sacrifice may be indicated. There will be few instances where graft replacement of the artery is feasible, particularly in the face of a composite resection with contamination of the operative field with mouth organisms, the risk of subsequent pharyngeal fistula with carotid hemorrhage, or thrombosis. In the previously irradiated patient such vascular substitution would seem to be even less appropriate. If the risks of such sacrifice seem excessive, then it is probably wiser to dissect as much tumor from the artery as possible without vascular injury and to give the patient postoperative radiation therapeutically. Often when dissecting in the appropriate subadventitial plane, beginning at a point distant from the adherent disease, the plane seems to develop rapidly and readily and the disease can be safely removed, admittedly with narrow margins, without vascular compromise. An occasional patient will be fortunate enough to be cured by such dissection. It should be pointed out that removal of that adventitia predisposes the carotid to greater jeopardy of rupture if exposed in the postoperative period as a result of skin necrosis (Swain et al. 1974).

After the resection, the wound should be meticulously inspected for the completeness of hemostasis. Forced hyperventilation by the anesthetist or placing the patient in reverse Trendelenburg position to produce venous hypertension will help to identify residual bleeding points. The wound should be thoroughly irrigated to wash out clots, loose debris, and residual cancer cells, and then after changing gowns, gloves, drapes and instruments (to avoid any possible recontamination by residual tumor cells), be closed airtight over two adequate-sized suction catheters. These catheters should be so positioned as to avoid any possible contact with, and compression of, the carotid arterial system, while insuring adequate drainage of the entire operative bed. It is appropriate to debride any traumatized, nonviable, or redundant portions of the skin flaps to assure approximation of only healthy, well-vascularized tissue. If hemostasis is adequate, the wound dry, and the flaps well approximated to the operative bed by the catheter suction, then external compression dressings are unnecessary. If, however, there was previous surgery with old scar and troublesome oozing, or if complete hemostasis was otherwise impossible to obtain, then a snugly applied, appropriately bulky, external compression dressing, circumferentially wrapping the head and neck for 24 to 36 hours, may be helpful in preventing postoperative hematoma. With appropriate care and meticulous hemostasis, it has been our experience that complete neck dissection in the average patient not previously irradiated or operated can be performed with minimal blood loss, necessitating no replacement.

### Complications

Any operative procedure, no matter how carefully planned and meticulously executed, may be accompanied by postoperative complications. Experience suggests that the better the choice of operative candidate, the more careful the surgical technique, and the more meticulous the attention to detail, the less the likelihood of complications. Most complications are best treated by prevention, especially hemorrhage, chyle fistula, flap elevation, and necrosis with carotid artery exposure and possible hemorrhage. Proper choice of incision, careful handling of tissues, debridement of nonvital flaps, and avoidance of wound approximation under tension will minimize wound slough. Meticulous hemostasis and attention to suction catheter placement and function will prevent hematoma/seroma. Flaps that do not promptly become fixed to the wound bed will frequently be accompanied by serum collections requiring drainage. Such serum or chyle accumulation in the presence of suction catheters indicates their malfunction and necessitates their removal and the establishment of adequate open drainage. The inexperienced head and neck surgeon will frequently wait too long adequately to open the operative wound under these circumstances. Almost all such wounds, no matter how widely open, will heal by secondary intention without need of graft or flap coverage. The adverse effect of previous radiotherapy on the incidence of postoperative complications has been well documented (Smithdeal, Corso, and Strong 1974; McGuirt, McCabe, and Krause 1979).

## Results

The justification of any treatment is measured by its ultimate results. Local recurrence of metastatic cancer in the treated neck is the ultimate complication and usually results in the patient's death (Pearlman 1979) from uncontrolled local cancer. Recurrence following radical neck dissection has been recorded (Beahrs and Barber 1962; Mustard and Rosen 1963; Strong et al. 1966). It is apparent that such recurrence varies directly with the extent of metastatic disease present at the time of surgery (Spiro et al. 1974; Kalnins et al. 1977). The current system of staging of cervical lymph node metastases acknowledges this fact by quantitating the extent of metastatic disease in the neck (American Joint Commission 1978). This system (table 17.2) has a distinct advantage over previous staging schemes by virtue of uniformity for all anatomic sites and histologic varieties of head and neck cancer. All neoplastic disease should be staged for the purpose of careful documentation, to assist in establishing prognosis, and to enable comparison of treatment results with other series. When histologically proved metastases are plotted in accordance with the leveling system used at Memorial Sloan-Kettering Cancer Center and are correlated with the ultimate prognosis, it is readily apparent that the lower in the neck the metastatic disease occurs, the poorer the ultimate prognosis. This is illustrated in table 17.3, which is based on our experience and also correlates roughly with the extent of metastatic disease in the neck (Farr and Arthur 1972; Spiro et al. 1974).

Detailed pathologic studies of neck dissection specimens have shown a tendency toward local proliferation of metastatic tumor within a limited area rather than widespread, early nodal dissemination, but skip lesions—absence of involvement of one anatomic group of lymph nodes situated along the lymphatic drainage pathway between primary and involved regional lymph nodes—occur in a significant number of specimens. More ominously, multiple foci of seemingly independent metastatic cancer involving the soft tissues occur without direct extension from neighboring metastatic lymph nodes (Toker 1963). This is more common in those neck specimens containing

**Table 17.2**
American Joint Commission: Staging of Cervical Lymph Nodes (1978)

| | |
|---|---|
| Nx | Nodes cannot be assessed. |
| N0 | No clinically positive node(s). |
| N1 | Single clinically positive homolateral node 3 cm or less in diameter. |
| N2 | Single clinically positive homolateral node more than 3 but not more than 6 cm in diameter, or multiple clinically positive homolateral nodes, none more than 6 cm in diameter. |
| $N2_a$ | Single clinically positive homolateral node more than 3 cm but not more than 6 cm in diameter. |
| $N2_b$ | Multiple clinically positive homolateral nodes, none more than 6 cm in diameter. |
| N3 | Massive homolateral node(s), bilateral nodes, or contralateral node(s). |
| $N3_a$ | Clinically positive homolateral node(s), one more than 6 cm in diameter. |
| $N3_b$ | Bilateral clinically positive nodes (in this situation each side should be staged separately). |
| $N3_c$ | Contralateral clinically positive node(s) only. |

**Table 17.3**
Surgical Pathologic Node Levels and Cure

| Pathologic Status of Lymph Nodes | Number of Patients | Percentage Five-Year Cure |
|---|---|---|
| Negative | 250 | 51 |
| Positive level I | 44 | 43 |
| Positive level II | 180 | 30 |
| Positive level III | 169 | 22 |
| Positive level IV | 133 | 19 |
| Positive level V | 26 | 4 |
| All positive neck dissected | 552 | 25 |

extensive metastatic tumor, but certainly suggests that incomplete resections may carry an unacceptably high risk of local recurrence. Although clinical studies of the distribution of nodal metastases from the various primary head and neck sites show reasonably predictable involvement of certain lymph node groups, while usually sparing others (Lindberg 1972), these are generalizations based on studies of groups of patients which may not pertain to the individual situation. While the posterior triangle lymph nodes may not be commonly involved by metastatic cancer, thus suggesting that preservation of the spinal accessory nerve may be safe, the course of that nerve in its uppermost portion is not in the posterior triangle, but passes through the upper third of the internal jugular chain. Macro- and microscopically involved lymph nodes occur in this area with no less frequency than in the remainder of the internal jugular chain, and routine blind preservation of the spinal accessory nerve may compromise complete resection of this nodal disease, leading to disastrous local recurrence (Schuller, Platz, and Krause 1978).

The ominous significance of extranodal and soft tissue involvement in the neck has been well documented (Shah et al. 1976; Kalnins et al. 1977). Recurrence following partial neck dissection for metastatic tumor is excessive (Chu and Strawitz 1978). While the precise mechanism of local recurrence is unknown, it is presumed to result from incomplete tumor removal. Apparently viable cancer cells have been isolated from washings of the operative wound (Harris and Smith 1960) and from postoperative wound drainage (Sako and Marchetta 1966), but there appears to be no direct correlation with their recovery and subsequent local recurrence. A suggestion of increased local recurrence in those patients whose specimens demonstrated vascular invasion supports the principle of performing the most radical surgical resection possible. In those patients at high risk of local failure (multiple involved lymph nodes, extracapsular or soft tissue extension, vascular invasion, involvement of lower neck nodes) subsequent adjuvant therapy to improve local control appears to be indicated (Vikram et al. 1980) with the hope of reducing disease morbidity. If one is to rely upon surgical excision alone for the treatment of cervical lymph node metastases, then the most complete excision possible would seem to offer the best chance of local control. There appears to be no place for less than classical radical neck dissection for bulky or multiple nodal involvement, soft tissue or extranodal tumor. With more advanced metastatic disease, failure rates will increase regardless of therapy (Spiro et al. 1974; Jesse and Fletcher 1978; Razack et al. 1978). Combined therapy has apparently lessened—but not eliminated—local recurrences, but overall cure has not been improved (Strong 1969; Jesse and Lindberg 1975). In fact, one study of a nonrandomized retrospectively analyzed group of patients comparing results of surgery alone with those for combined therapy found that survival for the surgery alone group was better than that of the combined therapy group, even when comparing stage for stage. While local and neck recurrences were similar in the two groups, the incidence of distant metastases was higher in the combined therapy group, negating any benefit from improved local control (Schuller et al. 1979). The morbidity of classical radical neck dissection has been documented (Ewing and Martin 1952). The cosmetic results are usually quite acceptable (fig. 17.4), even

**Figure 17.4**

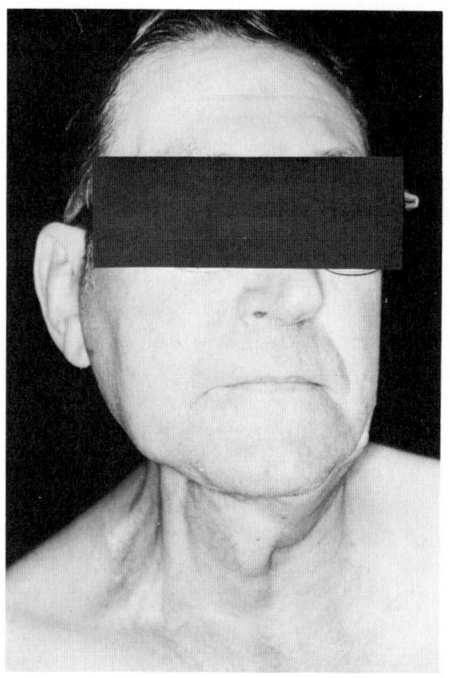

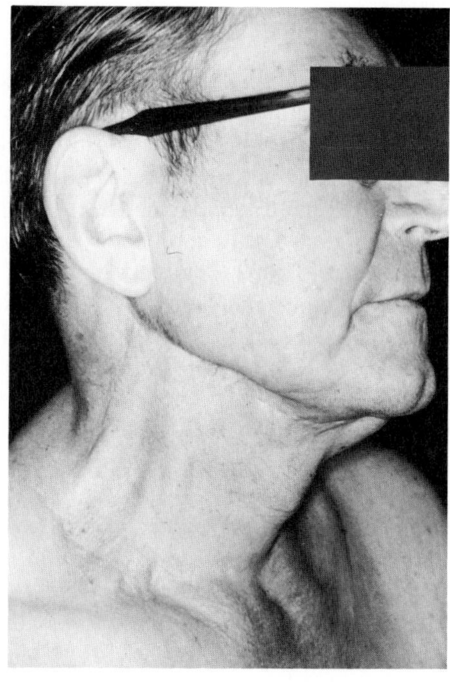

*Frontal and lateral photographs after unilateral radical neck dissection.*

when the procedure is performed bilaterally (fig. 17.5). The functional disability, mainly characterized by inability to abduct the arm completely, is real and not to be underestimated, but varies in severity from patient to patient, and apparently is not necessarily related to variations in the operative technique. Various surgical procedures to alleviate the shoulder instability have been described (Dewar and Harris 1950) but have not met with uniform success or wide application. Shoulder rehabilitation is facilitated by a very positive attitude on the part of the surgeon and the patient and by judicious postoperative physiotherapy, which will lessen the morbidity (Saunders and Johnson 1975; Schuller, Platz, and Krause 1978).

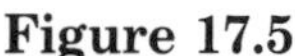

**Figure 17.5**

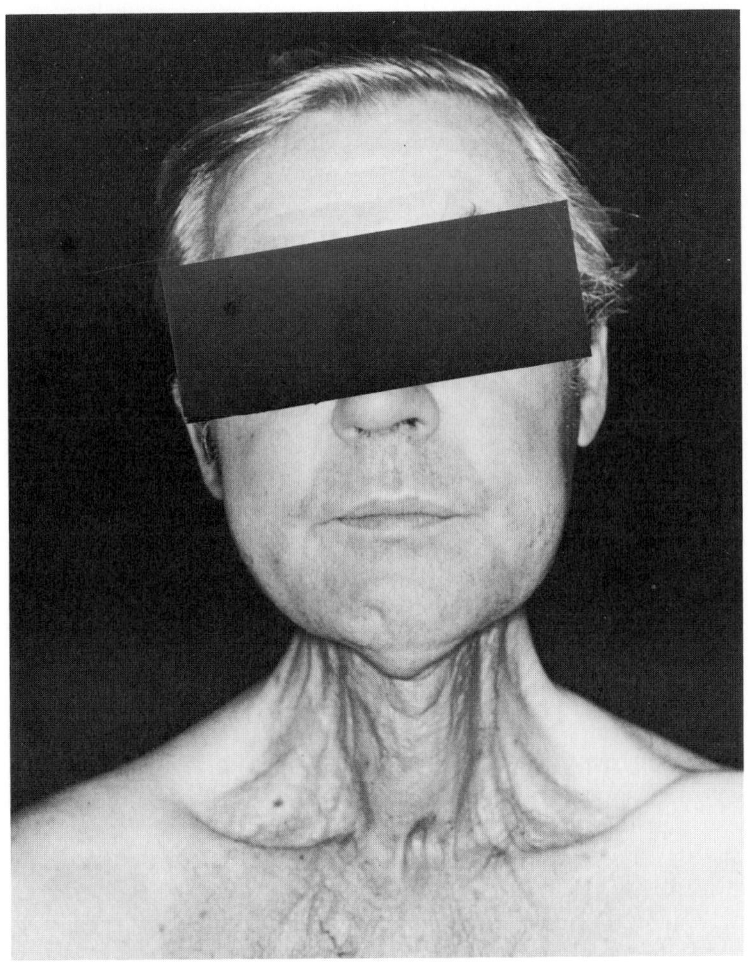

*Frontal photograph after bilateral radical dissection.*

## Nonepidermoid Tumors

Patients with tumors other than squamous or epidermoid carcinoma comprise a small proportion of those who come to radical neck dissection. Histologic varieties here include melanoma, adenocarcinoma of major and minor salivary gland and thyroid origin, soft part sarcoma, lymphoma, and other rarer malignant tumors. Radical neck dissection is the treatment of choice for metastatic melanoma and salivary gland carcinoma. Modified neck dissection usually effectively controls metastatic well-differentiated thyroid cancer, but classical radical neck dissection appears indicated for metastatic medullary thyroid cancer because of its propensity to extend beyond lymph node capsules and to invade adjacent structures, and its resistance to other therapeutic modalities. In view of the propensity of some soft part sarcomas to invade adjacent muscle and to extend along fascial planes, classical radical neck dissection is indicated for more adequate resection of these tissues at risk. Rarely is any neck dissection indicated in the treatment of malignant lymphoma. Only when the disease is recurrent after previous therapy and confined to the cervical lymph nodes is consideration of such a procedure justified. Each patient's treatment must be individualized based upon patient and tumor factors and upon the availability of, indications for, and anticipated results of that treatment.

## Summary

Cervical lymph nodes are frequently involved by metastases from malignant head and neck tumors. The location of such metastatic deposits will vary with the location of the primary tumor, while the incidence and extent of such metastases vary with the location, size (stage), and histologic differentiation of the primary. The prognosis following treatment of such metastases varies directly with the number and location of involved lymph nodes, the degree of invasion beyond the node capsule, and the extent of soft tissue involvement. The increased incidence of distant metastases accompanying extensive regional nodal involvement and/or failure of treatment at the primary site and/or neck has been documented. Classical radical neck dissection offers the widest possible resection of cervical tissues at risk and the best possibility of local control by surgery alone. Newer combinations of treatment may improve overall survival of those unfortunate patients with advanced disease. The prognostic significance of cervical lymph node metastases on the clinical course of head and neck cancer cannot be underemphasized. Their early detection is to be urgently sought and their prompt, adequate, and appropriate treatment must be accomplished.

## References

American Joint Commission for Cancer Staging and End-Results Reporting. *Manual for staging of cancer*, eds. O. Beahrs, D. Carr, and P. Rubin. Chicago: The Commission, 1978.

Bakamjian, V. Y.; Miller, S. H.; and Poole, A. G. A technique for radical dissection of the neck. *Surg. Gynecol. Obstet.* 144:419–424, 1977.

Beahrs, O. H., and Barber, K. W. The value of radical dissection of structures of the neck in the management of carcinoma of the lip, mouth, and larynx. *Arch. Surg.* 85:49–56, 1962.

Beahrs, O. H.; Gossel, J. D.; and Hollinshead, W. H. Technique and surgical anatomy of radical neck dissection. *Am. J. Surg.* 90:490–516, 1955.

Bocca, E. Conservative neck dissection. *Laryngoscope* 85:1511–1515, 1975.

Chu, W., and Strawitz, J. G. Result in suprahyoid, modified radical, and standard radical neck dissections for metastatic squamous carcinoma: recurrence and survival. *Am. J. Surg.* 136:512–515, 1978.

Crile, G. Excision of cancer of the head and neck. With special reference to the plan of dissection based upon 132 operations. *JAMA* 47:1780–1786, 1906.

Dayal, V. S., and DaSilva, A. J. Functional and radical neck dissection. *Arch. Otolaryngol.* 93:413–415, 1971.

Dewar, F. P., and Harris, R. I. Restoration of function of the shoulder following paralysis of the trapezius by fascial sling fixation and transplantation of the levator scapulae. *Ann. Surg.* 132:1111–1115, 1950.

Ewing, M. R., and Martin, H. Disability following "radical neck dissection." An assessment based upon the postoperative evaluation of 100 patients. *Cancer* 5:873–883, 1952.

Farr, H. W., and Arthur, K. Epidermoid carcinoma of the mouth and pharynx 1960–1964, *J. Laryngol.* 86:243–253, 1972.

Fisch, U. P., and Sigel, M. E. Cervical lymphatic system as visualized by lymphography. *Ann. Otol. Rhinol. Laryngol.* 73:869–883, 1964.

Freeland, A. P., and Rogers, J. H. The vascular supply of the cervical skin with reference to incision planning. *Laryngoscope* 85:714–725, 1975.

Gee, W.; Mekigan, J. T.; and Wylie, E. J. Measurement of collateral cerebral hemispheric blood pressure by ocular pneumoplethysmography. *Am. J. Surg.* 130:121–127, 1975.

Harris, A. H., and Smith, R. R. Operative wound seeding with tumor cells. Its role in recurrence of head and neck cancer. *Ann. Surg.* 151:330–334, 1960.

Heller, K. S., and Strong, E. W. Carotid arterial hemorrhage after radical head and neck surgery. *Am. J. Surg.* 138:607–610, 1979.

Huvos, A. G.; Leaming, R. H., and Moore, O. S. Clinicopathologic study of the resected carotid artery. *Am. J. Surg.* 126:570–574, 1973.

Jesse, R. H.; Ballantyne, A. J.; and Larson, D. Radical or modified neck dissection: a therapeutic dilemma. *Am. J. Surg.* 136:516–519, 1978.

Jesse, R. H., and Lindberg, R. D. The efficacy of combining radiation therapy with a surgical procedure in patients with cervical metastases from squamous cancer of the oropharynx and hypopharynx. *Cancer* 35:1163–1166, 1975.

Kalnins, I. K. et al. Correlation between prognosis and degree of lymph node involvement in carcinoma of the oral cavity. *Am. J. Surg.* 134:450–454, 1977.

Kennedy, J. T.; Krause, C. J.; and Leavy, S. The importance of tumor attachment to the carotid artery. *Arch. Otolaryngol.* 103:70–73, 1977.

Lee, J. G., and Krause, C. J. Radical neck dissection: elective, therapeutic, and secondary. *Arch. Otolaryngol.* 101:656–659, 1975.

Lindberg, R. Distribution of cervical lymph node metastases from squamous cell carcinoma of the upper respiratory and digestive tracts. *Cancer* 29:1446–1449, 1972.

Lingeman, R. E. et al. Neck dissection: radical or conservative. *Ann. Otol. Rhinol. Laryngol.* 86:737–744, 1977.

Martin, H. The treatment of cervical metastatic cancer. *Ann. Surg.* 114:972–986, 1941.

Martin, H. et al. Neck dissection. *Cancer* 4:441–499, 1951.

McFee, W. F. Transverse incisions for neck dissection. *Ann. Surg.* 151:279–284, 1960.

McGavran, M. H.; Bauer, W. C.; and Ogura, J. H. The incidence of cervical lymph node metastases from epidermoid carcinoma of the larynx and their relationship to certain characteristics of the primary tumor. *Cancer* 14:55–66, 1961.

McGuirt, W. F., and McCabe, B. F. Significance of node biopsy before definitive treatment of cervical metastatic carcinoma. *Laryngoscope* 88:594–597, 1978.

McGuirt, W. F.; McCabe, B. F.; and Krause, C. J. Complications of radical neck dissection: a survey of 788 patients. *Head Neck Surg.* 1:481–487, 1979.

McQuarrie, D. G. et al. A physiologic approach to the problems of simultaneous bilateral neck dissection. *Am. J. Surg.* 134:455–460, 1977.

Merino, O. R.; Lindberg, R. D.; and Fletcher, G. H. An analysis of distant metastases from squamous cell carcinoma of the upper respiratory and digestive tracts. *Cancer* 40:145–151, 1977.

Moore, O. S., and Frazell, E. L. Simultaneous bilateral neck dissection. *Am. J. Surg.* 107:565–568, 1964.

Mustard, R. A., and Rosen, I. B. Cervical lymph node involvement in oral cancer. *Am. J. Roentgenol.* 90:978–989, 1963.

Naham, A. A.; Bone, R. C.; and Davidson, T. M. The case for elective prophylactic node dissection. *Trans. Am. Acad. Ophthalmol. Otolaryngol.* 82:603–612, 1977.

Pearlman, N. W. Treatment outcome in recurrent head and neck cancer. *Arch. Surg.* 114:39–42, 1979.

Razack, M. S. et al. Significance of site and nodal metastases in squamous cell carcinoma of the epiglottis. *Am. J. Surg.* 136:520–524, 1978.

Sako, K. et al. Fallibility of palpation in the diagnosis of metastases to cervical nodes. *Surg. Gynecol. Obstet.* 118:989–990, 1964.

Sako, K., and Marchetta, F. C. Radioautography of in vitro labelled tumor cells in postoperative wound drainage. *Cancer* 19:735–737, 1966.

Saunders, W. H., and Johnson, E. W. Rehabilitation of the shoulder after radical neck dissection. *Ann. Otol. Rhinol. Laryngol.* 84:812–816, 1975.

Schuller, D. E. et al. Symposium: adjuvant cancer therapy of head and neck tumors. Increased survival with surgery alone vs combined therapy. *Laryngoscope* 89:582–594, 1979.

Schuller, D. E.; Platz, C. E.; and Krause, C. J. Spinal accessory lymph nodes: a prospective study of metastatic involvement. *Laryngoscope* 88:439–450, 1978.

Shah, J. P. et al. Carcinoma of the oral cavity: factors affecting treatment failure at the primary site and neck. *Am. J. Surg.* 132:504–507, 1976.

Shah, J. P., and Tollefsen, H. R. Epidermoid carcinoma of the supraglottic larynx. Role of neck dissection in initial surgical treatment. *Am. J. Surg.* 128:494–499, 1974.

Shear, M; Hawkins, D. M.; and Farr, H. W. The prediction of lymph node metastases from oral squamous carcinoma. *Cancer* 37:1901–1907, 1976.

Silliphant, W. M; Klinck, G. H.; and Levitin, M. S. Thyroid carcinoma and death—a clinicopathological study of 193 autopsies. *Cancer* 17:513–525, 1964.

Skolnick, E. M. et al. The posterior triangle in radical neck surgery. *Arch. Otolaryngol.* 102:1–4, 1976.

Smithdeal, C. D.; Corso, P. F.; and Strong, E. W. Dermis grafts for carotid artery protection: yes or no? A ten year experience. *Am. J. Surg.* 128:484–489, 1974.

Spiro, R. H. et al. Cervical node metastasis from epidermoid carcinoma of the oral cavity and oropharynx. *Am. J. Surg.* 128:562–567, 1974.

Spiro, R. H., and Strong, E. W. Epidermoid carcinoma of the mobile tongue. Treatment by partial glossectomy alone. *Am. J. Surg.* 122:707–710, 1971.

Spiro, R. H., and Strong, E. W. Epidermoid carcinoma of the oral cavity and oropharynx: elective vs therapeutic radical neck dissection as treatment. *Arch. Surg.* 107:382–384, 1973.

Strong, E. W. Preoperative radiation and radical neck dissection. *Surg. Clin. North Am.* 49:271–276, 1969.

Strong, E. W. et al. Preoperative x-ray therapy as an adjunct to radical neck dissection. *Cancer* 19:1509–1516, 1966.

Swain, R. E. et al. An experimental analysis of causative factors and protective methods in carotid artery rupture. *Arch. Otolaryngol.* 99:235–241, 1974.

Toker, C. Some observations on the distribution of metastatic squamous carcinoma within cervical lymph nodes. *Ann. Surg.* 157:419–426, 1963.

Vikram, B. et al. Elective postoperative radiation therapy in stages III and IV epidermoid carcinoma of the head and neck. *Am. J. Surg.*, 1980.

# Chapter 18

# *Radiation-Induced Cancer of the Head and Neck: The Surgeon's Viewpoint*

William Lawson and
Max L. Som

The oncogenic effect of ionizing radiation within the head and neck results from conventional and megavoltage beam radiation and the topical application, interstitial implantation, intracavitary installation, and injection and ingestion of radioactive substances (e.g., bone-seeking radionuclides). The cutaneous and hematologic consequences of exposure to radioactivity were soon recognized from the medical complications appearing in early workers. The total extent of the tissues and organs at risk and the dose required to induce neoplastic changes continue to be clarified, however. Retrospectively, it has become apparent that the amounts of radiation delivered for the treatment of benign conditions were excessive, and dosimetric monitoring was poor by present standards. Epidemiologic studies in humans and experimentation with animal models have shown that doses as low as 100 rad may be tumorigenic to a susceptible host. Moreover, the delayed nature of radiation oncogenesis carries future risks for the development of second primary tumors after high-dose radiotherapy for malignant lesions.

The problem of head and neck radiation oncogenesis will be discussed topographically, as various anatomic regions and tissues differ markedly in their susceptibility to neoplastic transformation, the doses required for tumor induction, and the histologic types of the tumors produced.

## Skin

The development of cancer of the skin of the head and neck following radiation for such benign conditions as dermatosis (acne, eczema), facial hirsutism, cutaneous tumors (hemangioma, nevi), cervical adenitis, and thyroid disorders is a well-documented phenomenon. Pack and Davis (1965) found a

24% incidence of carcinoma on review of 700 cases of radiodermatitis collected from the literature.

Martin, Strong, and Spiro (1970) reviewed 368 patients who had developed skin cancer of the head and neck following radiation. These patients received treatment by both medical specialists (principally dermatologists) and by lay institutions, generally with low-energy equipment. More than two-thirds of the lesions that developed were basal cell carcinomas, the remainder being squamous cell carcinomas. There was generally a female predominance in the ratio of 3 to 1. The latent period until the development of the skin tumor ranged from 1 to 64 years, with a median of 21 years. In 6% of the cases the interval was under 10 years and in 20% it was 30 to 50 years. Moderate to marked radiodermatitis was present in 72% of the cases. While the lesions generally arose in the heavily radiated central areas, they not infrequently appeared at the margins. The radiation-induced lesions tended to be multiple and ulcerative in character, often producing serious deformity. Pack and Davis (1965) found a 40% incidence of multicentricity in their series of cases. The incidence of regional and distant metastases appears to be greater for radiation-induced squamous carcinoma as compared to those of other etiologies. The tumor was lethal in 10% (35 cases) in the series of Martin, Strong, and Spiro (1970).

Lapidus (1976) reported on five women who had developed basal and squamous carcinomas following radiation epilation of facial hair 30 to 40 years previously. Three of the patients required massive head and neck resections in an attempt to control the tumor.

## Skeletal and Soft Tissue

Osseous tumors have been experimentally induced in animals with a variety of bone-seeking radioactive isotopes which include the following elements: strontium, calcium, phosphorus, plutonium, indium, thorium, americum, neptunium, and cerium (Casarett 1973). Histopathologically, the carcinogenic activity of the radionuclide on bone appears to result from a direct and localized damaging effect on osteogenic tissues present at the bone surface or near zones of endochondral bone formation and at epiphyseal and metaphyseal regions. The resultant neoplasms developed in or near areas of proliferating atypical osseous and fibrous tissue. In humans the development of malignant tumors in irradiated bone is relatively rare. Malignant skeletal and soft tissue tumors have arisen in patients receiving high-dose therapeutic radiation and in individuals contaminated by radium and thorium. Parker and Berry (1976) suggested the following criteria for radiation-induced osseous neoplasms: (1) the bone was normal before radiation; (2) the presence of a relatively long latency between radiation and neoplasm formation; (3) histologic confirmation of a primary bone tumor. The threshold dose required for bone tumorigenesis appears to be substantial, generally several thousand rad.

The areas at which malignant tumors have been reported to arise following radiation include the skull, cervical spine, temporal bone, orbit, facial bones, and the jaws. No bone shows a predilection for tumor formation, and the relative incidence of reported cases reflects the times a given region has been irradiated directly or to which bone-seeking radionuclides have access. The conditions for which radiation was delivered include such diverse entities as benign soft tissue or bone tumors (hemangioma, chemodectoma, ossifying fibroma, cyst), other malignancies (retinoblastoma, astrocytoma), chronic infection (mastoiditis, sinusitis), osseous disorders (fibrous dysplasia, tuberculosis), and miscellaneous conditions (acne, osteoarthritis).

Cahan and associates (1948) reviewed the literature concerning the experimental production of bone sarcomas by ionizing radiation in a variety of animals and their occurrence in humans after treatment of osseous tuberculosis and concluded that there was a causal relationship. They also reported 11 patients of their own in whom skeletal tumors arose after radiation of a benign condition. Among these were three facial bone lesions, including an osteogenic sarcoma of the mandible (7 years after 4500 R for ossifying fibroma); an osteogenic sarcoma of the maxilla (13 years after 3600 R for maxillary sinusitis); and an osteogenic sarcoma of the ethmoid (7 years after 2500 R for retinoblastoma).

Sim and colleagues (1972) analyzed 34 patients with postradiation sarcomas and found six lesions of the skull and jaws and two of the cervical spine. These included three fibrosarcomas of the skull (two for benign tumors and one for a chemodectoma), an osteosarcoma of the malar (for acne), a fibrosarcoma of the orbit (for a vascular tumor of the orbit), an osteosarcoma of the maxilla (for fibrous dysplasia), an osteosarcoma of the cervical spine (for bone cyst), and a fibrosarcoma of the cervical spine (for osteoarthritis). They found no differences in the length of latent period whether radiation was received in infancy or childhood.

Dowdle, Winter, and Dehner (1977) also reported an osteosarcoma of the cervical spine arising 11 years after radiation for a spinal cord astrocytoma.

A significant number of radiation-induced malignant tumors have been reported arising in the bones and soft tissues about the orbit following curative therapy for retinoblastoma. Soloway (1966) collected 22 such cases on review of the literature and added three of his own. While the majority of the resultant malignancies were mesenchymal tumors, epithelial lesions also appeared. The latent period ranged from 4 to 30 years, the majority appearing within 10 years. The latency was the same whether radiation was delivered in childhood or adulthood. The appearance of epithelial tumors seemed to be somewhat later, however. All sarcomas were generally fatal within one year. Rowe, Lane, and Snow (1980) concluded that 8.5% of patients with bilateral retinoblastoma receiving radiotherapy developed a second lethal tumor which was unrelated to age and dose. Histologically, more than half of the tumors were osteogenic sarcomas; however, fibrosarcomas, chondrosarcomas, angiosarcomas, mesenchymomas, and basal and squamous carcinomas also occurred. Rowe, Lane, and Snow reported an adenocarcinoma of the ethmoid arising in one of their patients.

Mindell, Shah, and Webster (1977), on reviewing the records of the Roswell Park Memorial Institute (1950–1971), found only 20 of 1169 patients with soft tissue and bone sarcomas to meet the criteria for radiation-induced tumors. The latent period ranged from 1 to 29 years, averaging 12.5 years. Only three cases occurred in the head and neck area: a leiomyosarcoma of the lower neck following radiotherapy for breast carcinoma (six years later); a fibrosarcoma of the palate following radiation for gingival carcinoma (seven years later); and a sarcoma on the orbit following radiotherapy for basal cell carcinoma of the eyelid (seven years later).

In the early part of this century the contamination of individuals by radium occurred accidentally, in watch-dial painters, or by the intentional ingestion of nostrums sold to the public or the injection of psychiatric patients with preparations containing radium salts. Martland (1931) reported 10 cases of sarcomas of the jaws arising in watch-dial painters. This resulted from placement of radium-contaminated paint brushes into the mouth with concentration of the radioactive substance within the bones. Medullary or periosteal osteogenic sarcomas and fibrosarcomas developed 7 to 12 years after exposure. Malignant tumors also developed, however, in watch-dial painters at sites remote to the jaws (Beal, Lindsay, and Ward 1965; Finkel, Miller, and Hasterlik 1969). The Center for Human Radiobiology at the Argonne National Laboratory, which has compiled data on these radium-contaminated individuals, collected 82 cases of bone sarcomas and 33 cases of nasopharyngeal, paranasal sinus, and temporal bone carcinomas (Brues and Kirsh 1976). Radium within the body tends to localize in areas of new bone formation. It is believed that this observed predilection for tumor formation in the paranasal sinuses and mastoids represents anatomic regions where a large mucosal surface is closely applied to alpha-particle–emitting bone (Applebaum 1979). Nilsson (1971) was also able experimentally to induce carcinomas of the external ear in mice with radiostrontium. Histopathologically, principally squamous cell carcinoma but also adenocarcinoma and adenosquamous carcinoma arose in a matrix of osteonecrosis (Littman 1973).

Temporal bone tumors have also been reported following the therapeutic use of radioactive substances and external beam radiation. Fuller and associates (1967) reported a fibrosarcoma arising in the mastoid after treatment of a glomus jugulare tumor with intracavitary radium. Ruben, Thaler, and Holzer (1977) reported the occurrence of a squamous cell carcinoma 24 years after radiation for a posterior fossa astrocytoma. These workers cited a communication with the Armed Forces Institute of Pathology relating two cases of squamous cell carcinoma following radiation for chronic ear disease and a fibrosarcoma after radiotherapy for a pituitary adenoma.

Malignant tumors of the soft supporting tissues have also been reported following local and beam radiation for benign and malignant conditions, or after radionuclide contamination. Pettit, Chamness, and Ackerman (1954) described two fibrosarcomas of the neck following radiation for goiter and metastatic carcinoma and one arising in the lip after radiotherapy for squamous carcinoma. Chasmar, Robertson, and Farmer (1957) reported two postradiation fibrosarcomas of the nose after treatment for basal cell carcinoma and one of the cheek after therapy for actinomycosis. The radiation dose to local tissues in these cases has been considerable, with marked radiodermatitis generally present. Radiation fibromatosis may precede sarcomatous transformation. Malignant mesenchymal tumors, however, have been reported following relatively low-dose radiation. Shore, Albert, and Pastemack (1976) reported two cervical schwannomas occurring in a group of over 2000 patients studied who had received radiation for tinea capitis. Mischler and colleagues (1978) reported a synovial sarcoma arising in the soft tissues of the neck 14 years after radiation for acne.

We have two patients with connective tissue malignancies following high-dose therapeutic radiation. One is a 54-year-old man who received 9500 R of orthovoltage therapy to the nasopharynx for a squamous cell carcinoma and developed a periosteal sarcoma of the mandible within the portal of radiation two years later. He was free of disease on follow-up 15 years after resection. The other is a 62-year-old man with a spindle cell sarcoma of the nose after curative orthovoltage therapy delivered to an antral carcinoma 32 years previously. This patient succumbed to the tumor within a year.

The use of Thoratrast, a colloidal solution of thorium dioxide, in diagnostic radiology has resulted in the production of inflammatory granulomas (thorotrastomas) as well as a variety of soft tissue tumors. The half-life of thorium 232 is so long ($1.4 \times 10^{10}$ years) that once introduced it is essentially trapped forever in the reticuloendothelial system or soft tissues. In the head and neck, lesions resulting from the introduction of Thoratrast occur at two principal sites. Extravasation of Thoratrast into the soft tissues of the neck after injection for carotid angiography has resulted in the formation of fibrosarcomas, neurofibrosarcomas, spindle cell sarcomas, and extraskeletal chondrosarcomas and osteosarcomas (Hasson et al. 1975). Entrapment of Thoratrast in the antrum following contrast sinography has produced various epithelial tumors. This will be discussed later.

## Oral Cavity

Reports of malignant tumors arising within the soft tissues of the oral cavity following radiation for benign conditions or malignant neoplasms are uncommon. The multicentric occurrence of squamous cell carcinoma within the oral cavity makes it difficult to determine whether a lesion appearing after radiotherapy for malignant tumor is indeed radiation-induced. The new lesion should be of a different histologic type (such as a sarcoma) and should arise within the portal of radiation; otherwise it may represent a new spontaneous epidermoid carcinoma. With benign tumors, the lesion itself should undergo malignant transformation following radiation, or a malignant tumor should arise in the irradiated overlying mucosa or adjacent connective tissues. Moreover, a sufficient time interval must elapse between the radiation and the appearance of the new lesion.

Deller (1951) reported a fibrosarcoma arising in the tongue at a site which had received an interstitial radium implant for carcinoma 19 years previously. Fredrickson, Haight, and Noyek (1979) described a carcinoma arising in the buccal mucosa of a patient repeatedly treated by the topical application of radium for an hemangioma present there. Slaughter and Southwick (1957) reported six cases of mucosal carcinoma involving the oral cavity (three), hypopharynx (two), and esophagus (one) following radiation. The two cases with tongue involvement may represent multiple primary epidermoid neoplasms; however, the buccal carcinoma, developed 21 years after local radium application and teleradiation of an ossifying fibroma of the maxilla, appears to be radiation-induced.

## Nasal Cavity, Paranasal Sinuses, Nasopharynx

Reports supporting a role for radiation oncogenesis within the upper respiratory tract are more numerous. Aanesen and Olofsson (1979) reported three cases of squamous carcinoma of the buccal mucosa arising 9, 17, and 21 years after radiation of a previous buccal carcinoma (two cases) and lupus vulgaris. As already noted, radionuclide contamination has a predilection for the development of epithelial malignancies within the paranasal sinuses. A bone-seeking radioisotope such as radium appears to induce carcinomas within the mucosal lining of the paranasal sinuses and nasopharynx (Brues and Kirsh 1976; Finkel, Miller, and Hasterlik 1969). The installation of Thoratrast into the maxillary sinus and its subsequent retention there has also resulted in the formation of malignant epithelial tumors secondary to the activity of an alpha-particle–emitting substance. Kligerman, Lattes, and Rankow (1960) and Feldman, Seaman, and Wells (1963) reviewed two cases of Thoratrast-induced tumors of the maxillary sinus found in the literature and reported six additional cases from their institution. The eight tumors consisted of five squamous cell carcinomas, two mucoepidermoid carcinomas, and one adenocarcinoma. The latent period ranged from 10 to 21 years, averaging 14 years. The resultant tumors were highly aggressive and rapidly lethal in the majority of cases. One of our patients was a 58-year-old man who developed a squamous cell carcinoma in the right maxillary sinus following entrapment of Thorotrast within the antrum 20 years previously.

Malignant tumors have also been reported within the nasopharynx following radiotherapy for benign and malignant tumors. The sarcomatous transformation of the juvenile nasopharyngeal angiofibroma has been reported following radiation (Batsakis, Klopp, and Newman 1955; Gissesson, Lindgren and Stenram 1958). Southwick (1977) cites two patients developing malignant histiocytoma of the posterior nasal cavity following radiotherapy for retinoblastoma.

A patient of ours, an eight-year-old child, developed a fibrosarcoma of the right antrum after receiving cobalt radiotherapy for a rhabdomyosarcoma of the ethmoid three years previously.

## Larynx, Hypopharynx, and Esophagus

Evidence supporting a role for radiation carcinogenesis within the larynx and laryngopharynx falls into three categories: (1) malignancies developing following radiation for benign extralaryngeal conditions; (2) malignancies developing after radiation for benign laryngeal neoplasms; (3) second malignancies developing after therapeutic radiation for laryngeal cancer.

In 1951 Goolden proposed criteria for radiation-induced cancer based on four cases of his own and five collected from the literature of laryngeal and hypopharyngeal malignancies developing in patients radiated for benign disease. These included (1) a history of radiation for a benign condition; (2) sufficient time lapse for the development of the malignancy (latent period); (3) evidence of radiation injury (e.g., radiation dermatitis); (4) histologic proof of a new malignant tumor. In 1955 Som and Peimer reviewed 18 cases, and by 1957 Goolden collected 25 cases reported in the world literature of malignant neoplasms of the larynx, hypopharynx, and esophagus following radiation for benign conditions. Lawson and Som (1975) discovered another 20 cases published from 1957 to 1974. Study of these 45 cases revealed all to be histologically squamous cell carcinoma except for two fibrosarcomas (Goolden 1951; Holinger and Rabbett 1953). The lesions arose in the larynx in 12, in the hypopharynx in 33, and in the esophagus in 2 patients. The radiotherapy was generally administered for benign thyroid disease (goiter, thyrotoxicosis) and tuberculous cervical adenitis. These patients also showed evidence of radiodermatitis (telangiectasia, atrophy, ulceration) within the portal of radiation. In five patients multicentric malignancies appeared. McGraw and McKenzie (1965) reported three patients each with an adenocarcinoma of the thyroid and a squamous carcinoma of the laryngopharynx; one patient also developed a skin cancer. The patients of both Cronin (1971) and Baker (1959) developed a carcinoma of the larynx and the hypopharynx, the latter case also forming basal and squamous skin cancers. All of these patients received orthovoltage therapy, with the latent period for the development of the malignancy ranging from 8 to 51 years, with a mean of 27 years.

There is also evidence that radiation of benign intralaryngeal lesions may induce malignant transformation. Rabbett (1965) collected nine cases of laryngeal carcinoma following orthovoltage radiation for juvenile papillomatosis. The latent period ranged from 4 to 28 years, averaging 12 years.

The oncogenetic effect of radiotherapy has also been implicated in the occurrence of second primary malignancies in the larynx and laryngopharynx following therapeutic radiation for laryngeal carcinoma. Som and Peimer (1955) were the first to describe carcinoma arising in the hypopharynx in two patients 17 and 20 years after such treatment, and implicated radiotherapy in their pathogenesis. Thomas (1964) reported as late recurrences two instances of laryngeal carcinoma appearing many years after curative radiotherapy to the larynx. Schindel and Castoriano (1965) reported five cases of hypopharyngeal carcinoma appearing 7 to 12 years after curative radiotherapy of intralaryngeal malignancies. They believed that these lesions were radiation-induced rather than multicentric tumors because they all arose in the postcricoid region in men, an uncommon site for primary malignancies in this sex, and all developed within the portal of radiation. We similarly observed a patient who developed a postcricoid carcinoma 12 years after successful radiation of a cordal carcinoma. All 10 cases cited received orthovoltage therapy, with a latent period of 7 to 30 years, averaging about 15 years. Baker and Weissman (1971) also treated seven patients with laryngeal malignancies who had been irradiated 5 to 25 years previously for another laryngeal carcinoma. Donaldson (1978) described a fibrosarcoma arising in a larynx 11 years after it received 5600 R for a squamous cell carcinoma.

In an attempt to demonstrate that the occurrence of multiple malignant tumors within the larynx was more than a fortuitous occurrence, two populations of treated patients with cordal carcinoma were compared (Lawson and Som 1975). The incidence of second primary laryngeal cancer in the operated group receiving partial laryngeal surgery (310 cases) was 3.9%, whereas in the irradiated group (225 cases) it was 8%. This rose to 9% in the latter group when the laryngopharynx was included. Twice as many new carcinomas occurred in the subgroup receiving supervoltage therapy as compared to the orthovoltage group. The latent period until the appearence of the second laryngeal primary ranged from 5 to 21 years, averaging about 7 years. The incidence of extralaryngeal malignancies was the same in both the operated and irradiated groups (3%). Radiation-induced carcinogenesis offers an explanation for this statistically significant difference in incidence in new malignancies observed within the larynx. Gates and Warren (1968) were able to induce experimentally esophageal carcinomas in mice with radioactive cobalt.

The latent period for the appearance of a laryngeal or hypopharyngeal malignancy following orthovoltage radiation of the neck for benign disease averaged 27 years. This decreased to an average of 12 to 15 years with orthovoltage therapy and to 7 years with supervoltage therapy when the radiation was directed to the laryngeal mucosa. These data suggest that it may be preferable to treat younger individuals under 50 years with laryngeal carcinoma by surgery rather than with primary radiotherapy.

## Salivary Gland

Retrospective studies of large series of patients irradiated for benign conditions reveal the occurrence of salivary gland neoplasms. In each series there was a control group of nonirradiated siblings who failed to develop any lesions. Saenger and associates (1960) found one mucoepidermoid carcinoma of the parotid developing seven years after 600 rad for adenoiditis and one adenocarcinoma of the submaxillary gland developing 11 years after 450 R for cervical adenitis among 1644 irradiated patients. No salivary gland tumors arose among 3777 controls. Hazen and colleagues (1966) noted two mixed tumors of the parotid arising among 971 children irradiated for lymphoid hyperplasia and ear infections. They concluded that radiation was oncogenic to the radiosensitive ductal epithelium. Each patient received about 900 rad with a mean latency of seven years. Hempelmann and associates (1967) found four salivary gland tumors among 2878 children receiving radiation for thymic enlargement. There was no case among 5006 nonirradiated siblings. Modan and colleagues (1974) reported seven parotid tumors (four malignant and three benign) among 12,000 Israeli children receiving 1750 to 2000 R for tinea capitis. The latent period averaged 13.3 years.

Schneider and associates (1977) found 27 tumors (19 benign and 8 malignant) among 1922 patients who received radiation to the tonsils and nasopharynx, with a latent period of 7 to 32 years. They found no correlation between age at initial therapy or dose and the occurrence of a salivary gland tumor. Age, dose, sex, and latency were also the same for patients with benign and malignant lesions.

Epidemiologic studies of Japanese patients exposed to atomic-bomb radiation also showed an increased incidence of salivary gland neoplasms. Belsky and colleagues (1972) reported a risk for developing a salivary gland tumor five times greater among the 109,000 survivors of atomic bomb explosions at Hiroshima and Nagasaki. Prevalence correlated with age and exposure. They found no relationship, however, between dose and tumor type or latency. The latent period ranged from 10 to 24 years. They found 8 malignant (3 parotid) and 14 benign (11 parotid) tumors in this group. Takeichi, Hirose, and Yamamoto (1976) confirmed this increased incidence in atomic bomb survivors and calculated a tenfold increase in the prevalance of malignant tumors.

Experimentally, Gross (1958) was able to induce parotid tumors in mice using whole-body radiation.

Other reports confirmed the association between radiation of the head and the neck and the development of salivary gland tumors. Ju (1968) reported seven patients irradiated for facial acne, eczema, or hirsutism who developed the triad of radiation dermatitis, skin cancers (10 to 20 years later), and salivary gland tumors (15 to 20 years later). There were five parotid (two benign and three malignant) and two submaxillary (one benign and one malignant) tumors in this group. Swelstad and associates (1978) reported 13 salivary gland neoplasms, 8 parathyroid adenomas, and 8 thyroid lesions arising in 18 patients receiving radiation for benign conditions. There were 10 parotid and 3 minor salivary gland tumors, 70% of which were malignant. The latency ranged from 3 to 60 years, averaging about 32 years. In their series 11 patients had two glandular tumors and 1 patient had three tumors. This prompted them to suggest the concept of polyglandular neoplasia and to recommend a complete and careful head and neck examination in any patient with a history of prior regional radiation. Similar observations were made by Katz (1979).

An instance of familial radiation tumorigenesis was reported by Smith and Levitt (1974) in which two parotid tumors (one benign and one malignant) developed among five siblings who had eight solid tumors. Isolated reports of salivary neoplasms following radiation for benign conditions have been made (Smith 1976; Rice, Batsakis, and McClatchey 1976; Becker and Economou 1975; Sogg 1977).

A survey of the 97 radiation-induced salivary gland neoplasms reported shows that 80% arose in the parotid, with the remainder occurring in the submaxillary and minor salivary glands. Malignant tumors accounted for 47% (46 cases) and benign tumors for 53% (51 cases) of the total. In 70 cases in which the histology was specified at each anatomic site, it was noted that 47% of the parotid tumors (26 of 55 cases) were malignant, with the mucoepidermoid carcinoma the most common type, followed by the adenocarcinoma. The mixed tumor was the commonest benign lesion (26 of 29 cases) and comprised 47% of all parotid tumors. Among the submaxillary and minor salivary gland tumors 73% (11 of 15 cases) were malignant, the majority of which were mucoepidermoid and adenocarcinomas.

## Thyroid

Radiation exposure has been implicated as a causal factor in the increased incidence of thyroid carcinoma observed during the last several decades. The presumed sources of the ionizing radiation include therapeutic external beam radiation, the internal administration of radioactive isotopes, and exposure to atomic explosions and their fallout. Experimental studies in animals support an oncogenic effect of external and internal ionizing radiation on thyroid tumor formation. Benign and malignant neoplasms were produced by radiation and $^{131}$I in rats (Doniach 1958; Nichols et al. 1965; Lindsay 1968) and dogs (Michaelson, Lu, and Quinlan 1973) after a latency of 1 to 2 years and 4 to 10 years, respectively. Doida, Hoke, and Hempelmann (1971) demonstrated chromosomal abnormalities in thyroid cells grown in tissue culture from glands removed from patients who had been irradiated in infancy.

Duffy and Fitzgerald (1950) noted that 10 of the 28 children in their series of thyroid carcinomas, an uncommon neoplasm within the pediatric age group, had an antecedent history of radiation for thymic enlargement. Winship (1951) made a similar observation at about the same time. A number of retrospective studies were performed which demonstrated the oncogenic potential of low-dose external beam radiation delivered in infancy and early childhood for such benign conditions as thymic enlargement and hyperplastic tonsils (Clark 1955; Simpson, Hempelmann, and Fuller 1955; Southwick, Slaughter, and Majarakis 1959; Wilson and Asper 1960). A worldwide questionnaire study by Winship and Rosvoll (1961) found that more than 80% of the children with thyroid carcinoma (562 cases) had received radiotherapy in infancy or early childhood.

In 1955 Simpson, Hempelmann, and Fuller began a questionnaire study of persons living in the Rochester, New York area, who had received radiation in infancy for thymic enlargement, which was subsequently carried through four surveys over a 20-year period (Hempelmann et al. 1967, 1975). They found on study of 2872 irradiated subjects an increased incidence of benign and thyroid neoplasms in the treated population when compared with 5005 sibling controls. There were 24 malignant and 52 benign thyroid neoplasms in the irradiated group as compared to no malignant and 6 benign lesions in the control group. An unusually high incidence was noted in a subgroup that had received high-dose radiation. While there appeared to be a dose-response relationship for the development of tumors, it could not be correlated with latent period or histologic type. The relative proportion of affected women to men was in the ratio of 2 to 1. Ethnic analysis also revealed a significant increased incidence of thyroid cancer in persons of Jewish derivation, especially young adult women. The minimal latent period was 5 years for cancer in men and 10 years for cancer in women and benign tumors in both sexes.

In 1955 Clark made similar observations in the Chicago area. He reported a series of 15 children with thyroid carcinoma, all of whom had received head, neck, and mediastinal radiation. DeGroot and Paloyan (1973) found 40% of 50 consecutive patients with thyroid carcinoma to have received neck radiation. Refetoff and colleagues (1975) detected palpable abnormalities of the thyroid in 26 of 100 patients seeking medical attention because of a history of childhood radiation. Among 15 patients undergoing surgery, 7 had carcinoma, 5 had adenomas, and 3 had other benign conditions. Favus and associates (1976), at the Michael Reese Hospital, detected thyroid nodules clinically in 16.5% and nonpalpable lesions by technetium scanning in another 10.7% of 1056 young adults screened with a history of nasopharyngeal and tonsillar irradiation. Thyroid carcinoma was present in one-third of the operated cases. Patients with benign and malignant tumors did not differ in the total dose, latency, or age at which they were irradiated. Becker and colleagues (1975) and Southwick (1977), at the Rush-Presbyterian–St. Luke's Medical Center, found a 37% incidence of thyroid carcinoma among 95 patients irradiated for thymic or tonsillar enlargement and facial dermatosis. Forty percent of these malignant tumors were multifocal. The mean latency between radiation and diagnosis of the tumor was 24 years. Among the 14 patients having only an abnormal thyroid scan, 4 were found to have carcinoma in association with thyroiditis or sclerosis. Paloyan and associates (1976) obtained a 54% incidence of carcinoma on total thyroidectomy in 70 patients with nodular thyroids and a history of radiation exposure. The latent period ranged from 6 to 44 years, with a mean of 22.4 years. In 14 patients cervical node metastases developed; in 4 patients distant metastases developed.

Janower and Miettinen (1971) conducted a questionnaire study of 466 patients in the Boston area irradiated in infancy for thymic enlargement. There were two malignant and nine benign thyroid tumors in the irradiated group, whereas there occurred no malignant and 10 benign tumors among 2604 control subjects. The average radiation dose was 400 rad.

Cerletty and colleagues (1978) found 19.6% of 1825 subjects from the Milwaukee area with a history of head and neck radiation to have thyroid abnormalities: 9% single or multiple nodules; 8.4% thyroidmegaly; and 2.2% prior thyroid surgery. Among 113 operated subjects with nodules, 30.1% had carcinoma, and 14 patients had lymph node metastases. These workers did not find thyroid imaging to increase nodule detection significantly. Determinations of thyroxine, thyroid-stimulating hormone, and thyroid antibodies were also not useful in screening for nodules or cancer. The average age of the patients was 30 years, with men and women equally affected. The mean latency was 22 years.

Using serial sections Komorowski and Hanson (1977) found thyroid carcinoma in 12 of 18 patients with a history of head and neck radiation in childhood who had nodules detected by physical examination or thyroid scanning; metastases developed in 6.

It next became apparent that external beam radiation of the head and neck of adults also carried a significant risk for the development of thyroid carcinoma. Block, Miller, and Horn (1969) found that 9 of 100 adults irradiated for benign conditions (including sinusitis, tonsillar hypertrophy, cervical lymph adenitis, and dermatologic conditions) developed thyroid carcinoma. The interval between radiation and clinical evidence of disease was 3 to 30 years, averaging 13 years. These authors collected from the literature numerous reports of thyroid carcinoma following radiation of adolescents and adults for such conditions as acne, tuberculous adenitis, medulloblastoma, thyrotoxicosis, and goiter. The development of thyroid carcinoma in individuals irradiated during the sixth and seventh decades showed that age provided no immunity to neoplasm induction.

Albright and Allday (1967) reported the association of thyroid carcinoma and radiotherapy for adolescent acne in five patients. The interval between radiation and surgery ranged from 5 to 40 years, the majority of cases appearing at about 20 years. Paloyan and Lawrence (1978) observed a 60% incidence of thyroid cancer among 20 patients operated on for thyroid nodules who had received radiation for acne in adolescence. The latent period was from 9 to 41 years.

Other dermatologic conditions in which low-dose radiotherapy has been given to the head and neck region of children and adults, placing the thyroid gland at risk, include facial hirsutism, hemangiomas, nevi, keloids, and fungal infections. Modan and associates (1974) reported 12 cases of thyroid carcinoma among 10,902 patients receiving scalp radiation for tinea capitis in childhood. Webber (1977) also called attention to the possible risk of thyroid cancer in children irradiated for pertussis during the 1920s and cited personal knowledge of one case.

Concerning the tumorigenic potential of internally administered radioactive isotopes, Seydel (1973) collected from the literature reports of two children and seven adults with biopsy-proved thyroid carcinoma arising 2 to 12 years after administration of radioactive iodine. McDougal and associates (1971), however, found only one patient to develop thyroid carcinoma 13 years after treatment for hyperthyroidism among 3570 patients treated with $^{131}$I and 200 patients treated with $^{125}$I.

An increased prevalence of thyroid carcinoma has also been reported in atomic-bomb survivors. Among the Hiroshima-Nagasaki population, Wood and colleagues (1969) found a higher incidence in younger versus older patients, in women versus men, and in patients exposed to 200 rad or more. The actual incidence of thyroid carcinoma, however, may be significantly greater than clinically apparent. In an autopsy study of this population, Sampson and associates (1969) found 536 tumors among 1971 consecutive autopsies, 97% of which were occult. Jablon and colleagues (1971) reported a substantial relative risk of thyroid carcinogenesis among Japanese exposed to atomic radiation as children, calculated as 1.23 after exposure to 10 to 99 rad and 6.1 with exposure over 100 rad. Parker and associates (1974) confirmed these findings and showed that the risk for women developing thyroid carcinoma continued for 26 years after exposure to atomic radiation. A dose of 50 rad separated those with a relatively increased risk from the lower-risk population.

Conrad and colleagues (1966, 1970) also noted a significantly increased incidence of thyroid carcinoma in Marshall Islands inhabitants exposed to iodine radionuclides (doses as large as 1200 rad) in fallout from atomic bomb tests performed in 1954.

Not all studies, however, support a causal relationship between radiation and thyroid carcinoma. Epidemiologic studies from Michigan (Pifer et al. 1968) and Pittsburgh (Conti et al. 1960) failed to demonstrate an increased incidence of thyroid carcinoma in thymus-irradiated children. Concerning the effect of high-dose radiotherapy, Seydel (1973) found only 1 case of thyroid carcinoma arising among a series of 458 patients irradiated for head and neck cancer and could not determine a statistically significant increased incidence. Also, this same patient was the only one who received radiation among 100 adults operated on for thyroid disease at the American Oncologic Hospital. A controlled study of recalled patients with a history of head and neck radiation by Royce, MacKay, and DiSabella (1979) failed to detect a significant increased incidence of thyroid abnormalities. They felt that the studies previously cited suffered from examiner bias, sampling errors, and lack of adequate controls.

It has also been suggested that thyroid carcinoma following radiation is an indirect result of the injured and hypofunctioning gland's causing an excessive thyroid-stimulating hormone production which actually produces the nodules and tumors (Block, Miller, and Horn 1969).

The natural history of radiation-induced thyroid carcinomas is no different from that of spontaneously arising neoplasms. While they have the capacity to produce local and distant metastases, they are no more aggressive clinically and respond similarly to surgical and medical management. The prevalance of women found with spontaneous neoplasms, however, is not seen in the irradiated group. Here it more often involves men and appears at an earlier age. Histologically, the same patterns are found in both irradiated and nonirradiated glands, with a predominance of papillary and mixed papillary-follicular types. Spindle cell tumors have also been reported (Hempelmann et al. 1975). The types of benign tumors reported arising in irradiated glands include colloid, follicular, fetal, and Hürthle cell adenomas (Albright and Allday 1967; Komorowski and Hanson 1977). The occurrence of both multiple benign and malignant nodules within irradiated thyroid glands has been observed by numerous authors and strongly influences surgical management. Refetoff and associates (1975) found 5 of 7 carcinomas to be multifocal; Komorowski and Hanson (1977) observed 8 of 12 carcinomas to be multifocal; Cerletty and colleagues (1978) noted 9 of 34 carcinomas to be multifocal; Favus and associates (1976) reported 28 of 60 carcinomas to be multifocal; and Paloyan and colleagues (1976) noted bilateral carcinoma in 17 of 38 cases. Komorowski and Hanson (1977) found 8 of 12 malignancies in their series to be in an area other than the gross nodule and often only 2 to 3 mm in diameter. This underscores the unreliability of frozen sections in establishing an operative diagnosis of malignancy in irradiated cases. Consequently, thyroid multinodularity does not signify a decreased probability of malignancy among irradiated patients but rather has led most surgeons to employ total thyroidectomy in such cases (Paloyan et al. 1976). In addition to being multinodular, the irradiated gland also shows lymphocytic thyroiditis, and interstitial fibrosis (Cerletty et al. 1978; Komorowski and Hanson 1977; Hempelmann et al. 1975, Swelstad et al. 1978).

As already noted in the section on salivary gland tumors, the codevelopment of thyroid, salivary, and parathyroid neoplasms has been observed in irradiated subjects by Swelstad and associates (1978) and by Katz (1979). The simultaneous occurrence of thyroid and salivary lesions following radiation was also noted by others (Becker and Economou 1975; Saenger et al. 1960; Hazen et al. 1966; Hempelmann et al. 1967.)

## Parathyroids

The parathyroids are another gland complex at risk for neoplastic transformation following head and neck radiation. The relatively small size and location of the resultant tumors, however, does not permit detection by clinical examination but results from investigation of symptomatic or asymptomatic hypercalcemia. In addition to producing hyperfunctioning adenomas and hyperplasia, radiation has also been shown to cause cellular abnormalities within the parathyroids. An experimental model for radiation-induced parathyroid neoplasia exists in rats. Lindsay and colleagues (1963) and Triggs and Williams (1977) were able to produce parathyroid adenomas and hyperplasia with radioactive iodine.

Rosen, Strawbridge, and Bain (1975) reported the first instance of hyperparathyroidism in a patient who had received radiation for facial hirsutism 40 years previously in whom radiodermatitis, a mixed tumor of the sublingual glands, and a parathyroid adenoma developed. They speculated that the parathyroid tumor was radiation induced. Other sporadic reports of hyperparathyroidism occurring in irradiated patients appeared (Albrechtson et al. 1977; Schachner and Hall 1978). Schachner and Hall reported two instances of hyperfunctioning parathyroid adenomas appearing 25 and 35 years following radiotherapy for facial acne and thymic enlargement, respectively.

Several retrospective studies were performed which showed an increased incidence of hyperparathyroidism in patients with head and neck radiation, confirming that the association was more than a fortuitous occurrence. Tissell and associates (1976) found 14% of 170 patients studied with proved hyperparathyroidism to have received prior radiation. They later (1977) found 11% of 100 neck radiation subjects to develop hyperparathyroidism. Four of six individuals receiving greater than 1200 R developed hypercalcemia. There were eight adenomas and three hyperplasias found on surgical exploration. The latent period between radiation and the development and hyperparathyroidism averaged 38 years. Paloyan and colleagues (1977) claimed that as many as 30% of hyperparathyroid patients (27 of 89) had a history of head and neck radiation. Christensson (1978) found 8 of 58 (14%) patients with hyperparathyroidism and parathyroid adenoma to have received radiation in childhood. All were irradiated for tuberculous adenitis in the range of 200 to 600 R, an average of 46 years previously. Prinz and associates (1977a, 1977b) reported that among 27 cases of hyperparathyroidism that had received head and neck radiation there were 13 adenomas and 14 hyperplasias or multiglandular disease. The latent period ranged from 10 to 47 years, with a mean of 30 years.

There is evidence that radiation-associated multiglandular tumorigenesis also involves the parathyroids. Swelstad and colleagues (1978) showed the occurrence of 8 parathyroid adenomas, 13 salivary tumors, and 8 thyroid neoplasms among 18 patients receiving prior head and neck radiation. Among the eight patients with parathyroid lesions the latency ranged from 23 to 33 years, with a mean of 27 years. Prinz and associates (1977a, 1977b) reported 4 thyroid carcinomas and 6 benign thyroid tumors among 27 irradiated patients with hyperparathyroidism secondary to adenoma or hyperplasia. Katz (1979) reported 59 thyroid carcinomas, 14 parathyroid tumors, and 6 salivary gland tumors among 151 patients with a history of childhood radiation. LiVolsi, LoGerfo, and Feind (1978), however, found only 1 patient in their series of 38 cases of coexisting nonmedullary thyroid carcinoma and parathyroid adenoma to have a history of head and neck radiation.

## References

Albrechtsen, R. et al. Parathyroid adenomas induced by radiation (letter). *Lancet* 1:854–855, 1977.

Albright, E. C., and Allday, R. W. Thyroid carcinoma after radiation therapy for adolescent acne vulgaris. *JAMA* 199:280–281, 1967.

Aanesen, S. P. and Olofsson, J. Irradiation-induced tumors of the head and neck. *Acta Otolaryngol. Suppl.* 360:178–181, 1979.

Applebaum, E. L. Radiation-induced carcinoma of the temporal bone. *Otolaryngol. Head Neck Surg.* 87:604–609, 1979.

Baker, D. C. Pseudosarcoma of the pharynx and larynx. *Ann. Otol. Rhinol. Laryngol.* 68:471–477, 1959.

Baker, D. C., and Weissman, B. Post irradiation carcinoma of the larynx. *Ann. Otol. Rhinol. Laryngol.* 80:634–637, 1971.

Batsakis, J.; Klopp, C.; and Newman, W. Fibrosarcoma arising in a juvenile nasopharyngeal angiofibroma following extensive radiation therapy. *Am. Surg.* 21:786–793, 1955.

Beal, D. D.; Lindsay, J. R.; and Ward, P. H. Radiation-induced carcinoma of the mastoid. *Arch. Otolaryngol.* 81:9–16, 1965.

Becker, F. O. et al. Adult thyroid cancer after head and neck irradiation in infancy and childhood. *Ann. Intern. Med.* 83:347–351, 1975.

Becker, F. O., and Economou, S. G. Parotid tumor and thyroid cancer. *JAMA* 232:512–514, 1975.

Belsky, J. L. et al. Salivary gland tumors in atomic bomb survivors. Hiroshima-Nagasaki, 1957–1970. *JAMA* 219:864–868, 1972.

Belsky, J. L. et al. Salivary gland neoplasms following atomic radiation: additional cases and reanalysis of combined data in a fixed population 1957–1970. *Cancer* 35:555–559, 1975.

Block, M. A.; Miller, M. J.; and Horn, R. C. Carcinoma of the thyroid after external radiation to the neck in adults. *Am. J. Surg.* 118:764–769, 1969.

Brues, A. M., and Kirsh, I. E. The fate of individuals containing radium. *Trans. Am. Clin. Climatol. Assoc.* 88:211–218, 1976.

Cahan, W. G. et al. Sarcoma arising in irradiated bone. *Cancer* 1:3–29, 1948.

Casarett, G. W. Pathogenesis of radionuclide tumors. In *Radionuclide carcinogenesis, proceedings of the twelfth annual Hanford Biology Symposium.* Washington, D. C.: U. S. Atomic Energy Commission, 1973.

Cerletty, J. M. et al. Radiation-related thyroid carcinoma. *Arch. Surg.* 13:1072–1076, 1978.

Chasmar, L. R.; Robertson, D. C.; and Farmer, A. W. Irradiation fibrosarcoma. *Plast. Reconstr. Surg.* 20:55–61, 1957.

Christensson, T. Hyperparathyroidism and radiation therapy. *Ann. Intern. Med.* 89:216–217, 1978.

Clark, D. E. Association of irradiation with cancer of the thyroid in children and adolescents. *JAMA* 159:1007–1009, 1955.

Conrad, R. A.; Dobyn, B. M.; and Sutow, W. W. Thyroid neoplasia as late effect of exposure to radioactive iodine in fallout. *JAMA* 214:316–324, 1970.

Conrad, R. A.; Rall, J. E.; and Sutow, W. W. Thyroid nodules as a late sequela of radioactive fallout in a Marshall island population exposed in 1954. *N. Engl. J. Med.* 274:1397–1399, 1966.

Conti, E. A. et al. Present health of children given x-ray treatment to the anterior mediastinum in infancy. *Radiology* 74:386–391, 1980.

Cronin, J. Radiation-induced cancer of larynx and pharynx. *J. Laryngol. Otol.* 25:621–622, 1971.

DeGroot, L., and Paloyan, E. Thyroid carcinoma and radiation—a Chicago endemic. *JAMA* 225:487–491, 1973.

Deller, P. Fibrosarcoma of the tongue after interstitial irradiation. *Lancet* 1:1159–1160, 1951.

Doida, Y.; Hoke, C.; and Hempelmann, L. H. Chromosomal damage in thyroid of adults irradiated with x-rays in infancy. *Radiat. Res.* 45:645–656, 1971.

Donaldson, I. Fibrosarcoma in a previously irradiated larynx. *J. Laryngol. Otol.* 92:425–428, 1978.

Doniach, I. Experimental induction of tumors of the thyroid by radiation. *Br. Med. Bull.* 14:181–183, 1958.

Dowdle, J. A.; Winter, R. B.; and Dehner, L. P. Postradiation osteosarcoma of the cervical spine in childhood. *J. Bone Joint Surg.* 59A:969–971, 1977.

Duffy, B. J., and Fitzgerald, P. J. Thyroid cancer in childhood and adolescence. Report of 28 cases. *Cancer* 3:1018–1030, 1950.

Favus, M. J. et al. Thyroid cancer occurring as a late consequence of head and neck irradiation. *N. Engl. J. Med.* 294:1019–1025, 1976.

Feldman, F.; Seaman, W. S.; and Wells, J. S. Residual thorotrast in the paranasal sinuses. *Am. J. Roentgenol.* 89:1147–1154, 1963.

Finkel, A. J.; Miller, C. E.; and Hasterlik, R. J. Radium-induced malignant tumors in man. In *Delayed effects of bone-seeking radionuclides*, eds. C. W. Mays et al. Salt Lake City: University of Utah Press, 1969.

Fredrickson, J. M.; Haight, J. S.; and Noyek, A. M. Radiation-induced carcinoma in a hemangioma. *Otolaryngol. Head Neck Surg.* 87:584–585, 1979.

Fuller, A. M. et al. Chemodectomas of the glomus jugulare. *Laryngoscope* 77:218–238, 1967.

Gates, O., and Warren, S. Radiation-induced experimental cancer of the esophagus. *Am. J. Pathol.* 53:667–685, 1968.

Gissesson, L.; Lindgren, M.; and Stenram, U. Sarcomatous transformation of a juvenile nasopharyngeal angiofibroma. *Acta Pathol. Microbiol. Scand.* 42:305–312, 1958.

Goolden, A. W. Radiation cancer of the pharynx. *Br. Med. J.* 2:1110–1112, 1951.

Goolden, A. W. Radiation cancer. A review with special reference to radiation tumors in the pharynx, larynx, and thyroid. *Br. J. Radiol.* 30:626–640, 1957.

Gross, L. Attempts to recover filterable agent from x-ray induced leukemia. *Acta Haematol.*. 19:353–361, 1958.

Hasson, J. et al. Thorotrast-induced extraskeletal osteosarcoma of the cervical region. Report of a case. *Cancer* 36:1826–1833, 1975.

Hazen, R. W. et al. Neoplasms following irradiation of the head. *Cancer Res.* 26:305–311, 1966.

Hempelmann, L. H. et al. Neoplasms in persons treated with x-rays in infancy for thymic enlargement. A report of the third follow-up study. *J. Natl. Cancer Inst.* 38:317–341, 1967.

Hempelmann, L. H. et al. Neoplasms in persons treated with x-rays in infancy: fourth survey in 20 years. *J. Natl. Cancer Inst.* 55:519–530, 1975.

Holinger, P. H., and Rabbett, W. F. Late development of laryngeal and pharyngeal carcinoma in previously irradiated areas. *Laryngoscope* 63:105–112, 1953.

Jablon, S. et al. Cancer in Japanese exposed as children to atomic bombs. *Lancet* 1:927–932, 1971.

Janower, M. L., and Miettinen, O. S. Neoplasms after childhood irradiation of the thymus gland. *JAMA* 215:753–756, 1971.

Ju, D. M. Salivary gland tumors occurring after radiation of the head and neck area. *Am. J. Surg.* 116:518–523, 1968.

Katz, A. D. Thyroid and associated polyglandular neoplasms in patients who received head and neck irradiation during childhood. *Head Neck Surg.* 1:417–422, 1979.

Kligerman, M.; Lattes, R.; and Rankow, R. Carcinoma of the maxillary sinus following thorotrast instillation—report of three cases. *Cancer* 13:967–973, 1960.

Komorowski, R. A., and Hanson, E. A. Morphologic changes in the thyroid following low-dose childhood irradiation. *Arch. Pathol. Lab. Med.* 101:36–39, 1977.

Lapidus, S. M. The tricho system: hypertrichosis, radiation, and cancer. *J. Surg. Oncol.* 8:267–274, 1976.

Lawson, W., and Som, M. L. Second primary cancer after irradiation of laryngeal cancer. *Ann. Otol. Rhinol. Laryngol.* 84:771–775, 1975.

Lindsay, S. The experimental production of thyroid neoplasms in the rat by irradiation. In *Thyroid neoplasia*, ed. S. Young, New York: Academic Press, 1968.

Lindsay, S.; Potter, G. D.; and Chaikoff, I. L. Radioiodine-induced thyroid carcinomas in female rats. *Arch. Pathol.* 75:20–24, 1963.

Littman, M. S. Characteristics of radium-induced malignant tumors of the mastoid and paranasal sinuses. Part 2. Argonne National Laboratory Radiological and Environment Research Division Annual Report, Center for Human Radiobiology, 1972–1973.

LiVolsi, V. A.; LoGerfo, P.; and Feind, C. R. Coexistent parathyroid adenomas and thyroid carcinoma. Can radiation be blamed. *Arch. Surg.* 113:285–286, 1978.

Martin, H.; Strong, E.; and Spiro, R. H. Radiation-induced skin cancer of the head and neck. *Cancer* 25:61–71, 1970.

Martland, H. S. The occurrence of malignancy in radioactive persons. *Am. J. Cancer* 15:2435–2515, 1931.

McDougall, I. R.; Kennedy, J. S.; and Thomson, J. A. Thyroid carcinoma following iodine-131 therapy. *J. Clin. Endocrinol.* 33:287–292, 1971.

McGraw, R. W., and McKenzie, A. D. Carcinoma of the thyroid and laryngopharynx following irradiation: a report of three cases. *Cancer* 18:692–696, 1965.

Michaelson, S. M.; Lu, S. T.; and Quinlan, W. J. Ionizing-radiation-induced thyroid carcinogenesis in the dog. In *Radionuclide carcinogenesis, proceedings of the twelfth annual Hanford Biology Symposium.* Washington, D. C.: U. S. Atomic Energy Commission, 1973.

Mindell, E. R.; Shah, N. K.; and Webster, J. H. Postradiation sarcoma of bone and soft tissues. *Orthop. Clin. North Am.* 8:821–834, 1977.

Mischler, N. E. et al. Synovial sarcoma of the neck associated with previous head and neck radiation therapy. *Arch. Otolaryngol.* 104:482–483, 1978.

Modan, B. et al. Radiation-induced head and neck tumors. *Lancet* 1:277, 1974.

Nichols, C. W. et al. Induction of neoplasms in the rat thyroid glands by x-irradiation of a single lobe. *Arch. Pathol.* 80:177–183, 1965.

Nilsson, A. Radiostrontium-induced carcinomas of the external ear. *Acta Radiol.* 10:321–328, 1971.

Pack, G. T., and Davis, J. Radiation cancer of the skin. *Radiology* 84:436–442, 1965.

Paloyan, E. et al. Total thyroidectomy and parathyroid autotransplantation for radiation-associated thyroid cancer. *Surgery* 80:70–76, 1976.

Paloyan, E. et al. Radiation-associated hyperparathyroidism (letter). *Lancet* 1:949, 1977.

Paloyan, E., and Lawrence, A. M. Thyroid neoplasms after radiation therapy for adolescent acne vulgaris. *Arch. Dermatol.* 114:53–58, 1978.

Parker, L. N. et al. Thyroid carcinoma after exposure to atomic radiation. A continuing survey of a fixed population, Hiroshima and Nagasaki, 1958–1971. *Ann. Intern. Med.* 80:600–604, 1974.

Parker, R. G., and Berry, H. C. Late effects of therapeutic irradiation of the skeleton and bone marrow. *Cancer* 37:1162–1171, 1976.

Pettit, V. D.; Chamness, J. T.; and Ackerman, L. V. Fibromatosis and fibrosarcoma following irradiation therapy. *Cancer* 7:149–158, 1954.

Pifer, J. W. et al. Neoplasms in the Ann Arbor series of thymus-irradiated children: a second survey. *Am. J. Roentgenol.* 103:13–18, 1968.

Prinz, R. A. et al. Radiation-associated hyperparathyroidism: a new syndrome. *Surgery* 82:296–302, 1977a.

Prinz, R. A. et al. Radiation exposure and hyperparathyroidism (abstr.). *Clin. Res.* 24:530, 1977b.

Rabbett, W. F. Juvenile laryngeal papillomatosis: the relation of irradiation to malignant degeneration in this disease. *Ann. Otol. Rhinol. Laryngol.* 74:1149–1163, 1965.

Refetoff, S. et al. Continuing occurrence of thyroid carcinoma after irradiation to the neck in infancy and childhood. *N. Engl. J. Med.* 292:171–175, 1975.

Rice, D. H.; Batsakis, J. G.; and McClatchey, K. D. Post-irradiation malignant salivary gland tumor. *Arch. Otolaryngol.* 102:699–701, 1976.

Rosen, I. B.; Strawbridge, H. G.; and Bain, J. A case of hyperparathyroidism associated with radiation to the head and neck area. *Cancer* 36:1111–1114, 1975.

Rowe, L. D.; Lane, R.; and Snow, J. B. Adenocarcinoma of the ethmoid following radiotherapy for bilateral retinoblastoma. *Laryngoscope* 90:61–69, 1980.

Royce, P. C.; MacKay, B. R.; and DiSabella, P. M. Value of post-irradiation screening for thyroid nodules. A controlled study of recalled patients. *JAMA* 242:2675–2678, 1979.

Ruben, R. J.; Thaler, S. U.; and Holzer, N. Radiation-induced carcinoma of the temporal bone. *Laryngoscope* 87:1613–1621, 1977.

Saenger, E. L. et al. Neoplasia following therapeutic irradiation for benign conditions in childhood. *Radiology* 74:889–901, 1960.

Sampson, R. J. et al. Thyroid cancer in Hiroshima and Nagasaki. I. The prevalence of thyroid carcinoma at autopsy. *JAMA* 209:65–70, 1969.

Schachner, S. H., and Hall, A. Parathyroid adenoma and previous head and neck irradiation. *Ann. Intern. Med.* 88:804, 1978.

Schindel, J., and Castoriano, I. M. Late-appearing (radiation-induced) carcinoma. *Arch. Otolaryngol.* 95:205–210, 1965.

Schneider, A. B. et al. Salivary gland neoplasms as a late consequence of head and neck irradiation. *Ann. Intern. Med.* 87:160–164, 1977.

Seydel, H. G. Thyroid neoplasms in therapeutically irradiated patients. In *Radionuclide carcinogenesis, proceedings of the twelfth annual Hanford Biology Symposium.* Washington, D. C.: U. S. Atomic Energy Commission, 1973.

Shore, R. E.; Albert, R. E.; and Pasternack, B. S. Follow-up study of patients treated by x-ray epilation for tinea capitis. *Arch. Environ. Health* 31:21–28, 1976.

Sim, F. H. et al. Post-radiation sarcoma of bone. *J. Bone Joint Surg.* 54A:1479–1489, 1972.

Simpson, C. L.; Hempelmann, L. H.; and Fuller, L. M. Neoplasia in children treated with x-rays in infancy for thymic enlargement. *Radiology* 64:840–845, 1955.

Slaughter, D. P., and Southwick, H. W. Mucosal carcinomas a result of irradiation. *Arch. Surg.* 74:420–429, 1957.

Smith, D., and Levitt, S. Radiation carcinogenesis. An unusual familial occurrence of neoplasia following irradiation in childhood for benign disease. *Cancer* 34:2069–2071, 1974.

Smith, S. A. Radiation-induced salivary gland tumors. *Arch. Otolaryngol.* 102:561–562, 1976.

Sogg, R. L. Parotid carcinoma and posterior fossa schwannoma following irradiation. *JAMA* 237:2098–2100, 1977.

Soloway, H. B. Radiation-induced neoplasms following curative therapy for retinoblastoma. *Cancer* 19:1984–1988, 1966.

Som, M. L., and Peimer, R. Postcricoid carcinoma as a sequel to radiotherapy for laryngeal carcinoma. *Arch. Otolaryngol.* 62:428–431, 1955.

Southwick, H. W. Radiation-associated head and neck tumors. *Am. J. Surg.* 134:438–443, 1977.

Southwick, H. W.; Slaughter, D. P.; and Majarakis, J. D. Malignant disease of the head and neck in childhood. *Arch. Surg.* 76:678, 1959.

Swelstad, J. A. et al. Radiation-induced polyglandular neoplasia of the head and neck. *Am. J. Surg.* 135:820–824, 1978.

Takeichi, N.; Hirose, F.; and Yamamoto, T. Salivary gland tumors in atomic bomb survivors, Hiroshima, Japan. *Cancer* 38:2462–2468, 1976.

Thomas, R. Late recurrence of laryngeal cancer. *J. Laryngol. Rhinol. Otol.* 78:1123–1124, 1964.

Tissell, L. E. et al. Autonomous hyperparathyroidism—a possible late complication of neck radiotherapy. *Acta Chir. Scand.* 142:367–373, 1976.

Tissell, L. E. et al. Hyperparathyroidism in persons treated with x-rays for tuberculous cervical adenitis. *Cancer* 40:846–854, 1977.

Triggs, S. M., and Williams, E. D. Irradiation of the thyroid as a cause of parathyroid adenoma (letter). *Lancet* 1:593–594, 1977.

Webber, B. M. Radiation therapy for pertussis: a possible etiologic factor in thyroid carcinoma. *Ann. Intern. Med.* 86:449–450, 1977.

Wilson, E. H., and Asper, S. P. The role of x-ray therapy to the neck region in the production of thyroid cancer in young people. *Arch. Intern. Med.* 105:244, 1960.

Winship, T. Carcinoma of the thyroid in children. *Trans. Am. Goiter Assoc.* 10:364, 1951.

Winship, T., and Rosvoll, R. V. Childhood thyroid carcinoma. *Cancer* 14:734–743, 1961.

Wood, J. W. et al. Thyroid carcinoma in atomic bomb survivors, Hiroshima and Nagasaki. *Am. J. Epidemiol.* 89:4–14, 1969.

## Chapter 19

# *Radiation-Induced Cancer as a Factor in Selection of Treatment for Patients with Head and Neck Cancers: The Radiation Therapist's Viewpoint*

Robert G. Parker

Clinical Medicine is the art of balancing risks to the benefit of the patient.

Ionizing radiations are recognized co-carcinogens. The first medically related, radiation-induced cancer, an epithelioma of the skin of the hand with metastases to regional lymph nodes in a 33-year-old roentgen-ray technician, was reported in 1902, within seven years of the discovery of man-made x-rays (Frieben 1902).

For many years, radiation-induced cancer was primarily an occupational hazard for those unsuspecting martyrs who had no knowledge of necessary protective measures. Even after protective measures minimized the risk of high-dose radiation damage to exposed parts, physicians using radiation sources continued to have an increased risk of leukemia and so-called life-shortening, attributed to low doses to the whole body received over many years (March 1950). Good practices, now available and even mandated, have minimized this occupational hazard (March 1961).

A second period of iatrogenic radiation-induced cancer followed. This unwelcomed consequence of the diagnostic and therapeutic use of ionizing radiations is a major concern today. Initially, almost all cancers attributed to radiation followed the treatment of benign lesions, many of which were not documented histologically. For example, in an early series reported by Cade (1957), 30 of the 34 patients developing cancer attributed to ionizing radiations were previously irradiated for benign lesions.

After studying this problem for many years, Cade, a surgeon, concluded that " . . . the elimination of all risks is unlikely in the medical uses of radiation and this applies equally to hazards of surgery, use of drugs, in fact, all therapeutic measures."

The questions to be addressed in this chapter are: (1) What are the risks of radiation-induced cancer relative to the major risks of surgery and chemotherapy for the patient with cancer arising in the head and neck? (2) What factors influence decision-making for the individual patient? (3) How should this information be presented to the patient so that it will support rather than deter rational decision-making?

# Radiation-Induced Cancer

It is a paradox that radiations both cure and cause cancer.
—Alexander (1957)

Although ionizing radiations have been identified as co-carcinogens in the human, "in cellular terms, radiation-induction of cancer must be a very rare phenomenon, so rare compared with cell sterilization or mutation-induction that the general corpus of radiobiological understanding may be inapplicable" (Mole 1975). This rarity of carcinogenic cellular transformation, which makes laboratory experimentation difficult, results in even greater difficulty in specifically identifying ionizing radiations as the carcinogen in the individual human when "the risks are many orders of magnitude less than the natural" (Mole 1975). This identification must rest on statistical evidence, inasmuch as there is no specific characteristic which unequivocally links an individual cancer with an etiologic agent.

In clinical medicine, the potential carcinogenicity of an effective therapeutic agent generates two questions: what is the risk of cancer induction in a specific situation and is the risk acceptable?

An attempt to answer the first question requires that the overall risk estimate be based on several component factors related to the radiations, basic biology, and the host.

## Radiation-Related Factors

### Total Radiation Dose

Although risk estimates usually assume a linear dose response without a threshold, the actual relationship is much more complicated. At least two components of this relationship have been identified: (1) the malignant transformation of cells (induction) which, at least for low linear energy transfer (LET) radiations, appears to be proportional to the total dose squared; and (2) cell-killing (sterilization), which reduces the number of cells at risk (Fry 1977). Thus the risk of radiation-induced cancer per rad increases to a maximum and then decreases as the total dose continues to increase (Mole 1975). This changing risk per rad differs for various cancers (Shellabarger 1976). The relatively high risk per rad at low doses may explain, at least partially, the disproportionately high number of cancers reported after the use of small doses for the treatment of benign disease compared to the paucity of tumors developing in tissues irradiated to much higher doses. For example, cancers of the thyroid (Kaplan and Taylor 1976), breast, and leukemia (Court-Brown and Doll 1965) have followed doses of a few hundred rad, while there has been no increase in the expected frequency of tumors following doses of 4500 to 20,000 rad used in the treatment of carcinoma of the cervix (Hutchison 1968). Dose-response data for tumorigenesis, however, are fortunately sparse within the dose ranges used in human radiation therapy (Fry 1977).

## Pattern of Application

Cancers have been attributed to single radiation exposures, as in the atomic-bomb survivors, have followed a few irregularly spaced increments, as in those youngsters receiving so-called thymic irradiation, have been noted following conventional use with daily fractionation over several weeks, and have been correlated with prolonged occupational exposure in radiation workers. Although there is no clinical evidence to correlate an increased risk with a specific pattern of application, based on data from animal experiments, fractionation of low-LET radiations probably reduces the incidence of induced tumors compared to similar doses delivered in a single or a few increments (Fry 1977).

## Dose Rate

If the induction of a tumor by ionizing radiations requires two or more events in a small volume within a short time to preclude repair of the initial damage, then for low-LET radiations low-dose rates could be less carcinogenic than high-dose rates (Shellabarger 1976). In an animal (mice) experiment testing for an excess of ovarian tumors, the nearly linear dose relationship had a decreasing slope as the dose rate decreased from 112 rad to 1.75 rad per day (Yuhas 1974). This cannot be extrapolated to the clinic, however, without considerable reservation, for in addition to species and tumor variations, these dose rates are far less than used in the treatment of cancer in the human. The relative paucity of cancers arising in tissues receiving low-dose rates from interstitial implants such as in the tongue or floor of the mouth (1000 rad per 24 hours or 40 to 45 rad per hour) should be noted, however.

## Dose Distribution

Although the risk of carcinogenesis must increase as the volume of tissue (number of cells) irradiated increases, other factors such as specific tissue susceptibility and total dose obscure this effect. Theoretically, the risks should be different for the high therapeutic doses in the irradiated volume compared to the lower doses outside this volume (Fry 1977). Nonhomogeneity of dose is maximal in interstitial implants most frequently used in the treatment of cancers of the head and neck. There are no clinical data, however, that can document the influence of this irregular dose distribution on risk of cancer induction.

### Radiation Quality

All types of ionizing radiations are carcinogenic (Hutchison 1972), but the dose-squared relationship for low-LET radiations and the linear relationship for high-LET radiations result in an increasing relative biological effectiveness (RBE) for high-LET radiations with decreasing dose until the first-power term describes the relationship for low-LET radiations (Fry 1977). The RBE for high-LET radiations for most tumor types studied in the laboratory ranges from one to five (Ullrich et al. 1976). Such variations in the RBE for carcinogenesis will require evaluation for each target organ as new types of radiations, such as fast neutrons (or pi-mesons) are introduced clinically.

## Biologic Factors

### Tumor Incidence

As noted by Mole (1975), an estimate of the risk of radiation carcinogenesis in clinical application "presupposes a remarkable confidence in the capacity to provide answers to questions about risks many orders of magnitude less than the natural." Hutchison (1972) proposed that the incidence of radiation-induced cancer in the human is about one to five cases per 1 million population per rad per year. This risk in the individual patient varies, however, with all the factors discussed in this chapter.

Even with a liberal working definition of radiation carcinogenesis, induced tumors are very rare. In an exhaustive recent review of the literature, inclusive of patients irradiated therapeutically with doses in excess of 3000 rad, Seydel (1975) found 12 carcinomas of the large bowel, 63 sarcomas of bone, 4 extraskeletal osteosarcomas, 12 malignant tumors of the skin and soft tissues, 3 thyroid cancers in patients treated for medulloblastoma, 5 carcinomas of the hypopharynx in patients treated for cancers of the larynx, and 54 patients who developed leukemia after treatment for Hodgkin's disease. Two-thirds of the latter group also had chemotherapy. Phillips and Sheline (1963) found 2 osteosarcomas 5 and 11 years after radiation of radiographically normal bone, for an incidence of 0.1% of the 2300 five-year survivors and 0.03% of the total of 6000 patients treated. In a review of 20 years' experience with supervoltage radiation (Parker, unpublished), from among several thousand patients treated, only 4 rectal cancers in patients treated for cancer of the cervix, an osteosarcoma developing in the clavicle of a patient treated for cancer of the esophagus, and leukemia developing in a patient treated for seminoma could be identified. Hutchison (1968) found no increase of leukemia or other malignant tumors in patients irradiated (60,000 person-years follow-up) for cancer of the uterine cervix.

Seydel's (1975) own data are usefully quantitated. Among 354 patients surviving from 5 to 39 years derived from 933 patients irradiated for cancer of the cervix, 3 patients (0.85%) developed adenocarcinomas of the endometrium and 3 (0.85%) developed adenocarcinomas of the rectum. In 611 patients surviving more than five years from 1464 patients irradiated for cancers of the oral cavity or oropharynx, 9 (1.14%) developed second malignant tumors. If the requirement for a latent period of several years following radiation is ignored and all 1464 patients are included, 23 patients (1.6%) developed second malignant tumors. In a comparable population at the same hospital, 8 of 407 patients (2%) treated by surgery alone developed second malignant tumors.

## Tumor Type

Nearly all histologic types of cancers, arising in all tissues, have been attributed to previous radiation (Hutchison 1972). That sarcomas are the most frequently reported radiation-induced tumors probably reflects the generous presence of connective tissue in all treatment volumes. For low-LET radiations, resultant leukemias are only about 20% as frequent as so-called solid cancers (Mole 1971). Based on data from survivors of atomic-bomb radiation (Fry 1977; Rossi and Kellerer 1974), however, fission neutrons seem to have a particularly high RBE for leukemogenesis.

## Latent Period

A prolonged interval between exposure to ionizing radiations and the clinical diagnosis of cancer is considered a prerequisite for the diagnosis of radiation-induced cancer. This characteristic, confirmed in the experimental laboratory, is of practical importance in separating posttreatment tumor persistence from a so-called new tumor arising from any cause. Latent periods have been reported for malignant thyroid tumors of 10 years (Kaplan and Taylor 1976); for skin cancer, 25 years (Pochin 1972); for head and neck cancers, 24 years (Kiguchi, Watanabe, and Abe); and for pharyngeal and laryngeal cancers, 27 years (Yoshizawa and Takeuchi 1974). Such long latent periods reduce the risk of radiation-induced tumors in the adult with head and neck cancer, who often exceeds 50 years of age at the time of treatment.

## Degree of Malignancy

Like the surgeon who intervened because the growing cancer was causing clinical problems, the radiation therapist has had treatment correlated with a seemingly increased adverse biologic behavior of a specific cancer. In both circumstances, the therapeutic intervention probably was a response to a clinical problem caused by an increasingly aggressive tumor. Thus, although in the laboratory animal the malignancy of a tumor, measured by lethality, has been increased by radiation (Fry and Ainsworth 1977), supporting data in human tumors are not available, except perhaps in the observed altered behavior of a few low-grade intraoral verrucous carcinomas (Ackerman 1948).

### Multiplicity of Tumors

As noted by Mole (1975), it is very difficult to detect the actual presence, let alone the etiology, of a very small increase of cancers, when there is a "high background noise" of frequently occurring cancers of "natural" origin. Patients with one cancer run a higher risk of additional cancers than the comparable population for all systems studied (Warren and Gates 1932). This is particularly true for patients with head and neck cancers, who have a high correlation with prolonged heavy smoking and high alcohol intake. In Seydel's (1975) data, the risk in Pennsylvania for primary cancer of the head and neck was 62 tumors per 1 million population per year, while 2% of those patients successfully treated surgically for cancers of the oral cavity or oropharynx developed additional cancers.

## Host Factors

### Age

The incidence, tumor type, latent period, and consequence of radiation-induced tumors are influenced by the age of the host at the time of radiation. These differences probably relate to differences in cellular proliferative activity, number of immunologically competent cells, and hormone levels (Fry 1977). For radiation-induced tumors of the thyroid, the young beyond infancy seem most vulnerable (Fry 1977). The susceptibility to radiation-induced leukemia increased with age for those treated for ankylosing spondylitis (Court-Brown and Doll 1965), while among the atomic-bomb survivors both the young and old were more affected than those of middle age (National Academy of Sciences 1972). Except for retinoblastoma, embryonal rhabdomyosarcoma, and selected brain tumors such as craniopharyngioma, medulloblastoma, optic tract and brain stem gliomas, and cystic astrocytomas of the cerebellum, which are predominant tumors of childhood, most head and neck cancers likely to be irradiated arise in older adult hosts.

### Sex

Tumor type and incidence can be related to the sex of the host. Cancers of the upper aerodigestive tract, except for an identified population of post-cricoid tumors (Lederman 1958), arise more frequently in men.

### Genotype

The host's genotype influences the susceptibility to cancer (Fry 1977). Identification of an initial cancer might indicate specific susceptibility to additional cancers. This influence, which may be detectable in children, is obscured in the adult with head and neck cancer by other identifiable etiologic associations, such as prolonged exposure to tobacco and alcohol and poor oral hygiene.

### Specific Tissues

Connective tissue, always at risk because of its presence in all volumes irradiated therapeutically, is the origin of sarcomas, the tumor type most frequently reported after conventional low-LET radiation therapy (Fry 1977). Yet there has been no reported increase of tumors arising in connective tissue or skin or the vasculature in Japanese atomic-bomb survivors who have had an increase above the expected of other tumors, such as leukemia and cancers of the breast and lung (Pochin 1972). The underlying reasons for such differences in susceptibility of various tissues to radiation carcinogenesis are unknown (Fry 1977).

### Exposure to Other Carcinogens, Including Treatment

Inasmuch as ionizing radiations are co-carcinogens, postradiation events may be influenced by exposure to other carcinogens, past, present, or future. This has been recently emphasized by the clear association of a marked increase of leukemia in survivors of Hodgkin's disease receiving combined radiation therapy and chemotherapy (MOPP), compared to those patients treated by either modality alone (Canellos et al. 1975). The complexity of this interrelationship is illustrated by contrasting evidence such as that presented by D'Angio and associates (1976), who noted a decrease in radiation-associated second malignant tumors in youngsters also receiving actinomycin D.

Although Mole (1975) has stated that a correlation between maintained tissue damage (by radiation) and tumor induction cannot be supported, the empirical experience of most clinicians is that a majority of the infrequent nonleukemic tumors attributed to the therapeutic use of high doses of ionizing radiations arise in grossly damaged tissues.

## Specific Tumors in the Head and Neck Attributed to the Therapeutic Use of Ionizing Radiations

Although cancers have been reported in nearly every anatomic structure following therapeutic radiation, the total number is anecdotal from among the millions of patients treated. The seriousness of this paradoxical development can interfere with a perspective necessary for the clinical evaluation of risks for an individual patient.

### Thyroid Cancer

Since 1950, when Duffy and Fitzgerald first suggested an etiologic relationship between external radiation and thyroid cancer in children, many such tumors have been identified. These multicentric papillary, follicular, or mixed carcinomas (Kaplan and Taylor 1976) usually are diagnosed 10 to 25 years after radiation to low doses (200 to 600 rad) and rarely can be associated with the high doses used in cancer therapy, although Seydel (1975) reported three cancers in patients receiving over 3000 rad in the treatment of medulloblastoma and Weshler and colleagues (1978) reported a carcinoma developing in the thyroid of a 22-year-old 16 years following radiation therapy for Hodgkin's disease. Beach and Dolphin (1962) estimated an incidence of about 1% following doses of 200 to 350 rad. The prognosis for patients developing these thyroid cancers has been highly favorable, with a reported 98% survival 10 years following surgical removal (Wilson, Platz, and Black 1970).

## Parathyroid Tumors

Fourteen percent of 170 patients with hyperparathyroidism received previous radiation therapy to the neck (Tissell et al. 1976). A few parathyroid adenomas, but no carcinomas, have been reported (Schachner and Hall 1978).

## Postcricoid Cancer

Epidermoid carcinomas of the postcricoid region, diagnosed from 7 to 17 years after successful radiation of epidermoid carcinomas of the larynx, have been reported in two men by Som and Peiner (1955) and in five men by Schindel, Castoriano, and Tikva (1972).

## Laryngeal Cancer

Kiguchi, Wanatabe, and Abe (1974) and Glanz (1976) have reported a total of 11 patients who developed epidermoid carcinomas in larynxes that had been irradiated more than five years previously.

## Cancers of the Oral Cavity and Oropharynx

Seydel (1975) reported eight epidermoid carcinomas and one fibrosarcoma arising within the irradiated volume of 611 survivors (1.14%) who had been treated more than five years previously. In a comparable population at the same medical center, eight second cancers were found in 407 patients (2%) treated surgically.

## Salivary Gland Tumors

Modan and associates (1974) found four malignant and three benign tumors of the parotid gland among the 10,902 children receiving 350 to 400 R (air) to the scalp as treatment for ringworm, although the parotid gland should not have been in a conventionally irradiated volume. This association had been reported previously (Saenger et al. 1960). Som (1975) reported a mucoepidermoid carcinoma of the parotid gland diagnosed eight years after radiation therapy of an epidermoid carcinoma of the nasopharynx.

### Bone and Soft Tissue Tumors

Malignant tumors arising in bone or soft tissue are the most frequent tumors attributed to therapeutic radiation. Although many of the malignant tumors in bone developed following radiation of presumed benign lesions, often the bone was considered normal. In an attempt to establish a perspective for clinical risk, Phillips and Sheline (1963) reviewed the radiation therapy of 5900 patients, including 2300 who survived more than five years, and found two osteosarcomas attributable to radiation; an incidence of 0.1% of the long-term survivors, or 0.03% of all patients treated.

In a review of 625 patients with retinoblastoma, Sagerman and colleagues (1969) estimated the incidence of radiation-induced osteosarcomas to be 1.5%, all diagnosed more than four years after the delivery of 3500 rad of megavoltage x-rays in 18 to 20 days. The incidence had been higher with the use of much larger doses. In a more recent study (Tretter 1979), it was noted that osteosarcomas also developed in the orbits of patients treated by surgery without radiation.

Osteosarcomas arising in other sites such as the skull (Sparagana et al. 1972) and sella (Abdul, Amine, and Sugar 1976) have followed therapeutic radiation.

Connective tissue, always at risk in the radiation therapy of cancer in humans, is the source of sarcomas, with the most frequent tumor attributed to low-LET radiations (Fry 1977). Although the latent period can be relatively short for these tumors, Hatfield and Schulz (1970) did not find a relationship between radiation dose and latent period.

Less common tumors such as hemangiopericytomas (Seydel 1975) and hemangiosarcomas (Ward and Buchanan 1977) have been reported in previously irradiated patients.

### Intracranial Tumors

A range of intracranial tumors including astrocytoma (Sogg, Donaldson, and Yorke 1978), pituitary sarcoma (Greenhouse 1964), and fibrous histiocytoma (Gonzalez-Vitale et al. 1976) have been attributed to ionizing radiations.

## Operative Mortality

Major complications related to surgery usually occur within a short interval after the operation. This contrasts to radiation-induced sequelae, which usually are recognized after a substantial posttreatment interval and increase in severity with time. Operative mortality, like radiation carcinogenesis, has an arbitrary definition. Postoperative death was defined by Martin and associates (1955) as death from any cause occurring within 30 days of surgery. This broad definition must include some deaths not incited by surgery, just as some cancers developing in radiated volumes, particularly in the head and neck, must be attributed to so-called natural causes.

While radiation carcinogenesis is inherent in use of the modality and seems unrelated to the skill of the physician, operative mortality varies with the skill of the surgeon (and the anesthesiologist). As noted by Merendino (1960), a surgeon, reports of surgically related complications, including treatment-related death, are likely to be from outstanding surgeons in major medical centers and so may not represent the experience of the majority.

Operative mortality is related to several other factors. There is a direct relationship to the extent of the surgical procedure, which should be dictated by the extent of the tumor. Despite major, and continuing, improvements in supportive care, the age and medical condition of the patient influence major complications of surgery more than those of radiation therapy. Actually age has a reciprocal influence, for with increasing age the risk of major surgical complications rises while the risk of radiation carcinogenesis falls.

In a recent report (Williams and Murtagh 1973) of 363 consecutive patients considered for primary surgical treatment of cancers arising in the head and neck, there were 18 postoperative deaths (6%) in the group of 278 patients who had definitive surgery (operability rate of 79%). Comparable postoperative mortality for the primary surgical treatment of head and neck cancer has been reported by others (Loewy and Huttner 1966).

Of these 18 postoperative deaths, two occurred in the seven patients who had laryngo-pharyngo-esophagectomy plus bilateral conservative or radical block neck dissections with mobilization and anastomosis of the stomach to the pharynx; 12 occurred in the 127 patients (9% mortality) who had resection of the primary tumor plus block dissection of the neck; four occurred among the remaining 144 patients (3% mortality), who underwent a range of operative procedures (Williams and Murtagh 1973). This relatively high mortality for laryngo-pharyngo-esophagectomy with transposition of the stomach into the neck has been reported by others (Stell 1970; Condon 1971).

There were no postoperative deaths in 57 patients under 49 years of age, 6% in 64 patients between 50 and 59 years, 5% in 78 patients between 60 and 69 years, 12% in 52 patients between 70 and 79 years, and 15% in 25 patients between 80 and 89 years (Williams and Murtagh 1973). This expected increase in risk in older patients has been noted by others (Martin, Rasmussen, and Perras 1955; Loewy and Huttner 1966; Herbst, Ulfelder, and Poskanzer 1971).

In the series of Williams and Murtagh (1973), the 18 postoperative deaths were attributed to the following causes: cardiac arrest during surgery, two; pulmonary embolus, two; inhalation of vomitus, two; failure to recover consciousness, two; coronary thrombosis, two; rupture of the carotid artery, two; bronchopneumonia, three; acute pancreatitis, one; respiratory obstruction, one; hematemesis, one. Theoretically, 7 of these 18 deaths might have been avoided, with a consequent irreducible postoperative mortality of 2% to 3%. There was no indication, however, of a reduction of these complications over the 10-year study period.

## Drug-Induced Cancer

Although chemical carcinogenesis may be environmental, occupational, or iatrogenic, only the latter is of concern in this discussion. In contrast to locoregional radiation, which places a limited number of normal cells at risk, systemic therapy with anticancer drugs, or immune modifiers, may place at risk a large number of cells throughout the body. Data are sparse for estimates of these risks.

A few drugs, such as Chlornaphazine, which causes bladder cancer, are well-documented carcinogens. Alkylating agents are usually carcinogenic in laboratory animals (Ryser 1971). An increase in acute leukemia has been reported in patients with myeloma treated with melphalan or cyclophosphamide (Kyle, Pierre, and Bayrd 1970). Canellos and colleagues (1975) reported that patients with Hodgkin's disease treated by MOPP and radiation had a higher incidence of leukemia than patients treated by either method alone. A link has been established (Herbst, Ulfelder, and Poskanzer 1971) between the therapeutic administration of stilbestrol during pregnancy and the development of adenocarcinoma of the vagina in the offspring. The similarity to the development of cancers in children receiving diagnostic doses of x-rays in utero is noteworthy.

As survival increases in patients treated with drugs or drugs and ionizing radiations, clinical risks will become more frequent and better defined.

## Conclusion

> Man lives with many risks and even the cure of many human diseases carries with it a risk.
>
> —Fry (1977)

The risk of cancer induced by either ionizing radiations or drugs is a reflection of therapeutic effectiveness, for such sequelae occur only in long-term survivors. In comparison with operative mortality, radiation carcinogenesis is inherent in the method and less related to the skill of the physician. Its development many years after treatment, rather than at the time of treatment, is advantageous for patients of all ages and may preclude the sequela in the elderly or medically compromised. Nearly all of the cancers attributed to the therapeutic use of ionizing radiations are themselves potentially curable, usually by surgery. Although the incidence of operative mortality for patients with head and neck cancers varies with a number of factors, it exceeds several fold the risk of radiation-induced cancer.

Therefore the risk of radiation carcinogenesis should be no greater a deterrent to properly indicated radiation therapy than the risk of operative mortality should be to the proper selection of surgery for the patient with head and neck cancer.

## References

Abdul, R. C.; Amine, M. D.; and Sugar, O. Suprasellar osteogenic sarcoma following radiation for pituitary adenoma. *J. Neurosurg.* 44:88–91, 1976.

Ackerman, L. V. Verrucous carcinoma of the oral cavity. *Surgery* 23:670–678, 1948.

Alexander, P. *Atomic radiation and life.* Baltimore: Penguin Books, 1957.

Beach, S. A., and Dolphin, G. W. A study of the relationship between x-ray dose delivered to the thyroids of children and subsequent development of malignant tumors. *Phys. Med. Biol.* 6:583–598, 1962.

Cade, S. Radiation-induced cancer in man. *Br. J. Radiol.* 30:393–402, 1957.

Canellos, G. P. et al. Second malignancies complicating Hodgkin's disease in remission. *Lancet* 1:947–949, 1975.

Condon, H. A. Anesthesia for pharyngo-laryngo-oesophagectomy with pharyngogastrostomy. *Br. J. Anaesth.* 43:1061–1065, 1971.

Court-Brown, W. M., and Doll, R. Mortality from cancer and other causes after radiotherapy for ankylosing spondylitis. *Br. Med. J.* 2:1327–1332, 1965.

D'Angio, G. J. et al. Decreased risk of radiation-associated second malignant neoplasms in actinomycin-D treated patients. *Cancer* 37:1177–1185, 1976.

Duffy, B. J., and Fitzgerald, P. J. Cancer of the thyroid in children: a report of 28 cases. *J. Clin. Endocrinol. Metab.* 10:1296–1308, 1950.

Frieben. Demonstration eines cancroid des recten handrückens, das sich nach langdauernder einwirkung von röntgenstrahlen entwickelt hatte. *Fortschr. Röntgenstr.* 6:106, 1902. Quoted by O. Petersen in *Acta Radiol.* 42:221–236, 1954.

Fry, R. J. M. Radiation carcinogenesis. *Int. J. Radiat. Oncol. Biol. Phys.* 3:219–226, 1977.

Fry, R. J. M., and Ainsworth, E. J. Radiation injury. Some aspects of the oncogenic effects. *Fed. Proc.* 36:1703–1707, 1977.

Glanz, H. Late recurrence or radiation induced cancer of the larynx. *Clin. Otolaryngol.* 1:123–129, 1976.

Gonzalez-Vitale, J. C.; Slavin, R. E.; and McQueen, J. D. Radiation-induced intracranial malignant fibrous histiocytoma. *Cancer* 37:2960–2963, 1976.

Greenhouse, A. H. Pituitary sarcoma. A possible consequence of radiation. *JAMA* 190:269–273, 1964.

Hatfield, P. M., and Schulz, M. D. Postirradiation sarcoma. *Radiology* 96:593–602, 1970.

Herbst, A. L.; Ulfelder, H.; and Poskanzer, D. C. Adenocarcinoma of the vagina: association of maternal stilbestrol therapy with tumor appearance in young women. *N. Engl. J. Med.* 284:878–881, 1971.

Hutchison, G. B. Leukemia in patients with cancer of the cervix uteri treated with radiation. A report covering the first 5 years on an international study. *J. Natl. Cancer Inst.* 40:951–982, 1968.

Hutchison, G. B. Late neoplastic changes following medical irradiation. *Radiology* 105:645–652, 1972.

Kaplan, E. L., and Taylor, J. Recent developments in radiation-induced carcinoma of the thyroid. *Surg. Clin. North Am.* 56:199–205, 1976.

Kiguchi, A.; Watanabe, C.; and Abe, M. Head and neck cancer following therapeutic irradiation. A brief review of those in Japan. *Nippon Acta Radiol.* 34:491–501, 1974.

Kyle, R. A.; Pierre, R. V.; and Bayrd, E. D. Multiple myeloma and acute myelomonocytic leukemia. Report of four cases possibly related to melphalan. *N. Engl. J. Med.* 283:1121–1125, 1970.

Lederman, M. Post-cricoid carcinoma. *J. Laryngol.* 72:397–405, 1958.

Loewy, A., and Huttner, D. J. Head and neck surgery in patients past 70. *Arch. Otolaryngol.* 84:523–526, 1966.

March, H. C. Leukemia in radiologists in a 20-year period. *Am. J. Med. Sci.* 220:282–286, 1950.

March, H. C. Leukemia in radiologists ten years later. *Am. J. Med. Sci.* 242:137–149, 1961.

Martin, H.; Rasmussen, L. H.; and Perras, C. Head and neck surgery in patients of the older age group. *Cancer* 8:707–711, 1955.

Mettler, F. A. et al. Breast neoplasms in women treated with x-rays for post-partum mastitis. *J. Natl. Cancer Inst.* 43:803–811, 1969.

Modan, B. et al. Radiation-induced head and neck tumors. *Lancet* 1:277–279, 1974.

Mole, R. H. Radiation effects in man: current views and prospects. *Health Phys.* 20:485–490, 1971.

Mole, R. H. Ionizing radiation as a carcinogen: practical questions and academic pursuits. *Br. J. Radiol.* 48:157–169, 1975.

National Academy of Sciences—National Research Council. *Report of advisory committee on the biological effects of ionizing radiations.* Washington, D.C.: U.S. Government Printing Office, 1972.

Parker, R. G. A review of 20 years experience of supervoltage roentgentherapy at the Tumor Institute of the Swedish Hospital, Seattle, 1938–1958, unpublished.

Phillips, T. L., and Sheline, G. E. Bone sarcoma following radiation therapy. *Radiology* 81:992–996, 1963.

Pochin, E. E. Frequency of induction of malignancies in man by ionizing radiations. In *Radiation biology*, eds. O. Hug and Z. Zuppinger. New York: Springer-Verlag, 1972.

Rossi, H. H., and Kellerer, A. M. The validity of risk estimates of leukemia incidence based on Japanese data. *Radiat. Res.* 58:131–140, 1974.

Ryser, H. J. Chemical carcinogenesis. *N. Engl. J. Med.* 285:721–734, 1971.

Saenger, E. L. et al. Neoplasia following therapeutic irradiation for benign conditions in childhood. *Radiology* 74:889–904, 1960.

Sagerman, R. H. et al. Radiation-induced neoplasia following external beam therapy for children with retinoblastoma. *Am. J. Roentgenol.* 105:529–535, 1969.

Schachner, S. H., and Hall, A. Parathyroid adenoma and previous head and neck irradiation. *Ann. Intern. Med.* 88:804, 1978.

Schindel, J.; Castoriano, I. M.; and Tikva, P. Late-appearing (radiation-induced) carcinoma. Carcinomas of the postcricoid and hypopharyngeal regions following successful irradiation therapy for laryngeal carcinoma. *Arch. Otolaryngol.* 95:205–210, 1972.

Seydel, H. G. The risk of tumor induction in man following medical irradiation for malignant neoplasm. *Cancer* 35:1641–1645, 1975.

Shellabarger, C. J. Radiation carcinogenesis. Laboratory studies. *Cancer* 37:1090–1096, 1976.

Sogg, R. L.; Donaldson, S. S.; and Yorke, C. H. Malignant astrocytoma following radiotherapy of a craniopharyngioma. *J. Neurosurg.* 48:622–627, 1978.

Som, M. L., and Peiner, R. Postcricoid carcinoma as a sequel to radiotherapy for laryngeal carcinoma. *Arch. Otolaryngol.* 62:428–431, 1955.

Som, Y. Radiation carcinogenesis. *Cancer* 36:941–945, 1975.

Sparagana, M. et al. Osteogenic sarcoma of the skull: a rare sequela of pituitary irradiation. *Cancer* 29:1376–1379, 1972.

Stell, P. M. Esophageal replacement by transposed stomach following pharyngolaryngo-esophagectomy for cancer of the cervical esophagus. *Arch. Otolaryngol.* 91:166–170, 1970.

Tissell, L. E. et al. Autonomous hyperparathyroidism. A possible late complication of neck radiotherapy. *Acta Clin. Scand.* 142:367–373, 1976.

Ullrich, R. L. et al. The influence of dose and dose rate on the incidence of neoplastic disease in RFM mice after neutron irradiation. *Radiat. Res.* 68:115–131, 1976.

Ward, C. M., and Buchanan, R. Haemangiosarcoma following irradiation of a haemangioma of the face. *J. Maxillofac. Surg.* 5:164–166, 1977.

Warren, S., and Gates, O. Multiple primary malignant tumors: survey of literature and statistical study. *Am. J. Cancer* 16:1358–1414, 1932.

Weshler, Z. et al. Thyroid carcinoma induced by irradiation for Hodgkin's disease. *Acta Radiol. Oncol.* 17:383–386, 1978.

Williams, R. G., and Murtagh, G. P. Mortality in surgery for head and neck cancer. *J. Laryngol. Otol.* 87:431–440, 1973.

Wilson, S. M.; Platz, C.; and Block, G. E. Thyroid carcinoma following irradiation. *Arch. Surg.* 100:330–337, 1970.

Yoshizawa, Y.; Kusama, T.; and Morimoto, K. Search for the lowest irradiation dose from literatures on radiation-induced bone tumor. *Nippon Acta Radiol.* 37:377–386, 1977.

Yoshizawa, Y., and Takeuchi, T. Search for the lowest irradiation dose from literature on radiation-induced cancer in pharynx and larynx. *Nippon Acta Radiol.* 34:903–909, 1974.

Yuhas, J. M. Recovery from radiation-carcinogenic injury to the mouse ovary. *Radiat. Res.* 60:321–332, 1974.

# Chapter 20

# *Combined Therapy (Radiation and Surgery)*

David Elkon and
William C. Constable

Every five years the pendulum swings back and we revert to treatment methods that have fallen into disfavor. We are currently in a phase where postoperative radiotherapy is being used more, with perhaps the notable exception of cancer of the bladder. The recent swing toward postoperative radiotherapy is not the result of conviction on the part of the radiotherapist that this is superior, but the consequence of a lack of adequate clinical trials, and changes in surgical procedures that might carry more morbidity, if performed in irradiated fields, for example, the various conservative laryngectomies.

There are two major modalities for treating primary head and neck cancer—radiotherapy and surgery. In many instances the use of one or the other of these results in a high cure, and the possibility of combining the modalities does not arise. On the other hand there are many cancers that are not cured because of (1) inadequate local control and (2) distant metastases. The combination of radiotherapy and surgery should logically be considered in the first group in an attempt to improve local control. There are five methods by which we may combine radiotherapy and surgery.

1. Immediate preoperative radiotherapy.
2. Immediate postoperative radiotherapy.
3. Radiotherapy with surgery for salvage.
4. Surgery with radiotherapy for salvage.
5. Sandwich techniques.

## The Radiobiologic Rationale for Immediate Preoperative or Postoperative Radiotherapy

There are well-recognized biologic reasons why preoperative or postoperative radiotherapy should improve local tumor control, and they provide an excellent reason for employing combinations even in the absence of clinical studies. The advantages attributed to preoperative radiotherapy are:

1. The elimination of outlying foci of disease that are the cause of recurrence following surgery if not excised. These small foci are more radiosensitive than the primary mass of tumor and can be eliminated by a dose of radiation that does not result in major changes in the normal tissues.
2. Reduction in bulk of the primary tumor, with the result that surgery is facilitated.
3. Reduction in the viability of cells that might be spread at surgery and result in distant metastases.

It will be seen that the latter two reasons will not result from postoperative radiation, but residual foci of disease may still be destroyed and recurrence prevented. This is achieved at a cost, however: these foci are likely to be less sensitive as a result of the surgical effects on blood supply, and the tolerance of the normal tissues is likely to decrease. When radiotherapy is used postoperatively, the reduction in the primary tumor mass is achieved by surgery, and the dissemination of distant metastases should stop at that time, although the surgical manipulation and anesthesia, both of which have been shown to increase metastases in experimental systems, may tend to negate this result (Cole 1973).

In an attempt to attain the advantages of both pre- and postoperative radiotherapy, so-called sandwich techniques have been designed wherein a certain amount of radiation is given prior to surgery and more is given postoperatively. Unfortunately, the consequences of the prolonged time period over which radiotherapy is given and the effect of the surgery on normal tissue tolerance to radiation have not been well defined, and these techniques have not found favor in most radiotherapy centers.

## The Clinical Advantages and Disadvantages of Preoperative Radiotherapy

The following advantages have been attributed to preoperative radiotherapy.

### Decrease in Local Recurrence

This is a consequence of the elimination of outlying radiosensitive foci during the preoperative course of radiotherapy. In our retrospective study comparing 151 patients with advanced cancer of the larynx treated by laryngectomy with a group of 72 patients receiving preoperative radiotherapy, the recurrence rates differed by 13% (29% for the laryngectomy alone group, 16% for the preoperative group) (Constable et al. 1972).

## Increased Survival

A reduction in the local recurrence rate does not necessarily imply increased survival. This has been well recognized, for example, in carcinoma of the breast, where reduction in the frequency of chest-wall recurrences with radiotherapy does not improve patient survival. In head and neck malignancies, however, many cases fail locally, and patients die of the local progression of the disease without evidence of distant metastases. It is therefore reasonable to assume that local control would be reflected in increased survival. This appeared to be so in the series described above where the determinate five-year survival was 78% for the preoperative group and 59% for the surgery alone group.

## Decrease in Distant Metastases

This is an extremely controversial point but is argued on the basis that cells that may be spread at the time of surgery have been damaged by the previous radiation and are therefore not viable. Again, in the study cited the incidence of distant metastases was just over one-third in the preoperative group compared with the laryngectomy group (5.6% vs 14%).

## Improved Resectability of the Primary Tumor

Where the tumor is resectable initially this question does not arise. It is in cases of borderline operability where the line of resection will presumably pass through areas involved in tumor that the radiation may contribute by sterilizing these extensions of disease. We would agree that this is not always the case, but inasmuch as the surgery is already at its limit there would appear to be an urgency not to disregard the possible sterilizing effect of radiation in these patients. Unquestionably, pathologic reports on many surgical specimens indicate that all the tumor has been eradicated and that therefore there must be instances where the margins of otherwise inoperable growths have been sterilized (Constable et al. 1974).

## Decrease in Postoperative Complications

Because of the variability between the extensive surgical procedures performed at many head and neck sites, comparison of complications with and without radiotherapy is extremely difficult. These complications are frequently related to the ability and experience of the surgeon. With a relatively simple and standard surgical procedure such as a wide field laryngectomy it is possible to compare the effect preoperative radiotherapy might have on morbidity. In the series that has been discussed there was no increase, and possibly a decrease, in morbidity and postoperative mortality in the preoperative group (Constable et al. 1972). When it is remembered that most tumors are infected when first seen, and that their presence has impaired nutrition, the removal of this infected mass by previous radiation can only be advantageous to any subsequent surgery.

### Improved Nutrition

Head and neck malignancies not infrequently result in a reduced nutritional intake and a negative nitrogen balance. The removal of the tumor bulk obviously aids in the patient's general nutrition, and during the period following radiotherapy and prior to surgery more active steps can be taken to enhance their nutritional status.

There are two main disadvantages that are cited in relation to preoperative radiotherapy: postoperative complications and delay before surgery. It is true that complications can be increased if an inappropriately high dose of radiation is used (Constable et al. 1975a). If the preoperative dose has been moderate, however, an increase in morbidity is not a necessary consequence (Constable et al. 1974). Healing of the tissues will be slower, although changes in surgical techniques (for example, the elimination of the notorious trifurcate incision) when dealing with irradiated tissues can largely obviate this problem.

The only instance in which delay in surgery may affect the outcome, inasmuch as the preoperative radiotherapy is already controlling the primary tumor, will be when distant metastases arise during the period of radiotherapy and the waiting period before surgery. Considering the large number of cells rendered nonviable by radiation during the first few treatments, it is hard to visualize that this is of any significance. On the other hand, metastases already present may become detectable during this period, and unnecessary surgery can then be avoided.

## Practical Considerations

Two questions raised by the surgeon when faced with preoperative radiotherapy concern the appropriate level of dose and when to operate.

Unquestionably, inadequate radiation has resulted in confusion as to the effect of preoperative radiotherapy. Certain low doses in a numerical sense given in a single or a few fractions, e.g., 2000 rad in five consecutive fractions, may be as effective as high doses given over longer periods; however, low doses over long periods are probably of no value at all. The advantages the radiotherapist sees in the longer period of treatment are that there is less assault on the normal tissues, improved recovery of the normal tissues, and less postoperative morbidity. Our personal preference has been a minimum dose of 4500 rad to a maximum of 5000 rad in five weeks. With this order of dose complications have been no greater than those associated with the comparable surgical technique only, that is, without preoperative radiotherapy. There are good radiobiologic reasons for the effectiveness of radiation at this level of dose in eradicating micrometastases.

The time of operation will depend on the type of preoperative regimen adopted. After short, intensive courses of treatment immediate surgery may be contemplated. If the tumor is bulky or of borderline operability, however, then one of the advantages of preoperative radiotherapy's improving tumor resectability has been lost. The reason these treatments have become popular with surgeons is that there is no delay before surgery, and therefore the hypothetical increase in distant metastases during this period will not take place. It is questionable, however, whether the latter is true. The advantages of the longer course of treatment and waiting period, such as the reduction in infection and improved nutrition and healing, more than justify the longer course of treatment and delay. Various studies have shown that the appropriate time to operate following a protracted course of treatment is between four and six weeks. We performed thermographic studies on patients receiving preoperative radiotherapy and showed that the hyperemia following radiation reverted to the baseline level during this four-to-six-week period (Scruggs et al. 1975).

## Clinical Applications

### Oral Cavity and Oropharynx

Radiotherapy or surgery alone is usually adequate for treatment of early lesions at these sites. For the advanced lesions (T3 and T4), combined therapy has become the rule. Where the resection of bone is anticipated, preoperative radiotherapy is not appropriate because the surgical trauma to the irradiated bone may result in osteonecrosis of the remnant. Where bony resection is not anticipated, preoperative radiotherapy is indicated.

### Paranasal Sinuses

There is currently very little disagreement that preoperative radiotherapy is the method of choice where there is involvement of the antrum and ethmoids and where the tumor is thought to be resectable. It is interesting to reflect on the point that although the usual preoperative dose at this site is often 6000 rad, complications are minimal after surgery. This is probably related to the fact that the surgery encompasses the entire radiated volume, and complicated closures are not undertaken.

## Larynx

Locally advanced cancers of the larynx are appropriately considered for preoperative radiation. Total or wide-field laryngectomy is no longer used as a standard approach in these cases; conservative laryngectomies with retention of a relatively normal voice are considered appropriate in certain instances. Preoperative radiotherapy does not interfere with the surgical options, and in fact may allow a conservative approach more frequently.

## Hypopharynx

The pyriform sinuses are the only sites where a combined approach can be regularly considered. In this instance we believe that preoperative radiotherapy is indicated because tumors here are frequently more extensive than appreciated. Good regression with these tumors may permit so-called cheating with the margins of resection. Inasmuch as nutrition is always impaired in hypopharyngeal tumors the waiting period before surgery following elimination of the tumor mass would seem to be a decided advantage.

## Cervical Lymph Nodes

Preoperative radiotherapy at a level of 5000 rad sterilizes undetected metastases in lymph nodes (Fletcher and Shukovsky 1975). If the nodes, therefore, are not clinically detectable the same preoperative dose to the primary will have achieved sterilization of latent metastases in the neck. When the nodes are grossly involved, even though there has been excellent regression following radiation, we recommend a radical neck dissection following the preoperative treatment. When there is gross bilateral involvement of lymph nodes, we consider the prognosis to be poor and bilateral neck dissection unjustified, and in this instance implantation of the lymph nodes would constitute the appropriate supplemental procedure following preoperative radiotherapy.

## Rare Tumors

Certain unusual tumors are amenable to a combined approach. This is particularly well illustrated by the success of combined therapy for advanced esthesioneuroblastoma (Elkon et al. 1979).

# The Clinical Advantages and Disadvantages of Postoperative Radiotherapy

In general, although the advantages of preoperative radiotherapy would appear to outweigh those of postoperative radiotherapy, there are certain situations where postoperative radiotherapy would appear to be the treatment of choice.

## Decrease in Local Recurrence

The radiobiologic basis for this is essentially the same as for preoperative radiotherapy in that residual foci of disease may be eradicated by a relatively moderate dose of radiation. Postoperative radiotherapy would appear to be applicable when the primary neoplasm, either because of the histologic type or large tumor size, is resistant to radiation. Recently this has been well demonstrated in malignant tumors of the salivary gland, where hitherto the value of radiation had been in question. In a series of malignant salivary gland tumors in which 17 patients were treated electively with postoperative radiotherapy, the local recurrence was 6%, compared with the usually reported surgical recurrence of between 25% and 38%, and over 50% for many histologic types (Elkon, Colman, and Hendrickson 1978). We have also demonstrated this for adenoid cystic carcinoma of the salivary gland (Elkon, Pope, and Constable 1980).

## Determination of Disease Extent

This has been considered an advantage at various sites outside the head and neck region, particularly the abdomen, where unsuspected extensions of the malignancy may be marked and then irradiated. This is of limited value in the head and neck region, however, and detection of any residual disease would imply that the tumor has been transected, and this must counterbalance any advantage.

The fact that radiation is delayed until healing is complete would indicate that immediate postoperative complications are reduced. Radiotherapy in this situation carries complications of its own, however.

## Delay to Surgery

Delay to surgery of course is minimal if surgery precedes radiotherapy. What may be more important in these advanced and often borderline resectable cases is the delay between surgery and radiotherapy, particularly when the tumor may have been cut through.

On the surface, the apparent disadvantages of postoperative radiotherapy would seem to mitigate against its use.

## Decreased Vascularity

Decreased vascularity increases radioresistance, and therefore higher doses will usually be required postoperatively to achieve results comparable to those achieved preoperatively. It is usual to give doses of 6000 rad postoperatively, and this will result in an increase in radiation reactions and complications as a consequence of the impaired tolerance of the tissues.

### Spread of Metastases

Margins on borderline operable lesions may be inadequate, leading to an increased chance of both local and distant metastases. In this regard it should be noted that unlike the situation following preoperative radiotherapy, any cells spread will be viable.

### Delay to Radiotherapy

Perhaps the major disadvantage of postoperative radiotherapy is that there is often considerable delay before the patient is referred. During this period rapid regrowth of the residual disease may negate the advantage obtained by the reduction of the primary bulk of the tumor.

### Volume Irradiated

The volume to undergo radiation treatment must encompass the operative field, inasmuch as recurrence may occur at any site within this region. This larger volume of treatment, together with the impaired blood supply and higher dose required, increases radiation complications.

### Nutrition

Patients with head and neck malignancies are often in a poor nutritional state. Efforts may be made to correct this with hyperalimentation, but, in the absence of this, surgery is being carried out in less than ideal circumstances, undoubtedly contributing to the rather prolonged periods of healing in these patients prior to initiating radiotherapy.

## Practical Considerations

With regard to the dose and time of initiating radiotherapy there would appear to be more agreement than there is concerning preoperative radiotherapy. Postoperatively it is felt that radiotherapy to gross residual disease must be on the order of 6000 rad in six weeks. In practice this means 5000 rad to the entire operative field and microscopic areas of extension, with an additional 1000 rad to the site of the primary tumor and sites of known residual disease. Ideally radiotherapy should be initiated within two to three weeks of the surgery if healing has occurred, although this is seldom realized.

# Clinical Applications

## Salivary Gland Tumors

With the single exception of low-grade mucoepidermoid carcinomas, postoperative radiotherapy is recommended in all cases of salivary gland tumor, on the basis of the dramatic reduction in postoperative recurrences observed when postoperative radiotherapy has been used. (Elkon, Pope, and Constable 1980). The recurrence after surgery of even low-grade tumors such as acinic cell carcinomas can be substantially reduced in this fashion. In adenoid cystic carcinoma the propensity for perineural extension is one of the major causes of recurrence, and this determines that large volumes should be encompassed by the radiation field. The dose, in accord with the principle outlined above, is 6000 rad in six weeks. It is worth noting that we have had no complications with facial nerve grafts treated to this dose level.

## Oral Cavity and Oropharynx

A conservative approach in early lingual cancer has proved to be local excision of the primary lesion and postoperative radiotherapy by means of a radium needle implant to the immediately adjacent area. This has the advantage of resulting in minimal deformity of the tongue and reducing the xerostomia associated with external radiation. In this situation the neck nodes are not treated in a prophylactic fashion but only when detected at follow-up, when they are treated by a radical neck dissection.

With large lesions where resection of the mandible is anticipated, postoperative radiotherapy is preferred to preoperative. Similarly, when temporal bone resection is undertaken, radiotherapy is preferably given postoperatively.

## Unplanned Radiotherapy

By far the largest number of patients receiving postoperative radiotherapy are in fact those whose surgery has been undertaken without consultation with the radiotherapist and whose pathologic specimens indicate that the surgery has probably been inadequate. Unfortunately in these cases, there has often been considerable delay before radiotherapy, the major cause of the poor results attributed to postoperative radiation. The surgical incision has often not been planned with a view to the patient's receiving radiotherapy, and more extensive volumes must therefore be treated, with the associated hazards.

## Sandwich Technique

The intention with this approach is to try to combine the advantages of both pre- and postoperative radiotherapy, but in practice it appears to combine the disadvantages, too. A certain proportion of radiation is given prior to surgery, with the balance, depending on the normal tissue tolerance, following the surgery. Unfortunately, it has proved difficult to determine what the normal tissue tolerances are in these circumstances. This approach is currently being explored in cancer of the rectum and bladder, but at the present time it is not being used in head and neck malignancies.

## Delayed Sequential Treatment of Recurrent Malignancy

Early cancer of the larynx is an example where radiotherapy can cure an exceedingly high percentage of patients and where almost all recurrent cases may be salvaged by subsequent surgery. Recent reports would indicate, particularly in cancer of the larynx, that late cases are also cured in substantial numbers, perhaps on the order of 40% to 50% (Constable et al. 1975b). If these patients are treated with radical radiotherapy, 40% to 50% would retain their larynx. The question then arises as to how the recurrent cases should be treated and whether, in fact, surgery in this delayed sequential fashion would achieve cures comparable to those of preoperative radiotherapy and immediate surgery. The indication from these reports is that there is no difference in local control where surgery has been delayed until recurrence is overt. It is possible that this approach could be extended to other sites such as early lesions in the oral cavity and oropharynx, with close follow-up determining the need for surgery should there be recurrence.

Unfortunately, when radiotherapy is delayed following surgery, control rates do not equal those for patients receiving immediate postoperative radiation. This is clearly shown regarding salivary gland tumors (Elkon, Colman, and Hendrickson 1978). Another classic example is the almost total resistance of stomal recurrences to treatment by radiation.

## Summary

We believe that there are a number of good indications for preoperative radiotherapy and a lesser number for postoperative radiotherapy. It is difficult to see how controlled clinical studies can resolve the problem as this would entail input from a large number of centers and an even larger number of surgeons. The physical factors of delivering radiation therapy are relatively standard, but the type and execution of the surgery varies considerably. In particular, clinical trials wherein a number of sites are lumped together to achieve significant accrual of patients must be treated with some skepticism—as, for example, when the surgery and complications following the treatment of the T3 or T4 lesion of the oral cavity are included with those following treatment of a similar lesion in the larynx, which are much less extensive. Delayed sequential (salvage) therapy should certainly be considered for cancer of the larynx, and it is not felt that those patients subsequently requiring surgery would be eliminated from consideration for conservative laryngectomy. This approach would seem to be the one exciting alternative to our present methods of combining radiotherapy and surgery.

## References

Cole, W. H. The mechanisms of spread of cancer. *Surg. Gynecol. Obstet.* 137:853–871, 1973.

Constable, W. C. et al. High dose pre-operative radiotherapy and surgery for cancer of the larynx. *Laryngoscope* 82:1–8, 1972.

Constable, W. C. et al. Intermediate dose pre-operative radiotherapy for cancer of the larynx—end results. *Can. J. Otolaryngol.* 4:246–250, 1975a.

Constable, W. C. et al. Radiotherapeutic management of cancer of the glottis, University of Virginia, 1956–1971. *Laryngoscope* 85:1–10, 1975b.

Constable, W. C. et al. Tumor sterilization with preoperative radiation in laryngeal cancer. *Arch. Otolaryngol.* 99:252–254, 1974.

Elkon, D. et al. Esthesioneuroblastoma. *Cancer* 44:1087–1094, 1979.

Elkon, D.; Colman, M.; and Hendrickson, F. R. Radiation therapy in the treatment of malignant salivary gland tumors. *Cancer* 41:502–506, 1978.

Elkon, D.; Pope, T. L.; and Constable, W. C. Adenoid cystic carcinoma of the salivary gland. *Arch. Otolaryngol.* 106:410–413, 1980.

Fletcher, G. H., and Shukovsky, L. J. The interplay of radiocurability and tolerance in the irradiation of human cancers. *J. Radiol. Electrol.* 56:383–400, 1975.

Harwood, A. R. et al. Management of advanced glottic cancer: a ten-year review of the Toronto experience. *Int. J. Radiat. Oncol. Biol. Phys.* 5:899–904, 1979.

Scruggs, H. J. et al. Use of thermography to evaluate the optimum time for surgery after preoperative radiation. *Laryngoscope* 85:1–8, 1975.

## Chapter 21

# *Misconceptions in the Management of Squamous Cell Carcinoma of the Aerodigestive Tract*

# Paul H. Ward

This chapter's style and content are based upon the requests of the volume editors, one of whom frequently attends the weekly UCLA interdisciplinary head and neck tumor conferences, which I moderate. Specifically, this chapter shares my experiences gained through extensive patient care, observation, and the teaching of residents in several university and university-affiliated hospitals over the last two decades. In some instances the conclusions I make may be erroneous, but they are expressed with the honest conviction that their validity has been tested repeatedly. The unique experience gained by supervising many residents and allowing them the opportunity to make almost predictable, but retrievable, mistakes provides for an intense and continued learning environment that cannot be conveyed in statistics. Thus citations of reported series of statistics are not used to substantiate the observations or statements herein.

The objective of this book is to call attention to, discuss, and elucidate various controversial areas in head and neck surgery. Let us therefore begin by examining closely some of the current so-called sacred cows. The popular trend is for the National Cancer Institute program committees, editors, and readers to be impressed by statistics (nearly always retrospective), particularly when the numbers are large. Preference is given to statistical papers on programs and in publications. These "series" results, repeatedly cited during conferences and tumor boards, play an influential part in the planning of treatment for patients. Unwarranted reliance upon such reports has led to the common misconception that statistical data formulated in retrospective studies and reported in the literature provide reliable information of considerable value in determining the most effective treatment of a patient with an epidermoid carcinoma of the aerodigestive tract. The major deficiencies undermining the validity of the majority of statistical retrospective studies are as follows: (1) the data are often incomplete, inaccurately acquired, misinterpreted, and/or fabricated; (2) staging by the TNM system as recommended by the Joint Commission for Cancer Staging and End-Results Reporting of the various epidermoid cancers according to their size, location, and extent of metastasis can be used as a guide to the selection of effective treatment of an individual patient; (3) similarly classified and staged cancers behave in the same manner; (4) many authors are consciously or unconsciously selling their preconceptions.

A brief discussion of each of these errors may provide elucidation of the problems. Deficiencies and inaccuracies in chart reviews and tabulation of statistical data are frequent. They commonly originate with the assignment of a busy resident or fellow to the task of reviewing the charts and tabulating the data. Many patients' charts provide little or no documentation of several areas under investigation. Since acceptable statistics can be obtained only if similar information is present for all cases under study, the reviewer follows the given instructions to check or devise the best possible answer based upon the information available. Once the "complete" data are available, the authors (senior and associate) tabulate, analyze, and neatly package in tables and slides the information for the report. At this stage the fabrications and underlying inaccuracies are easily overlooked or forgotten. Absence of factual information or incorporation of this type of data automatically biases the statistics and invalidates the majority of such studies.

Another common error is the attempt by inexperienced surgeons or radiotherapists to use the TNM classification and staging system as a basis for determining the treatment technique or modality for a specific patient with an epidermoid carcinoma of the aerodigestive tract. This was not the original intent of the Joint Commission, although changes in the classification and staging have been implemented by some to more closely match current treatment modalities. As a resident, I helped to review a large number of charts of patients with epidermoid carcinoma of the oral cavity (for the Joint Commission), which were used to determine the statistical results upon which the TNM classification and staging system is built. Without known personal biases, I followed meticulously the instructions to fill in the questionnaire based upon the best available information. No matter how dispassionately the information is formulated, however, weaknesses prevail. The TNM system of classification and staging is designed to assist in the meaningful description of tumors as to size, location, and extent of spread, and provide some type of common ground for comparison of the results reported by different investigators. It is not a framework for the formulation of treatment.

In carrying out the elected treatment modality, experience combined with technical capability is most important in managing malignancies of the head and neck. Unfortunately, experience requires many years to acquire. Residents are often told that by the time surgeons become sufficiently knowledgeable to manage the various types of tumors of the head and neck, they are often too old to stand by the table for the lengthy period of time needed to perform the surgery adequately. This is an exaggeration, of course, but it contains an important element of truth. Probably in no other area of the body is experience more valuable in the diagnosis, management, and prognostication of a cancer than in the head and neck.

Experience leads to recognition that all epidermoid cancers of the aerodigestive tract, even though similarly classified and staged, do not behave in the same fashion. This is another problem inherent in reliance upon the TNM classification and staging system and retrospective series statistics as a basis for treatment selection. The novice may make treatment decisions based upon such information; the veteran oncologist readily acknowledges this data but acquires a remarkably large additional amount of evidence from the moment the patient enters the examination room. The importance of the interaction and behavior of the cancer in each individual patient and the patients' responses to the tumor are acknowledged. The general health, habits, and nutritional status and the body's local and systemic responses to the cancer are observed and synthesized, along with perceptions of the gross appearance, degree of aggressive behavior, extension, and histologic characteristics of the tumor. Also noted are the presence or absence of either indolent or aggressive behavior, degree of invasiveness, surrounding induration, ulceration, and the extent or degree of necrotic breakdown. The experienced oncologist never blindly and uncritically accepts the pathology report but personally reviews the patient's slides, often discussing the findings with a trusted pathologist. These discussions provide a learning experience for both the oncologist and the pathologist. The clinician brings the vast amount of historical data and physical observation to combine with and enhance the pathologist's superior technical abilities in evaluating the histopathologic behavior of the tumor. The clinician will eventually acquire a new competence as an amateur pathologist, adding to his or her capabilities in the decision-making process. This background provides the experienced clinician with the "intuitive" knowledge necessary for a more accurate prognosis and for advising the patient as to the preferred treatment regimen.

There are several retrospective studies in the literature that suggest an absence of correlation between the prognosis and the histologic differentiation of a tumor. These articles emphasize that varying degrees of differentiation can be found in large epidermoid carcinomas. This helps to explain why these cancers have a poorer prognosis. As a general rule, however, denial of any correlation between histopathology and tumor behavior is a serious misconception. It is acknowledged that at times histologically well-differentiated tumors behave aggressively, metastasizing to regional lymph nodes and to distal sites, while an occasional poorly-differentiated carcinoma may remain localized. These, however, are the exceptions to the rule. After taking into consideration all the previously mentioned characteristics of the tumor and the status of the patient, the wise surgeon rarely elects to treat the poorly-differentiated tumor solely with the knife. The cancer may seem to have recurred or metastasized before healing is complete. Likewise, most knowledgeable radiotherapists recognize a degree of correlation with slow response, diminished sensitivity, and failure to eradicate the extremely well-differentiated and/or verrucoid-type epidermoid carcinomas.

The degree of differentiation of an epidermoid carcinoma and its location are often closely correlated and of prognostic significance as to potential for metastasis and for five-year survival. Cancers of the base of the tongue (of different embryologic origin from those of the anterior two thirds) are nearly always moderately- to poorly-differentiated epidermoid carcinomas. They behave aggressively because of the extensive, diffuse bilateral lymphatic distribution and the propensity for early metastases. A much greater degree of differentiation is usually present in epidermoid cancers of the anterior two-thirds of the tongue. The latter have fewer contralateral lymphatics, are less apt to metastasize early to the regional lymph nodes (although regional metastasis remains relatively high), and certainly have a much higher five-year survival when adequately treated than do cancers of the base of the tongue. These differences may lull the novice into inadequate treatment of carcinomas of the anterior two-thirds of the tongue. This is borne out in the reported series where T2N0M0 carcinomas have a higher five-year survival than T1N0M0 lesions. The results of injudicious, inadequate local resection are seen in a number of patients referred each year to a large medical center. The high incidence of local recurrence and/or metastatic neck disease in these inadequately-treated patients markedly reduces the chance of successful eradication and long-term survival for these unfortunate patients.

Another serious misconception promulgated in numerous statistical series occurs when small numbers of different cases of carcinomas in a regional area are grouped together. For example, it is common to see tonsillar, tonsillar pillar, palate, base of the tongue, retromolar trigone, and even buccal carcinomas grouped together in order to provide numbers sufficient for "statistically significant" results. Statistics obtained from these groupings are worthless and even misleading to the inexperienced physician. The behavior of these cancers may be as different as the appearance and taste of apples and oranges. As a general rule, the base of tongue, tonsillar, and palatal cancers are usually moderately to poorly differentiated and, because of the extensive distribution of lymphatic vessels, have a propensity to early homolateral and/or contralateral metastasis. Exceptions to this rule are the occasional, well-localized hyperkeratotic lesion with dysplasia (even showing superficial invasion), which can be effectively treated by local excision. In general, successful treatment for aggressive invasive cancers must be radical by surgery, radiation, or preferably by both therapeutic modalities. The treatment must include the regional lymphatic vessels and lymph nodes in the neck because of the high incidence of early metastasis (manifest or occult).

Clinical experience repeatedly demonstrates that retromolar trigone carcinomas are entirely different in their behavior. Characteristically, they are exophytic, more superficial, less invasive, show greater histologic differentiation, and have less surrounding reactivity and underlying induration than the more aggressive tonsillar and palatal cancers. They rarely metastasize to the neck; however, if neglected, extensive local growth can occur. Retromolar trigone carcinomas present a distinct treatment problem because they occur immediately overlying bone. Early involvement of the periosteum is, and must be, taken into consideration in planning treatment. The frequent, small retromolar trigone lesions are preferably treated by marginal resection of the mandible with wide local excision of the tumor and surrounding tissues. The defects can be closed with regional tongue flaps. Larger lesions require composite resection of the cancer, mandible and radical neck dissection, and/or postoperative radiation. The contrast in the behavior between the poorly-differentiated tonsil, base of the tongue, infiltrating palatal carcinomas, and the less aggressive yet more differentiated retromolar trigone lesion serves as an example to emphasize the futility in the grouping of different regional cancers together for statistical analysis.

Cancers located even more anteriorly, involving the buccal mucosa and/or alveolar ridge, are generally even less aggressive. These lesions usually are well circumscribed, superficially invasive, show little surrounding reactivity, and until reaching large proportions, rarely manifest lymphatic or vascular invasion. They are histologically well differentiated with keratinization. Wide local resection with sparing of the external facial skin (when it is not involved), marginal resection of the mandible (when indicated), and closure by regional tongue and mucosal flaps or split thickness skin grafts are preferred modalities of treatment. The rationale for preference of radiation (or combined surgery and radiation) for aggressive cancers and surgery for the more indolent, less aggressive cancers is immediately obvious.

Another common error in the reporting of cancers of the oral cavity is the grouping of anterior tongue with floor of the mouth cancers. There are significant dissimilarities, not only between the behavior of the cancers in these two areas, but even among epidermoid tumors in each of these locations. Except for the early superficial hyperkeratotic, leukoplakia with dyskeratosis, and/or superficial invasion, most of the floor of the mouth lesions are aggressive, infiltrative, moderately-differentiated epidermoid carcinomas that metastasize early to the regional nodes. They often encroach upon the alveolar ridge and mandible, requiring marginal and/or segmental resection. To mistakenly treat an aggressive floor of the mouth cancer that invades the mandible as a more indolent alveolar ridge carcinoma invites disaster. Invasive floor of the mouth cancers that involve the mandible often require segmental resection of the mandible. At times the patient injudiciously elects radiation in these surgical lesions to avoid surgical deformity. This usually delays the operation for six months to a year or more. A cancerocidal dose of radiation given to a high percentage of these unfortunate patients would result in radionecrosis of the mandible. The eventual surgical procedures and complications may surpass the magnitude and deformity of the originally proposed surgery. When there is no bone encroachment, aggressive floor of the mouth lesions may be preferably treated with radiation with equal survival rates and less deformity, although the prognosis is guarded when floor of the mouth cancers are treated with either radiation and/or surgery. Thus far, efforts to combine both modalities of therapy have not significantly improved the survival statistics of patients with these aggressive lesions. About one-third of all patients with epidermoid floor of the mouth carcinomas survive five years or longer.

By contrast, overall five-year survival of patients of anterior two-thirds of the tongue epidermoid cancers following appropriate radical surgery or radical radiation is 60% to 70%. Since the survival statistics are similar for both treatment modalities, radiotherapy is elected more frequently for these cancers because of the better functional results.

Factors other than survival statistics must be taken into consideration in helping each patient decide upon the appropriate treatment for his or her respective cancer.

The socioeconomic and behavioral patterns of patients are of considerable importance in the treatment. It is a misconception that the unreliable, self-destructive alcoholic with multiple nutritional deficiencies should be treated exactly the same as the reliable, compulsive professional. In the former patient, the only chance of achieving eradication of the tumor may be to perform radical resection of the cancer to heal the patient before his or her release from the hospital. Some of these patients are unable to discipline themselves long enough to complete a six-week course of radiotherapy even though it may be the preferred modality. In contrast, some reliable professional patients with cancers of the larynx might preferably be treated by radical surgery. After adequate information has been provided to them concerning the functional results of radiation and surgery, they may elect to receive radiation and be followed closely. This may be a calculated gamble on their part; however, their priorities are such that their need for an essentially normal voice may make the acceptance of eventual total laryngectomy or even a diminished chance of survival a rational choice. These priorities change with time and circumstances. People in their fifth and sixth decades reaching the peak of their career may have different priorities than older patients who have passed these hard-driving years. The treatment of these two groups of patients may be different; their survival statistics will most certainly be different. The "private type" patient who notices the common symptoms and seeks early diagnosis and treatment has a much greater chance of survival. Furthermore, because of the differences in their nutritional status, the grouping of these two types of patients together is of limited value.

Those physicians responsible for the care and management of patients with cancers of the head and neck must continually evaluate and assess promising new therapeutic modalities if they are to remain competent. The past two decades have seen significant changes in the approach to the treatment of patients with carcinoma of the larynx. Surgeons or radiotherapists who treat all "small" cancers with radiation and all others with total laryngectomy are obsolete. The merits of conservation surgery are now accepted, and yet many patients continue to undergo unnecessary total laryngectomy. The five-year survival statistics for judicial selection and performance of partial laryngectomy with reconstruction closely approach those for total laryngectomy. The tragic disability of total laryngectomy can be avoided in over one-half of the cases with cancer of the larynx. While the new voice restoration fistula procedures and devices are promising, they continue to have problems of unpredictable voice leakage of saliva and aspiration. In the near future it is doubtful that voice restoration procedures for total laryngectomies will surpass the superior functional results of the reconstructed partial laryngectomy. The use of the laser for the treatment of early glottic carcinoma of the larynx is currently being assessed and may find a useful place in the treatment of these cancers.

A common error of the inexperienced head and neck cancer surgeon or radiotherapist is inadequate knowledge of metastatic patterns. The probability of occult metastasis can be correlated roughly with each of the factors that have been previously mentioned. Metastasis from pyriform sinus, base of the tongue, lateral pharyngeal wall, retropharyngeal wall, and invasive palatal cancers is extremely frequent and warrants either radical neck dissection in continuity with the primary cancer or radiation that incorporates the primary lymphatics in the neck. The failure to initiate immediate adequate treatment results in a significant reduction in survival.

There are exceptions to the usual anticipated behavior of cancer. For example, a small T1 cancer of the vocal cord and anterior commissure, instead of being a well-differentiated epidermoid carcinoma with keratinization, may rarely prove to be a poorly-differentiated tumor with bilateral neck metastases. An occasional small retromolar trigone or even well-differentiated buccal mucosal cancer may present with early metastasis. These cases are not the common examples, but exceptions. Our understanding of the presence or absence of the individual's immune protective mechanisms has yet to be delineated. Even so, these anecdotal cases should not deter the head and neck surgeon from planning and conducting therapy based on high probabilities that the characteristics of the tumor, location, degree of differentiation, and appearance of the lesion would dictate. Absence of metastatic disease following composite resection of the primary and regional nodes unquestionably provides hope for a good prognosis. Metastatic lymph node involvement in the presence of a small primary tumor foretells a severely diminished probability of long-term survival.

The correlation of large tumors, degree of differentiation, and the likelihood of metastasis is more difficult and less accurate. Large cancers represent either neglect or loss of the body's immune response. Tumors that have grown 4 or 5 cm or greater in diameter behave more aggressively and have a high propensity to metastasize regardless of the degree of differentiation.

The head and neck surgeon is faced with difficult decisions that result from the cosmetic deformity and functional derangement that resection of the numerous important vessels, nerves, organs, and other structures frequently require. Erroneous decisions made with overdue concern for preservation of appearance or ability to close the wound may lead to the early demise of the patient. It is generally recognized that the cosmetically-oriented surgeon is oftentimes not the best cancer surgeon. A concern with cosmesis and reconstruction may bias judgement leading to inadequate resection of the cancer. The old adage "radical early and conservative late" has ultimate application in the management of cancer of the head and neck. Failure to resect adequately the tumor may result in a nice immediate cosmetic appearance and good functional capability. Early recurrence and the accompanying poor prognosis, even with attempted salvage using the second modality, negates the initial good result. Regardless of the extent of radical resection in advanced and recurrent cancers, success is limited. Preoperative planning of reconstruction is important but should never override adequate excision. The availability of a wide variety of skin flaps and grafts (regional, myocutaneous, and pedicle flaps) make appropriate resection of the cancer with immediate reconstruction feasible. The prosthodontist plays an important role in the preoperative planning and the postoperative rehabilitation of many surgical defects. It is a common oversight not to incorporate a competent prosthodontist into the team management of cancer of the head and neck.

The good head and neck surgeon has important responsibilities in addition to the preoperative and postoperative care of the patient. Compulsive attention to details perhaps beyond that expected of other physicians and surgeons is essential. It is difficult to accept the behavior of the surgeon who does not study the patient's specimens after surgery and, upon receiving a report that there is tumor at the margins, rationalizes that radiation will eradicate the few remaining cells. In actuality, if there is residual cancer the surgeon has merely performed a large biopsy. There is no such thing as *a touch of tumor;* if the original cancer was appropriate for surgical resection and additional tissue can be resected, then a return of the patient to the operating room is in order. The secondary resection can be followed by radiation if appropriate. The importance of the surgeon's study of the gross specimen, knowledge of surgical specimen processing, and personal review of the histopathologic slides cannot be overemphasized. This will prevent return to the operating room when the reported margins are not truly margins but rather an error in determining margins by new or inexperienced pathologists. The experienced head and neck surgeon can help reorient the pathologist if the surgeon is secure in his gross resection. The pathologist can then change his report or the surgeon can annotate the margins of the report. If there is tumor present, the surgeon learns a lesson and needs to return with the patient to the operating room.

A misconception that prevails with some surgeons and radiotherapists is, "I'll do what I can and if it doesn't work then something else can be tried." It is a tragic mismanagement to operate upon a patient with a cancer that would more appropriately have been treated by radiation. Likewise the patient is ill treated when radiotherapy is injudiciously administered for cancer which would have been better treated by surgery.

For years an adversary relationship existed between surgeons and radiotherapists in many institutions. To the disadvantage of the patient this persists in a few communities and hospitals. Interdisciplinary tumor conferences and boards have provided a better understanding of the contributions of each discipline in the combined use of radiotherapy, chemotherapy, and surgery.

The recent shift to performance of the surgery prior to radiation has diminished markedly the numerous significant complications that were encountered using preoperative radiation. The administration of radiation postoperatively has helped overcome another problem encountered with combined therapy. When radiation was given first there was sometimes significant improvement in the patient's symptoms resulting in withdrawal from the previously planned combined therapy. At other times the radiotherapist and surgeon responsible for the care of the patient saw such a dramatic response in the patient's tumor that they weakened in their resolve to encourage the patient to complete the full treatment. This attitude, while understandable, is irrational; experience has demonstrated that cancer can show early and significant shrinkage, only later to resume growth.

It is logical to expect an increase in the survival statistics of patients given both modalities of therapy prior to any evidence of recurrence. Based upon the rather poor current statistics, the only proven increase in survival resulting from combined radical surgery and radiation is for pyriform sinus lesions. There are some series suggesting that survival statistics for palatal and tonsillar lesions may also be improved by combined therapy. A failure of surgery followed by treatment with radiation, or a failure of radiation followed by attempted salvage, is not combined therapy. The misconception in determining statistics in the past was the inclusion of all cases that received both surgery and radiation. The failure of either modality to eradicate a tumor casts this tumor into an entirely new category and indicates a poor prognosis. Tumors surviving one modality have a high probability of failing to be eradicated by the second modality.

In the past it was generally considered preferable to irradiate poorly-differentiated tumors and to operate on the more differentiated tumors; this concept has some validity. Currently under evaluation is the use of both modalities of therapy in a planned combined form. The eventual success or failure of true combined therapy with surgery followed by postoperative radiation perhaps will be more effective than separate use of either modality.

Hope continues to spring eternal that new methods of immunotherapy (stimulation of the body's immune response against invasion and metastasis) and the development of effective chemotherapeutic agents will be successful in conquering head and neck cancers. These newer modalities of treatment may be adjunctive to and might even replace surgery and radiation therapy.

This is, however, only an ideal for which to strive, and magical thinking should not replace rational, judicious surgical and radiotherapeutic approaches to the management of cancer.

It is a tragic error for some well-meaning physicians, investigators, politicians, charlatans, and the press to raise false hopes for new miracle drugs before they have been proven and/or are available to patients. Presently some chemotherapy using single or multiple drugs has reduced tumor size. Often the side effects are of such severity as to raise the question of their merit. Until such a "magic bullet" becomes available there remains no substitute for the informed, experienced, and caring multidisciplined team approach to the diagnosis, treatment, and care of patients with head and neck cancer.

# INDEX

## Subject Index

## D

## I



## J



## K



## L

## P

## Q



## R

## S

## T

# Author Index

## C



## D



## E



## F



## G

## M



## N



## O



## P

## Q



## R



## S